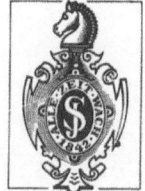

Hans-Rudolf Henche · Jörg Holder

Arthroscopy of the Knee Joint

Diagnosis and Operative Techniques

Second, Revised and Enlarged Edition

With Forewords by Robert W. Jackson and Erwin Morscher

Drawings by Franz Freuler and Manfred Jauch
Translated by David Le Vay

With 225 Figures Mostly in Color

Springer-Verlag
Berlin Heidelberg NewYork
London Paris Tokyo

Hans-Rudolf Henche, Dr. med.
Kreiskrankenhaus Rheinfelden, D-7888 Rheinfelden

Jörg Holder, Dr. med.
Friedberger Anlage 31, D-6000 Frankfurt 1

Translator:

David Le Vay, FRCS
Dewhurst Lodge, Wadhurst, East Sussex, TN5 6QB, England

Translation of the 2nd German edition:

Die Arthroskopie des Kniegelenks
© by Springer-Verlag Berlin Heidelberg 1988

Library of Congress Cataloging-in-Publication Data. Henche, Hans-Rudolf. 1940–   [Arthroskopie des Kniegelenks. English] Arthroscopy of the knee joint: diagnosis and operative techniques. Hans-Rudolf Henche, Jörg Holder; drawings by F. Freuler and M. Jauch; translated by D. Le Vay. — 2nd, rev. and enl. ed.   p.   cm.
Translation of: Die Arthroskopie des Kniegelenks. 2nd German ed. © 1988.
Bibliography: p.   Includes index.
ISBN-13: 978-3-642-72921-8   e-ISBN-13: 978-3-642-72919-5
DOI: 10.1007/978-3-642-72919-5

1. Knee—Examination. 2. Arthroscopy. 3. Endoscopic surgery. 4. Knee—Surgery. I. Holder, Jörg. II. Title. [DNLM: 1. Arthroscopy. 2. Joint Diseases—diagnosis. 3. Knee Joint—surgery. WE 870 H494a] RD561.H4513 1988   617′.582′0754—dc19

Reproduction of figures: Gustav Dreher GmbH, Stuttgart

2124/3130-543210 – Printed on acid-free paper

Foreword to the Second Edition

A quarter of a century has gone by since the Western orthopaedic world reawoke to the potential benefits of arthroscopy. In the early days of this awakening, diagnostic problems were the only indication for arthroscopy, as the master surgeons of that era were confident in their clinical diagnoses and in their ability to treat any disorder of the knee through a large incision.

Two important changes subsequently took place. Firstly, it became apparent that most clinical diagnoses, while not actually erroneous, frequently failed fully to elucidate the problems within the knee joint. Arthroscopic examination led to a marked increase in diagnostic accuracy.

The second important change consisted in the development of arthroscopic surgical techniques. The ability to see pathology was coupled with a desire to treat it under arthroscopic control. This led to the development of new instruments and new techniques that enabled a large variety of conditions to be treated. With the passage of time it has become abundantly clear that the minimal intervention techniques used in arthroscopic surgery are far superior to the traditional, massive, open arthrotomy techniques. For example, there is little doubt that partial meniscectomy gives better long-term results than total meniscectomy.

During this evolutionary period Dr. Henche continued the pioneering work of Bircher and developed the technique of gas arthroscopy to a high degree of proficiency. He also developed several surgical techniques and is regarded as one of the great teachers of arthroscopy. This textbook, originally published in German, is one of the most complete treatises on arthroscopy and arthroscopic surgery available today. The skilful translation results in a book that is readable and understandable. In addition, the illustrations are excellent and have been reproduced with great care. The result is a very pleasing and informative book.

It is an honour to write the foreword for this significant milestone in the history of arthroscopy and arthroscopic surgery. This beautiful book is a tribute to the hard work and pioneering activities of Dr. Henche and I congratulate him.

R.W. Jackson, MD, MS, FRCS (C)
Professor, Department of Surgery
University of Toronto
Chief of Staff/Surgery
Orthopaedic & Arthritic Hospital
Toronto, Canada

Foreword to the First Edition

In 1921 the Swiss surgeon Bircher published the first report on arthroscopy of the knee joint. The initial trials with the method revealed problems, mainly technical in origin, which caused it to be abandoned and forgotten until recently. Modern technical improvements, for which Japanese orthopaedic surgeons, above all Watanabe, were mainly responsible, have now led to a revival of interest in this method of investigation. The quality and versatility of the instruments currently available and the experience of the endoscopists who use them are such that arthroscopy of the knee joint is becoming an indispensable diagnostic aid. Arthroscopy is superior to arthrotomy in every respect; it is not only simpler but can be carried out on an ambulatory basis under local anaesthesia. In addition, it provides more information than arthrotomy, and the arthroscopic findings can be simply documented photographically. The complication rate is extremely low; cumulated statistics recently obtained from six clinics revealed no case of infection following nearly 4,000 arthroscopies. The main indication for arthroscopy is the "painful, diagnostically obscure knee joint" in the widest sense. The procedure is also useful for further investigation of knee joint lesions which have already been diagnosed, as it allows their type and extent to be diagnosed more precisely, and the indication for surgery in a given case can be assessed more clearly. Unnecessary surgery can often be avoided in this manner. Arthroscopic biopsy is simple, and a variety of operations (e.g. cartilage transplantation) can be followed up endoscopically.

Since 1971, arthroscopy of the knee joint has been carried out systematically at the Orthopaedic Clinic of the University of Basel by Dr. H.R. Henche, and the associated technique has gradually been improved. In particular, Dr. Henche has succeeded in perfecting endoscopy of the gas-filled joint and has developed it into a standard procedure. Dr. Henche has summarized his experience of over 500 arthroscopies in this manual, which provides an introduction to, and a practical description of the technique for the surgeon who has to deal with the diseased or injured knee joint.

Finally, it must be emphasized that the development of arthroscopy is continuing, and there is no doubt that the ability to perform endoscopic surgery will be included among the benefits which future technical advances will bring.

Basel   Professor Dr. Erwin Morscher

Preface to the Second Edition

Arthroscopy and arthroscopic surgery are achieving a prominence unimaginable a little over a decade ago. This rapid development has made a new edition of this book necessary. On careful examination, however, it can be seen that this is not merely a new edition, but that the whole book has been substantially modified and greatly expanded. To make it possible to present a complete overview of the various diagnostic and, in particular, operative techniques involved in arthroscopic procedures, Jörg Holder agreed to collaborate on this edition of the book, bringing with him his very wide experience. A further advantage is that Holder, as a great advocate of "fluid filling" goes into this technique in detail. Readers can inform themselves about the techniques of both gas and fluid filling and then make their own choice of method.

In comparison with the first edition, it is particularly noticeable that arthroscopy is no longer aimed primarily at diagnosis but is clearly focused on therapy – this tendency will become even more apparent in future years.

We are grateful to everyone who has contributed to the completion of this second edition of the book, and would especially like to thank both of our artists.

Rheinfelden-Frankfurt   Hans-Rudolf Henche
September 1988   Jörg Holder

Preface to the First Edition

The possibility of using a slender optical device to look into the knee joint and directly diagnose the causes of otherwise cryptogenic joint problems has fascinated surgeons since the beginning of this century. Eugen Bircher and Kenji Takagi took up this challenge independently at the beginning of the twentieth century. They earned no laurels from their contemporaries, as they were unable to document their findings and thus provide evidence with which to reassure the doubters.

Diseases of the cartilage of the knee joint are difficult to diagnose and assess clinically, and this explains the early interest in arthroscopy at an orthopaedic clinic such as that in Basel. My teacher, Prof. Erwin Morscher, had been convinced by Robert W. Jackson in Toronto that it was possible to inspect the inside of the knee joint by arthroscopy. On becoming Director of the Orthopedic Clinic in Basel in 1971 he asked me to study and develop the technique of knee joint arthroscopy, a commission which I regarded at that time as an unwelcome duty. In 1971 we began to carry out arthroscopy on patients whose diagnosis was clear and on those in whom arthrotomy was to be carried out immediately following the arthroscopy. The results of our first arthroscopies were frequently scanty. We followed the techniques described by Watanabe in his arthroscopy atlas, but nevertheless we seldom succeeded in precisely identifying an area of cartilage.

With the aid of all the members of the surgical team the technique described was developed in the years 1971–1972. I am particularly grateful to Professor Hugin, who assisted me in the solution of technical problems.

In recent years investigation of joints by arthroscopy has gained acceptance in many clinics. The questions and requests of colleagues who wished to start using the method gave me the idea of summarizing my experience in the form of a book. This monograph is also intended to encourage those who, like me, have been disappointed by the unsatisfactory initial results of this apparently simple method. For this reason an ample proportion of this "recipe book" is devoted to the complications and sources of error.

Dr. Franz Freuler contributed greatly to this book by furnishing the diagrams which accompany the photographs. I am very grateful to him for his collaboration. In preparing the photographic documentation I received considerable help from Mrs. Thierstein; the high quality of the documentation could not have been achieved without her skill and cooperation. Finally, I should like to thank Miss R. Wagner and her secretarial colleagues.

This book is being published at a time when arthroscopy is leaving the experimental phase and becoming a routine clinical method. There is no doubt that it will gain enormously in popularity in the coming years. If this book succeeds in fuelling the latter process it will have achieved its purpose.

Rheinfelden   H.-R. Henche

Contents

General

1	Historical Review	3
2	Instruments and Equipment	6
2.1	Caliber of the Arthroscope	6
2.2	Quality of the Optical System	6
2.3	Basic Equipment	7
2.4	Double Eyepiece Systems	12
2.5	Operating Arthroscopes	13
2.6	Photographic Equipment	13
2.7	Video Systems	14
3	How to Learn Arthroscopy	18
4	Documentation of Arthroscopic Investigation	21
4.1	Written Records	21
4.2	Photographic Documentation	21
4.3	Video Recording	21
5	Indications for Arthroscopy	24
6	Preparation of the Patient for Arthroscopy	25
6.1	Explanation and Appointment	25
6.2	Positioning	25
7	Theater Nurse's Preparations for Arthroscopy	39
8	Care of Equipment	30
9	Anesthesia for Arthroscopy	31
9.1	General Anesthesia	31
9.2	Regional Anesthesia	31
9.3	Local Anesthesia	32
9.4	Technique of Local Anesthesia	32
10	Approaches to the Knee Joint	35
11	Examination Using Fluid or Gas Media	38
11.1	Filling the Knee Joint with Fluid	38
11.2	Filling the Joint Cavity with Gas	40
11.3	Alternate Filling of the Joint Cavity with Fluid and Gas	42
12	Anatomic Considerations	43
13	Arthroscopic Procedure	46

13.1 Insertion of the Arthroscope into the Knee Joint 46
13.2 Systematic Inspection of the Knee Joint Using the Lateral Approach 50

14 Pathologic Changes in the Joint Cavity 66
14.1 Synovial Membrane 66
14.2 Pathologic Changes in the Medial Meniscus 66
14.3 Pathologic Changes in Lateral Meniscus 71
14.4 Lesions of the Articular Cartilage 74
14.5 Chondromalacia of the Patella 78
14.6 Osteochondritis Dissecans 80
14.7 Arthroscopic Appearance of Lesions of the Anterior Cruciate
Ligament 81
14.8 Arthroscopic Appearance of Lesions of the Posterior Cruciate
Ligament 83
14.9 Lesions of the Plicae – Previously Operated Knee Joints 85

15 Assessment and Appraisal of Problematic Internal Traumatic Lesions 88

Arthroscopic Operations

16 Conditions for Operative Arthroscopy 93
16.1 Anesthesia 94
16.2 Positioning 94
16.3 Tourniquet, Drapes 96
16.4 Gas Filling, Fluid Irrigation 96
16.5 Incisions 97
16.6 Operative Equipment 99

17 Removal of Loose Bodies 102

18 Arthroscopic Meniscus Operations 106

19 Technique of Arthroscopic Medial Meniscus Operations 108
19.1 Medial Bucket-Handle Tear 108
19.2 Longitudinal Tear of Posterior Horn 116
19.3 Flap Tear 123
19.4 Transverse Fissure 129
19.5 Tangential, Horizontal, and Incomplete Fissures 134
19.6 Degenerative Lesions and Fraying 136
19.7 Subtotal Medial Meniscectomy 139

20 Technique of Arthroscopic Lateral Meniscus Opertions 141
20.1 Lateral Bucket-Handle Tear 141
20.2 Lateral Posterior Horn Resection 147
20.3 Lateral Anterior Horn Resection 150
20.4 Discoid Lateral Meniscus 154

21 Procedures on the Articular Cartilage 158

22 Other Arthroscopic Operations 165
22.1 Procedures on the Synovial Membrane 165

22.2 Resection of a Hypertrophied Medial Plica 165
22.3 Cruciate Ligament Procedures 168
22.4 Meniscus Suture 168
22.5 Lateral Release 169
22.6 Removal of Metal and Foreign Bodies 173
22.7 Diathermy 173

23 Completion of Operation and Aftertreatment 175

24 Complications, Problems, and Hazards of Operative Arthroscopy 178

25 Practice of Operative Arthroscopy 180

26 Arthroscopic Operations with Gas Filling of the Knee Joint 180

27 Miniarthrotomy under Local Anesthesia 182

28 Perspectives 183

References 184

Subject Index 189

General

CHAPTER 1
Historical Review

The attempts of doctors to look into the human body cavities have a very long history. In the first half of the nineteenth century it became possible to visualize the larynx, the ear and the optic fundus. The names of Ludwig Thürk, Freiherr von Troeltsch and Herrmann Helmholtz are indelibly associated with these pioneer developments.

The creation of the white-hot platinum wire led to the invention of the electric light and made it possible to illuminate the body cavities. The first attempts at endoscopy of the urinary bladder and the stomach were carried out in the second half of the nineteenth century. Max Nitze is regarded as the father of cystoscopy. In May 1879, with the aid of a device developed by himself and the instrument maker Joseph Leitner, he was able to examine the interior of the bladder. The first successful gastroscopy was probably that carried out by Mikulicz in Breslau. By 1881 he had succeeded in visualizing individual features in the stomach, such as the activity of the pylorus.

The invention of the carbon-filament light bulb by Thomas Edison enabled considerable advances to be made in endoscopy of all kinds. At the turn of the century cystoscopy had already become a routine procedure. A few years later gastroscopes – still rigid at that time – became available. Laparoscopy was a more or less parallel development. Jacobaeus, together with the Georg Wolf Company, designed an instrument for the inspection of the peritoneal cavity. This was the instrument which was first used for endoscopy of the knee joint.

In 1919/1920 the Swiss surgeon, Eugen Bircher (Fig. 1), carried out the first experimental endoscopies of cadaver knee joints using the Jacobaeus laparoscope. In 1920/1921 the technique was used in living humans. In

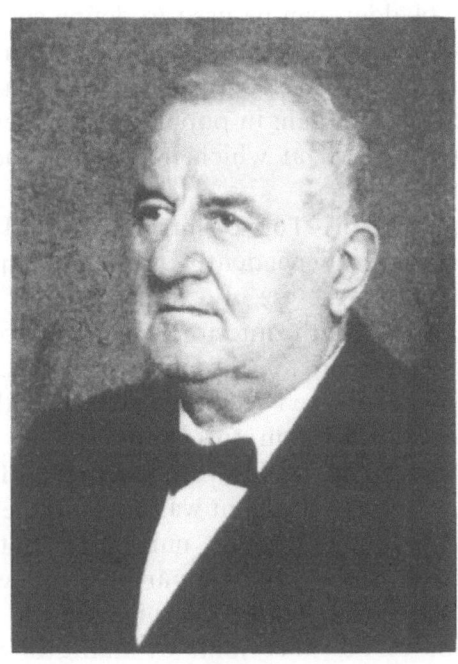

Fig. 1. Eugen Bircher

his famous paper – the first publication whatsoever on arthroscopy – in the *Zentralblatt für Chirurgie* in 1921 he reported the use of the laparoscope for arthroscopy of the knee joints of 18 patients. In 13 cases he was able to establish a correct diagnosis which was confirmed by the subsequent operation. In three cases the diagnosis was unsure. He reported only two incorrect diagnoses in tuberculous joints. Bircher carried out the investigation under general anesthesia in almost all cases. The joints were filled with oxygen and nitrogen.

One year later, in 1922, Bircher published an article on the pathology and diagnosis of meniscus injuries in 20 knee joints which had been investigated endoscopically. Even at that stage he succeeded in endoscopically diagnosing eight out of nine meniscus injuries, the diagnoses being confirmed during subsequent surgery. At the end of the paper Eugen Bircher wrote: "Arthroscopy allows us to examine the interior of the joint and identify pathologic changes, i.e., the diagnosis is made by direct visualization of the lesion. It is therefore superior to all other methods of investigation and, like endoscopy of the bladder, can be used to define certain indications for surgery. It will meet with resistance, as did cystoscopy, but, like the latter procedure, will gain in popularity and develop of the point at which it becomes indispensable."

In 1918 the Tokyo surgeon K. Takagi (Fig. 2) had, independently of Bircher, experimented with the use of a cystoscope for the visualization of the interior of the knee joint, or so his pupil, M. Watanabe, reports. In 1920 he developed a special device with a diameter of 7.3 mm for endoscopy of the knee joint (Fig. 3). However, because of its thickness this instrument was not suitable for practical use. It was not until 1931 that he succeeded in developing an arthroscope with a diameter of 3.5 mm. Takagi expanded the interior of the knee joint by filling it with saline. The first publication concerning his arthroscope appeared in 1933 in the *Japanese Journal of Orthopedic Surgery*.

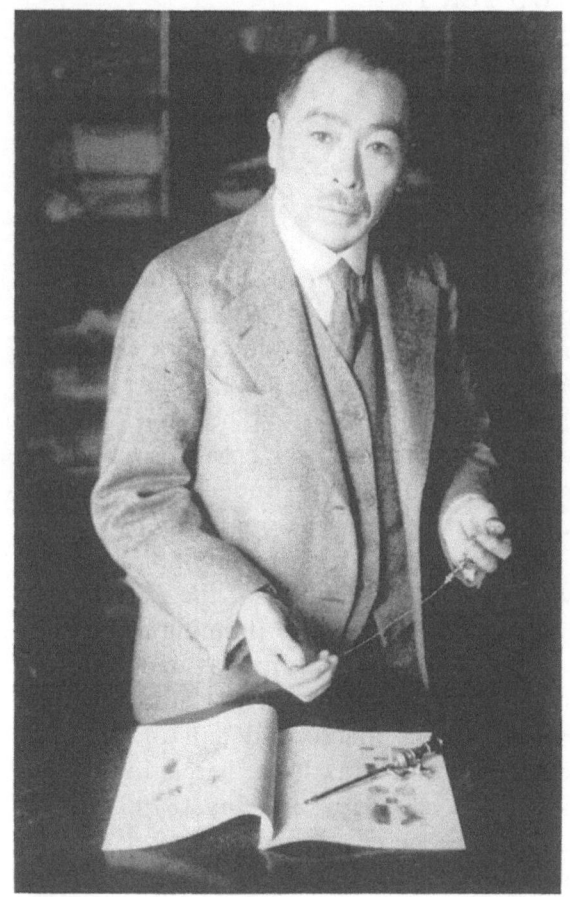

Fig. 2. K. Takagi

Fig. 3. Arthroscopy at the Kantonsspital, Aarau, 1920

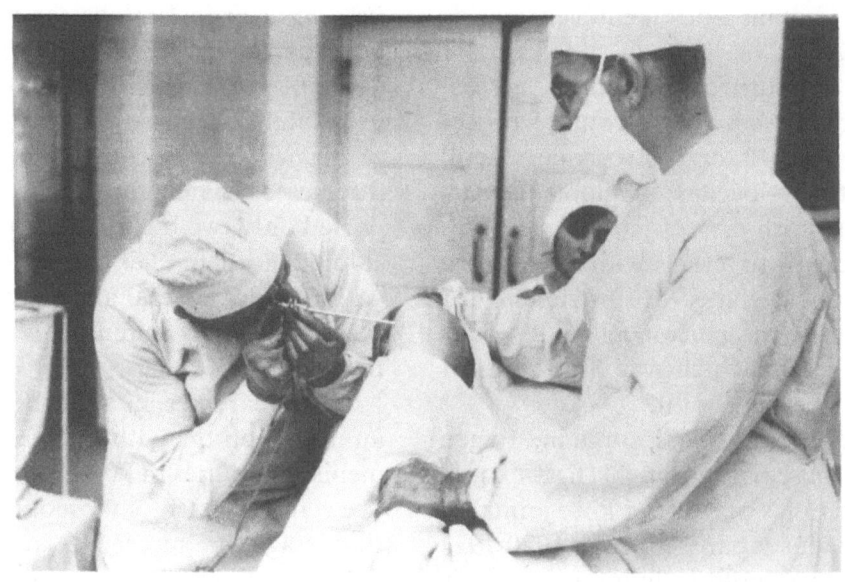

The first paper on arthroscopy of the knee joint in English was that by P.H. Kreuscher in 1925 in which he described an arthroscope of his own development. He considered arthroscopy to be especially suitable for the early detection of meniscus injuries.

In New York at the beginning of the 1930s M.S. Burman, H. Finkelstein, and L. Mayer at the Hospital for Joint Diseases were also working on an instrument for arthroscopy of the knee joint. Following a short publication in 1931, the current state of development was summarized in a paper in 1934. This article described for the first time a clearly defined technique of arthroscopy. The authors preferred local anesthesia. The irrigation was carried out with Ringer solution. A description of the systematic inspection of the knee joint was followed by a clear account of the complications which could arise during the procedure. They reported 30 cases which they had investigated, and concluded that arthritis of the knee joint and meniscus lesions were the main indications for arthroscopy of the knee joint.

The development of this investigative technique was continued in Germany. In 1937 R. Sommer reported several cases in which he had carried out arthroscopy, although his paper in the *Zentralblatt für Chirurgie* did not deal with the technique and complications in detail. Like Sommer, the rheumatologist J. Vaupel was only familiar with Bircher's initial work as he tried to introduce arthroscopy for the diagnosis of lesions of the knee joint. As a rheumatologist, Vaupel stressed the importance of the method in chronic arthritis. He arthroscoped individual knee joints as many as three times and hoped, by following the changes in the appearance of the synovial membrane, to gain insight into the course of the disease. Vaupel also tried to record his findings photographically. He used an arthroscope with a diameter of 3.1 mm for normal investigations and developed an instrument with a diameter of 4.7 mm for those cases which he wished to photograph. However, the underdeveloped state of photographic technology at that time prevented him from obtaining satisfactory pictures.

In 1939 K.H. Wilcke published a good review of the state of arthroscopic technology in the German- and English-speaking countries. Wilcke carried out his arthroscopies exclusively in cadavers. He described the technique of the investigation precisely. The colored photographs provide evidence of the technical inadequacy of the photographic methods available at that time. In his summary Wilcke wrote: "Endoscopy is, in suitable cases, a worthwhile addition to the methods which are available for the investigation and diagnosis of lesions of the knee joint, but its value is not such that it could be recommended for routine use in living patients."

After the Second World War the main impetus in the development of arthroscopy of the knee joint came from Japan. At the annual meeting of the Japanese Orthopedic Association in 1953 M. Watanabe, K. Sato, and W. Kawashima presented a report on the clinical use of the technique. Four years later, in 1957, the first edition of the *Atlas of Arthroscopy* by M. Watanabe, S. Taketa, and H. Ikeuchi was published. This atlas was the basis of the subsequent world-wide increase in interest in arthroscopy of the knee joint.

Arthroscopic surgery also began in Japan, where, on April 5, 1962, Watanabe did the first partial removal of a meniscus. Initially it was very difficult, and it was O'Connor's great achievement to have markedly improved the technique of operative arthroscopy. The publications of R. Jackson and L. Johnson also marked important steps in the development of many arthroscopic procedures. It was not until the 1970s that the Europeans acquired the technique from the Americans. From England (Dandy) and Sweden (Eriksson, Gillquist) the use of arthroscopy (initially diagnostic, but soon followed by operative methods) spread and became established in other European countries.

CHAPTER 2
Instruments and Equipment

When purchasing an arthroscope, the potential user should be familiar with the various advantages and disadvantages of the different systems. The main important features are outlined in the following sections.

2.1 Caliber of the Arthroscope

The caliber of the arthroscope, i.e., the external diameter of the trocar, is of considerable importance in inspection of the knee joint. Only a few years ago it was thought that a very narrow arthroscope made it easier to penetrate the posterior recess of the knee joint and a better view that was thereby provided. This has proved to be quite unimportant. A modern arthroscope of standard caliber has an external diameter of 4–6 mm. It has been shown in practice that, if the knee joint is adequately distended and the appropriate angle of view with such an arthroscope is chosen, all parts of the knee joint can be thoroughly and properly inspected. Thinner arthroscopes do not give a high-quality image. The argument that the use of the thinnest possible arthroscope carries less risk of damaging the articular cartilage does not ap-

ply if an experienced practitioner uses the standard procedure. A narrow arthroscope is more likely to be damaged. Bending of the glass fibers leads to opacity of the optical system and to a a greater chance of the endoscope breaking.

2.2 Quality of the Optical System

There are two basic types of optical systems: lens systems (Fig. 4) and glass fiber systems. The traditional lens system with a series of lenses has been abandoned in favor of the so-called rod-lens system. It is possible to combine glass fiber elements with rod-lenses and this is now employed almost universally (Storz, Olympus, Wolf). The quality of the image is determined by the resolving power of the optical system, and here a lens system is far superior to a fiberoptic system with its limited resolving power. This is most apparent in photographic documentation of the arthroscopic findings.

Fig. 4. Lens systems

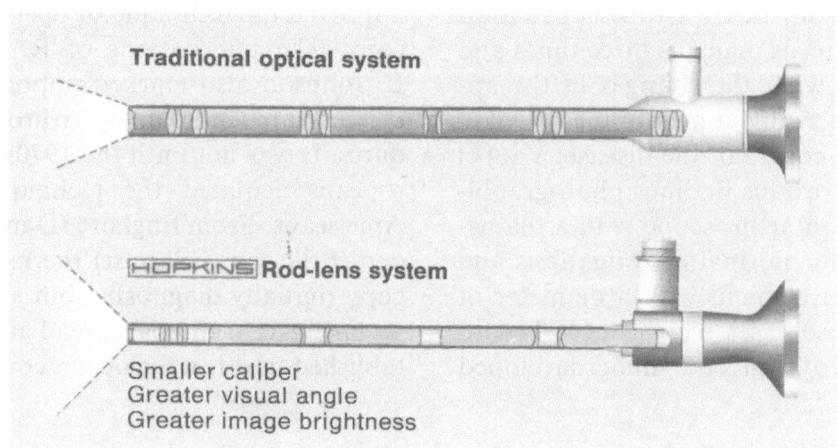

6

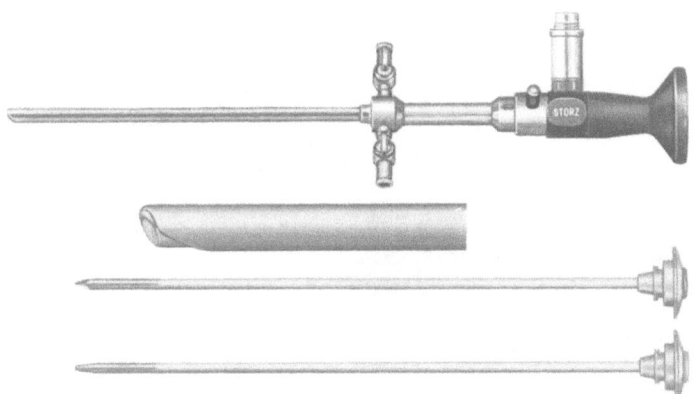
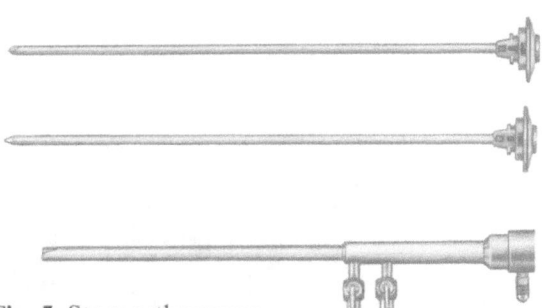

Fig. 5. Storz arthroscope

2.3 Basic Equipment

The arthroscope made by the Storz company (Tuttlingen) illustrates the basic instrument assembly (Fig. 5). The principal component of the instrument is the rod-lens optical system, which has better light-conducting properties than a conventional lens system. The standard pattern is a 4 mm × 15 cm optical system with a connection for the light-conducting cable close to the eyepiece. Like those of all other manufacturers, this optical system is available in several designs with various angles of view. The 30°-angled system is routinely preferred by nearly all practitioners (Fig. 6), but a 70° system, which is particularly indicated for inspection of the posteri-

or knee joint recess, and a straight-line system are also available. The advantage of the straight-line system is that the surgeon can advance the instrument exactly in the line of sight, and even with the 30° system it is still possible to see the space into which the instrument is entering. This is not so with the 70° optical system, which provides only a side view so that the instrument is advanced with difficulty and with constant change in the direction of view, or even blindly. This optical system calls for special experience on the part of the surgeon.

Fig. 6. Viewing angles and visual fields of optical systems

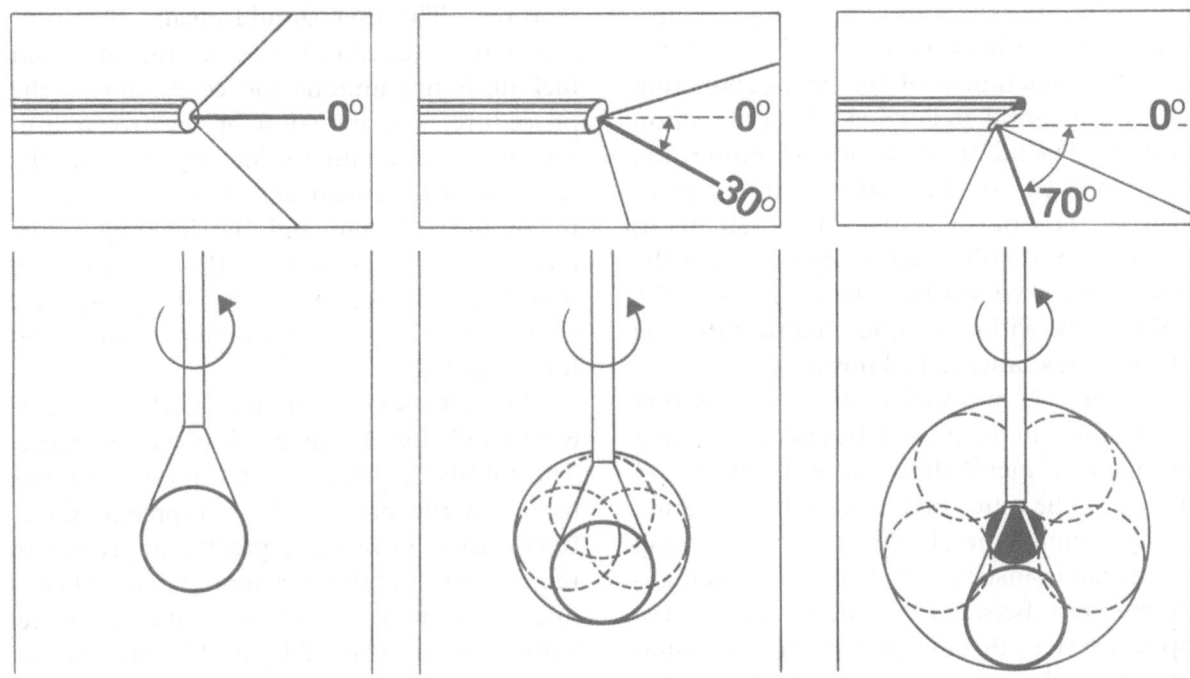

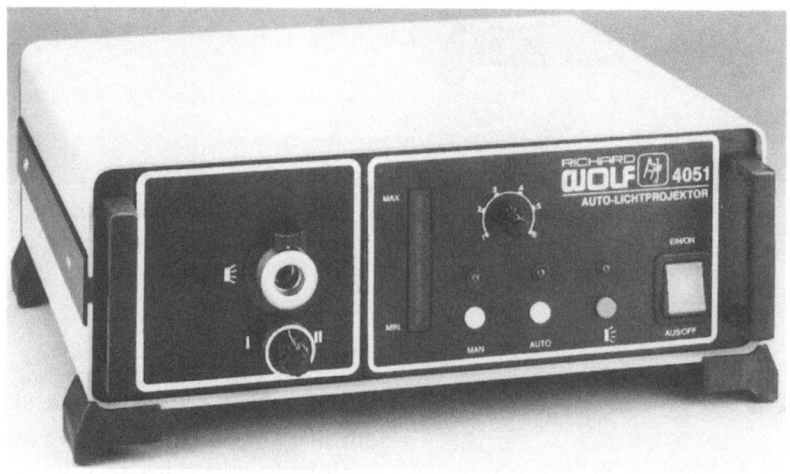

Fig. 7. Wolf light source

It is essential for the arthroscopist to understand that the visual field can be greatly expanded if the line of sight is altered by rotating the optical system (Fig. 6). One of the most important criteria for the mastery of arthroscopy is the appreciation and understanding of the possibility of this expansion of the visual field. Merely by rotating the arthroscope, without altering the position of the instrument, it is possible to obtain a panoramic view of the interior of the knee. However, the surgeon should always be aware of the direction in which he is looking, and the beginner is helped here by shining a light source through the skin or by using an external palpating finger. In all angled optical systems the attachment of the light-conducting cable is a useful indication of the direction of view; depending on the manufacturer, the cable may be attached either in direction of view of the optical system or at 180° to it. It cannot be emphasized enough that, for the less experienced worker, the position of the arthroscope within the knee and thus the line of sight must always be known.

During the procedure, the optical system is contained in the outer tube and is protected by this firm metal sheath from bending and damage. The outer tube usually has a diameter of around 6 mm, leaving a space – varying somewhat in instruments from different manufacturers – between the outer tube and the optical system through which irrigation fluid or gas can be introduced into the knee. The outer tube accomodates the sharp and blunt trocars which enable it to be inserted into the knee joint (see Chap. 13). One or two taps are usually fixed to the outer tube for the attachment of gas or fluid supply and suction systems. Easy control of these taps, if possible by one finger, should be ensured. The outer tube should also have an attached locking device for the optical system. This locking system again varies between manufacturers. The user should ensure that this, too, has an uncomplicated action and that locking is not undone too easily during the procedure. The insertion of the trocar into the outer tube and its locking therein, the removal of the trocar and its replacement by the optical system, and the locking of the latter must be practiced by the surgeon until they become second nature. Previous "dry runs," especially on a model knee, are therefore essential.

The attachment for the cold-light source is situated close to the black plastic eyepiece. The cold-light cable, about 1 m long, belongs to the sterile part of the equipment. Glass fiber cables have been greatly improved in recent years and they are now capable of conducting a great deal of light into the knee, without much loss of light. The attachment to the optical system must be secure and sim-

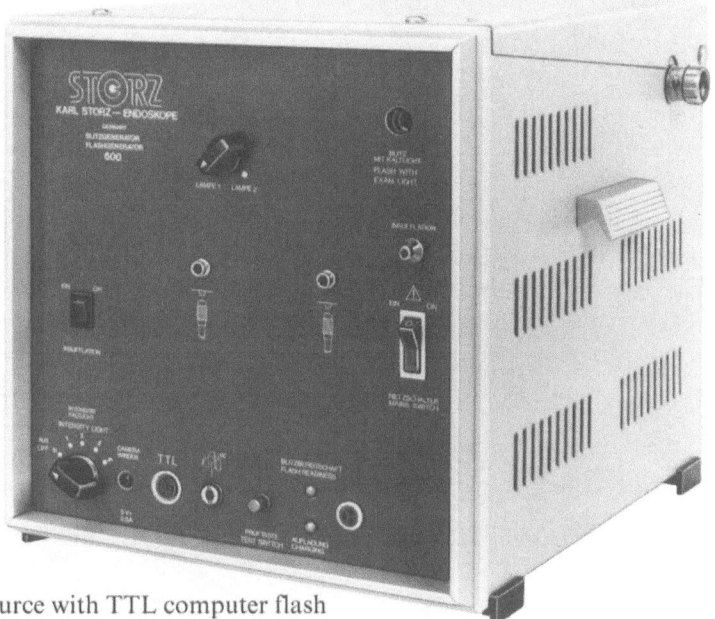

Fig. 8. Storz light source with TTL computer flash

ple. The nonsterile end of the glass fiber cable is connected to the cold-light source. If loss of light is found to occur after a few months, both the cable and the optical system must be checked. Changes at the ends of the cable in the form of burns due to severe heat build-up are frequently found.

The design of light sources is very varied, as is the intensity of illumination they provide (Figs. 7, 8). It is advantageous if an electronic flash is built into the apparatus for photodocumentation. The cold-light sources of similar size and quality supplied by all manufacturers give enough light to permit video recording; however, as there can hardly ever be too much light for such recording, it is sensible to use a very powerful light source, especially for inspection of non-reflecting surfaces in the knee joint. One possibility here is a xenon light source, which makes cinematography within the knee joint possible.

Some firms other than those that manufacture complete arthroscopy systems, including equipment for operative arthroscopy, have, in recent years, specialized in the manufacture of instruments for operation. Stille supplies high-quality instruments for operative arthroscopy. Akufe has developed special grasping systems for easy manipulation

during arthroscopic operations; the instruments of this firm are characterized by their high quality and durability. Olympus and Arthrex, likewise, manufacture arthroscopic operating instruments of individual design and high quality (Figs. 9, 10). The wide distribution of the products of these firms allows combination of inspection and operating instruments from different firms, according to the surgeon's requirements.

Aesculap was one of the first firms to develop a so-called arthroresector (Fig. 11), consisting of high-frequency equipment for diathermy resection of tissues in the knee joint. It is not yet possible to say whether diathermy resection can replace conventional operation techniques, at least in part. So-called motor-driven instruments are becoming increasingly important in operative arthroscopy, with motor-operated knives and reamers available for cutting and smoothing in the knee joint. These shaver systems are also supplied by various firms. The rotary instruments are particularly suitable for smoothing defects in cartilage surfaces; they are combined with a suction system and can be employed only under water (Fig. 12). The rotary knives can be used for smoothing and tidying the meniscal margins in degenerative meniscopathy. Because of the relative thick-

Fig. 9a, b. Storz basket forceps

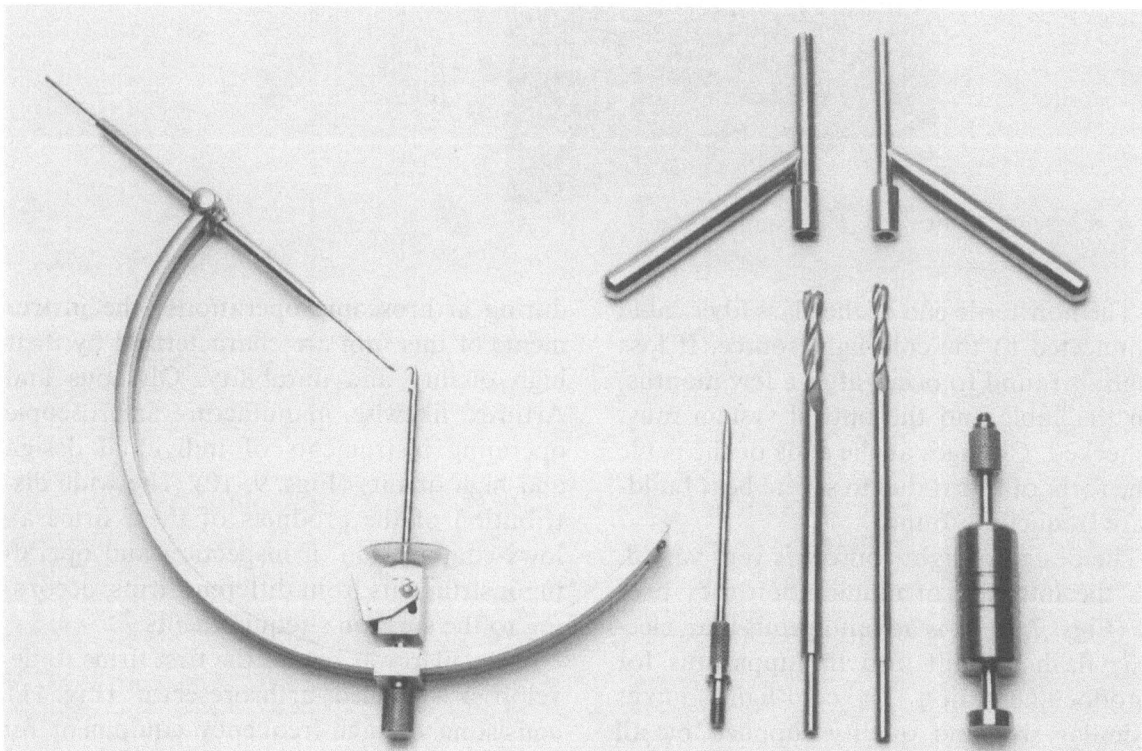

Fig. 10. Accessory instruments for arthroscopic cruciate ligamentoplasty (Arthrex)

ness of the shaver system, its use in the medial posterior horn region is very limited. Removal of the synovial membrane – endoscopic synovectomy – is also possible with the rotating knife. Only future experience will show whether this type of synovectomy has advantages over conventional procedures. However, with improvements in shaver systems and technical developments this seems very probable.

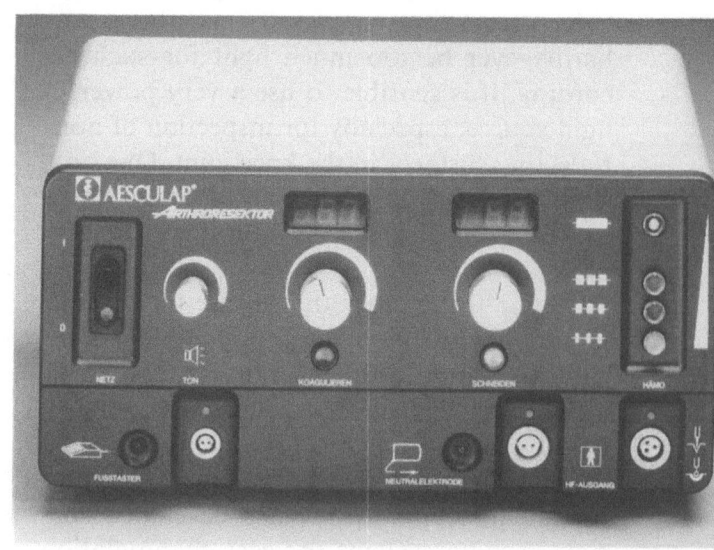

Fig. 11. Diathermy resector (Aesculap)   ▷

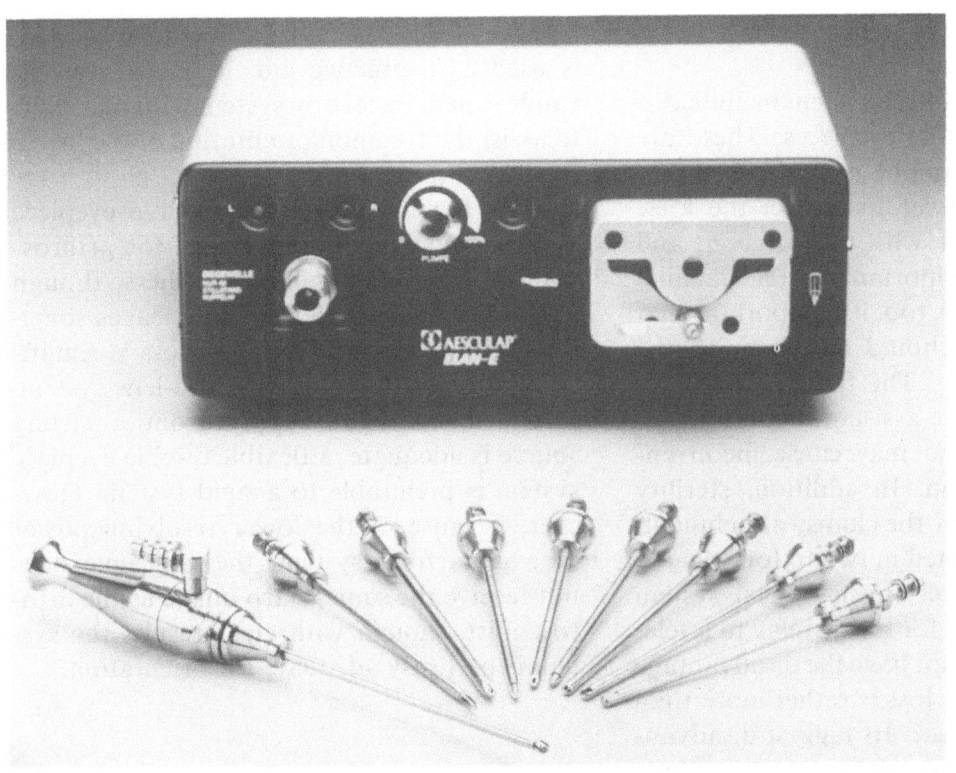

a

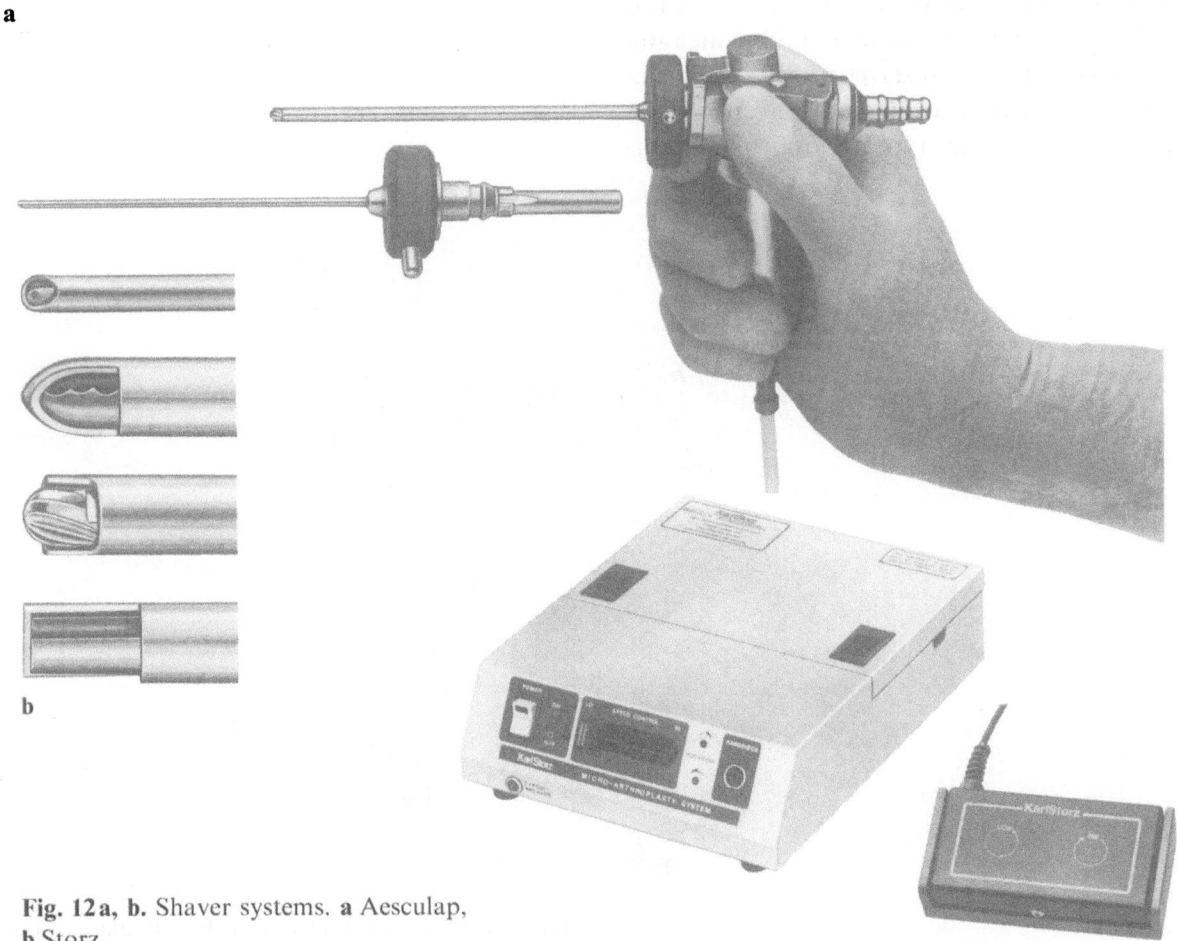

b

Fig. 12a, b. Shaver systems. **a** Aesculap, **b** Storz

2.4 Double Eyepiece Systems

Further accessories of the system include different types of double eyepieces. These are attachments to the optical system which enable a second observer to inspect the knee joint cavity together with the surgeon, and are of the greatest importance in the teaching of arthroscopy. Here, too, it is important that the optical system should not diminish the quality of the image. The fixed double eyepiece often places the assistant in an uncomfortable position and may cause inconvenience to the surgeon. In addition, sterility may be threatened by the clumsy attachment.

Because it is jointed in two to four places, the articulated viewer in an optical system originally developed for image relay to a television camera does not have the disadvantage of rigidity. The light loss is rather more than with the fixed eyepiece. Its biggest disadvantage is that the fellow-observer sees a quite different rotation of the image, i.e., when the results are unclear, surgeon and colleague cannot orientate themselves precisely. This is also the great disadvantage of screen projection used with this type of optical system.

If, nevertheless, such an articulated eyepiece is used as a practice aid, it is advisable to employ an arthroscopy system with markings to assist the common orientation of the investigators (Fig. 13).

The flexible glass fiber double eyepiece system is extremely convenient for arthroscopists, whether pupils or teachers, though its quality of light and imaging leaves something to be desired. The light loss is significantly higher than with the rod-lens system. Provided the light supply from a strong source is adequate, a flexible double eyepiece system is preferable to a rigid system. However, because of the lower resolving power of a glass fiber system, the colleague does not receive the same sharp image as the arthroscopist, though with clear results the system is perfectly adequate for orientation.

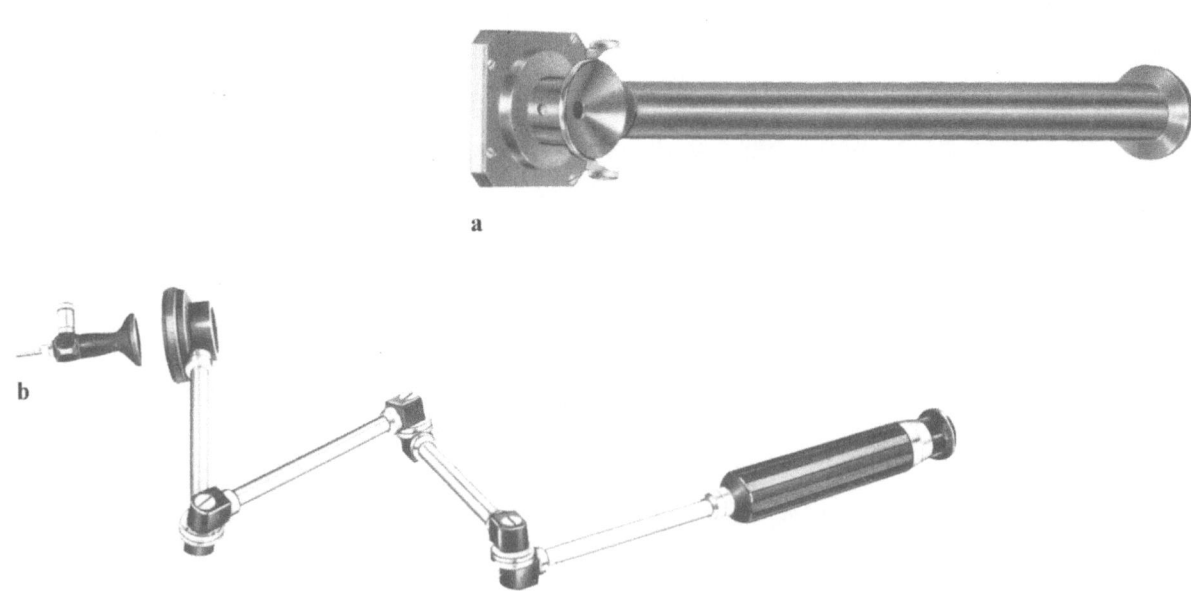

Fig. 13. a Rigid double viewer. b Articulated optical system

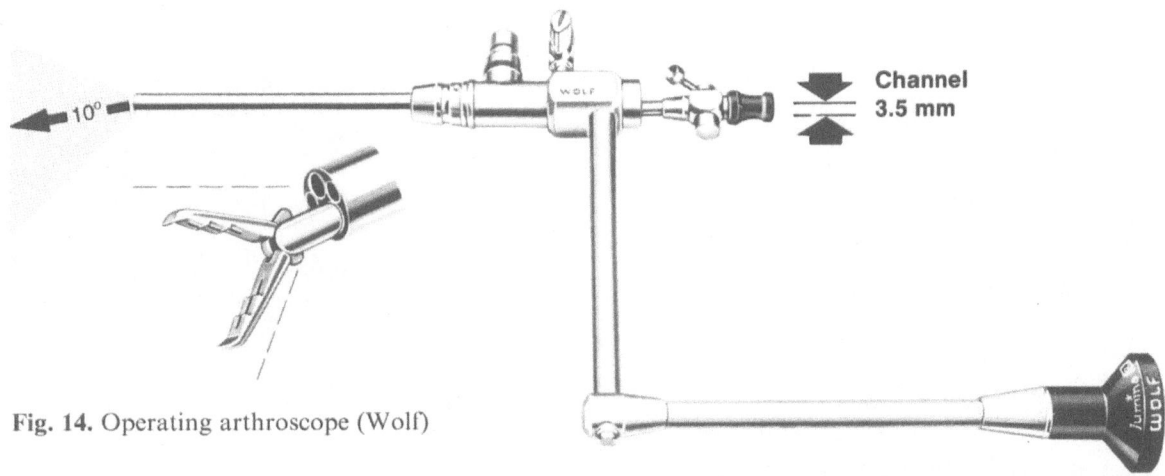

Fig. 14. Operating arthroscope (Wolf)

2.5 Operating Arthroscopes

The various arthroscopy systems produced by Storz, Wolf (Fig. 14), Aesculap, and Stryker have become increasingly harmonized in recent years. O'Connor, who elaborated his arthroscopy system with the Wolf company, distinguished between the diagnostic and the operating arthroscope. Operating arthroscopes are still supplied but have proved rather inadequate, as the operating channel lies parallel to the optical system and there is no freedom of movement for the instrument. Rod-lens systems from different firms are similar in principle, although they differ in angle and breadth of view. As far as is possible to judge, the quality of the optical systems from the leading companies does not vary.

2.6 Photographic Equipment

Documentation of the observed findings is as important as the photography itself. Olympus supply a Polaroid camera (Fig. 15) which, within minutes, reproduces the most important findings on an image surface 3 cm in diameter, the quality being thoroughly satisfactory. Olympus have set new standards with their OM 40 camera (Fig. 16); as well as having a data screen, the data on which can be included in the transparency, it now regulates the exposure automatically. Transparencies of the knee cavity, often difficult to obtain with earlier systems, are now available with greater reliability and better quality.

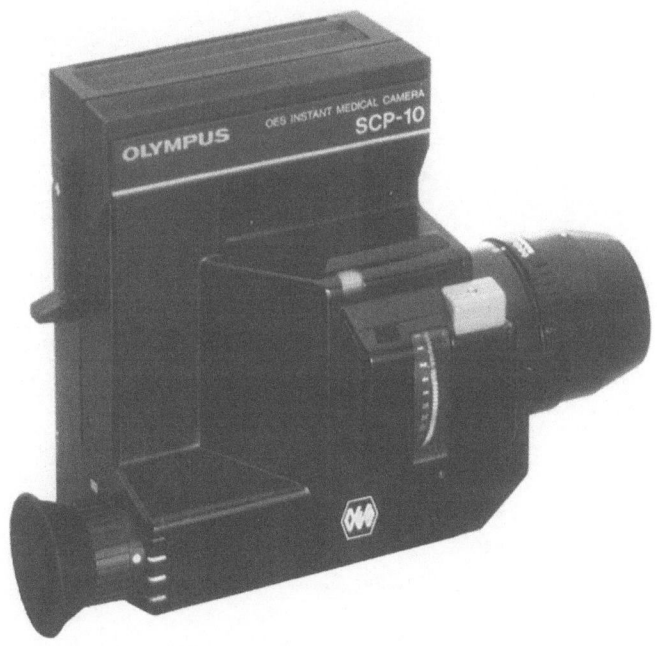

Fig. 15. Olympus Polaroid camera

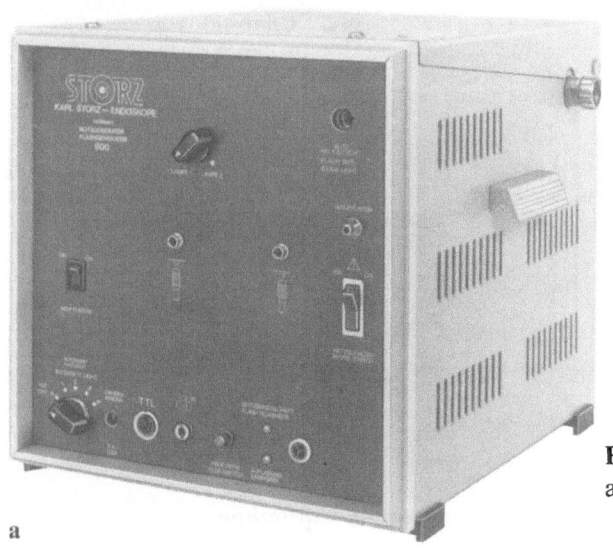

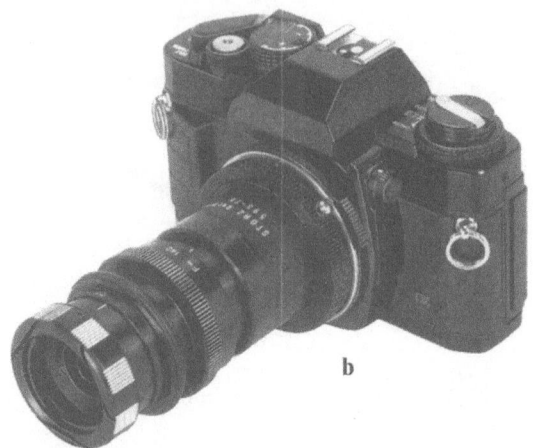

Fig. 16a, b. Recording unit computer flash (Storz) and Olympus OM 40 camera

A new development is under way. In the coming months it will probably become possible to take the most important images directly from the monitor with a newly developed Polaroid camera. Systems of this kind are in the process of development and are already producing satisfactory pictures. Taking photographs from the monitor has the great advantage that the nonsterile camera need no longer be attached to a side-arm of the system, so saving time and trouble.

2.7 Video Systems

Before it became technically possible to transfer the image to a television screen, the surgeon was only able to inspect the knee joint directly through the optical system. This was and is a "semisterile" procedure. The surgeon's eye came very close to the eyepiece and the optical component was always considered nonsterile. This is an essentially uncontrollable factor in long arthroscopic procedures and can lead to increased risk. Only transfer of the image to a television screen by means of a video camera permits complete sterility by appropriate draping. The large tube cameras have been greatly improved in recent years, and many manufacturers now supply small portable tube cameras. In addition, there are charge-coupled devices (CCD cameras) the size of a cigarette packet. With a normal light source it is possible to obtain good monitor pictures. Obviously, it will always be necessary for arthroscopy to be learnt by direct viewing within the knee, which gives students more of a three-dimensional impression than the monitor. Nevertheless, there are enormous advantages if several people can follow the television pictures of the knee joint cavity simultaneously.

Fig. 17. a Chip camera (Storz) and monitor. **b** Charge-coupled camera (Wolf)

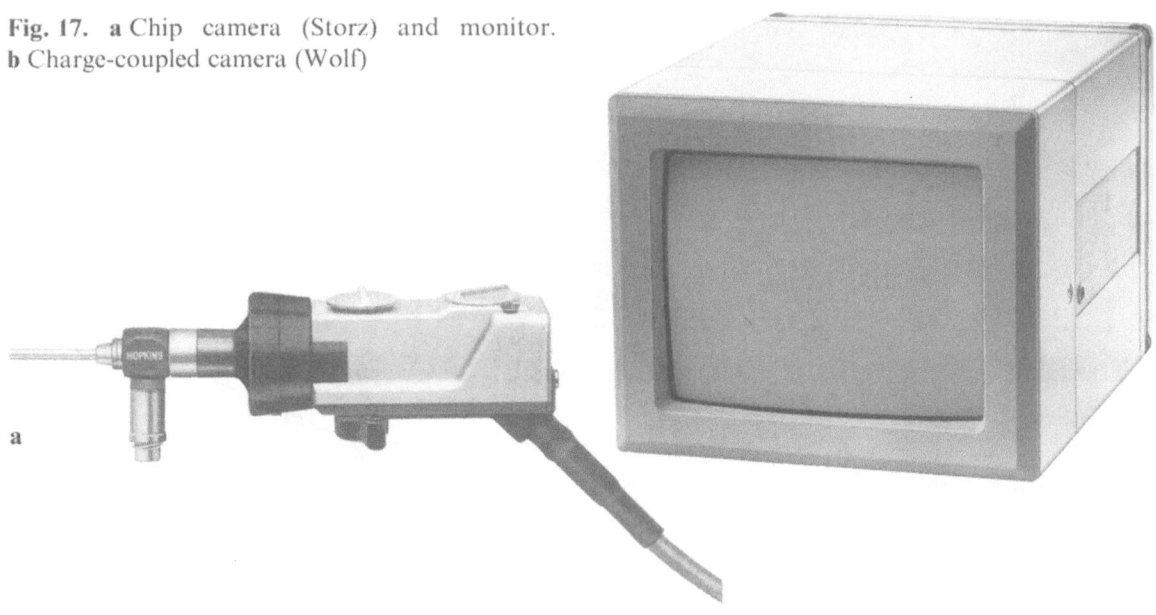

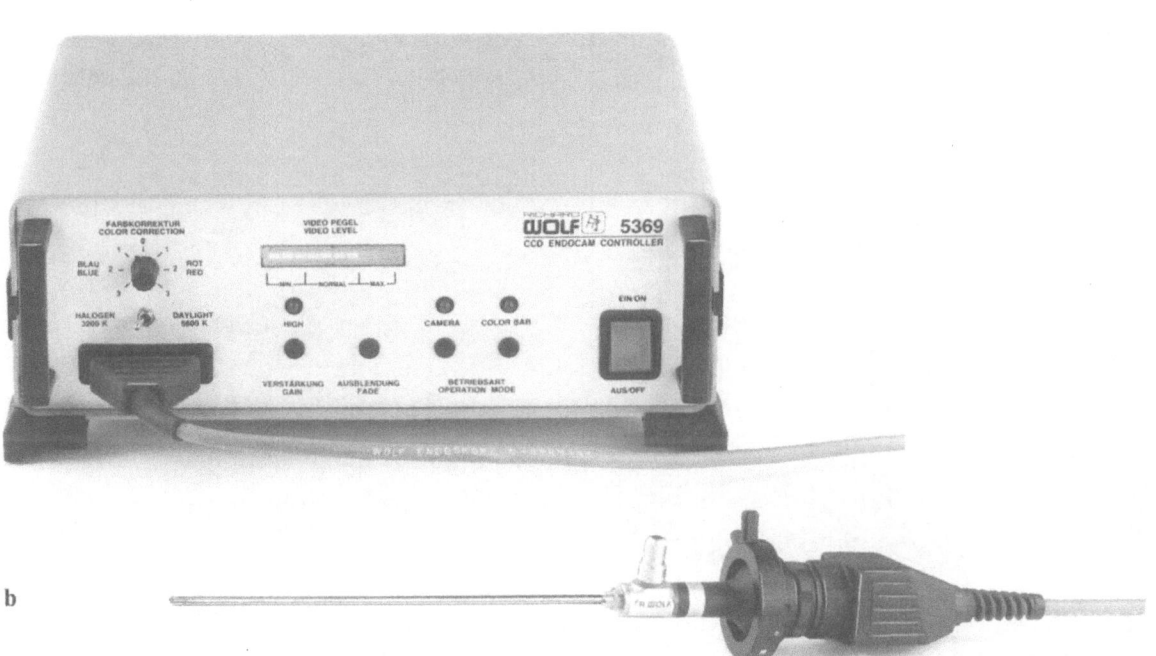

At present, the relatively small chip cameras (Fig. 17a) seem superior to the CCDs (Fig. 17b) in quality, though the latter are sterilizable. Before purchasing such a system, several models should be tested and a choice made on the basis of quality, price, and requirements. It is advisable for the television monitor to be placed on the far side so that the picture is visible to the surgeon and his assistants, while the patient can also follow the operation if he or she wishes. The cable of the television camera is supported in as high a loop as possible above the patient, possibly via a pulley system, to the opposite side, so that it can be attached to the arthroscope with the minimum of tension. Here again, practice on a model knee with this setup of camera and monitor is advantageous.

Obviously, a video recorder can be attached to such a television system. All systems are applicable for recording purposes. VHS, Betamax or similar systems are cer-

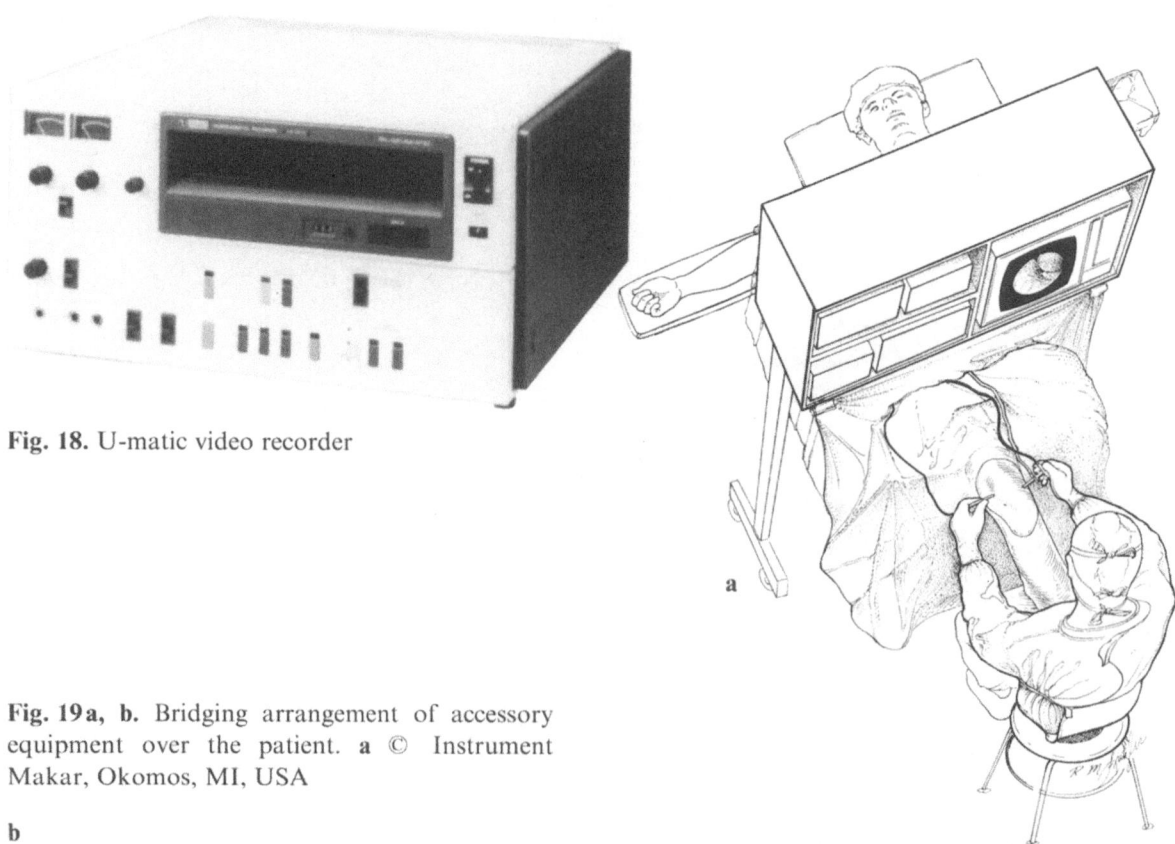

Fig. 18. U-matic video recorder

Fig. 19a, b. Bridging arrangement of accessory equipment over the patient. a © Instrument Makar, Okomos, MI, USA

b

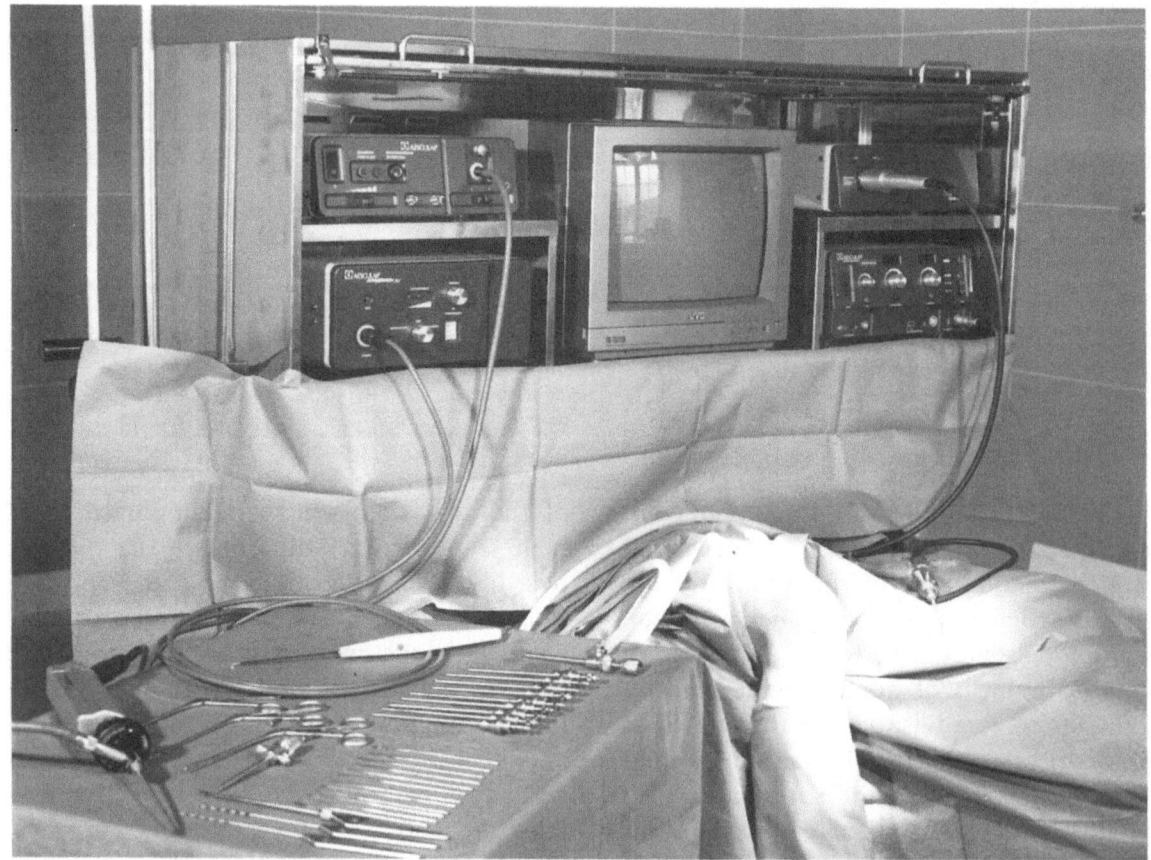

tainly adequate for routine work or documentation. If scientific tapes are to be made, the purchase of a U-matic system is recommended (Fig. 18), the system being widely used internationally. Playback on a normal system is always possible. What was foreseen years ago has now proved possible. Ultimately, arthroscopic operations can only be performed under safe and sterile conditions if the image is transferred to a monitor. In the relaxed atmosphere of an operating theater, where everyone is involved in the proceedings, the problems of sterility can be reliably solved only in this way. The grouping of the individual pieces of equipment, including the video system, around the patient and surgeon can be varied. It is desirable to arrange the system so that it forms a bridge over the patient (Fig. 19). The surgeon then sits at the foot-end of the operating table in front of the draped knee joint and has the monitor and the other instruments in front of him in his visual field. The disadvantage of this arrangement is that a conscious patient is unable to follow the operation. In this case the accessory equipment is arranged to the left and right of the operating table.

CHAPTER 3
How to Learn Arthroscopy

It is a prerequisite for arthroscopy that the investigation and possible operation take place in an operating theater. Those who wish to learn arthroscopy will already have had some experience in surgery of the knee joint. Further prerequisites are knowledge of endoscopic procedures and particularly of endoscopic operations. Accordingly, the surgeon must not be impatient. The operation takes place in a darkened theater and therefore in a quite different atmosphere from that when open arthrotomy is performed. It is not expected that every surgeon, however experienced, should have to learn this method and to replace hitherto successful procedures with this complicated and initially worrying "keyhole" method. Reading the relevant literature is obviously an important preliminary, and this should go together with a study of the equipment and observation of a colleague already practicing arthroscopy. Then the learner can decide whether the method is a suitable one for him.

In recent years, arthroscopy courses have spread worldwide. In a course lasting several days, the theoretic aspects are explained to trainees by experienced arthroscopists. However, the practical aspects should also not be neglected; practice on a model knee and instruction by experienced surgeons are effective aids for beginners. They can become familiar with the equipment and can learn systematic investigation of the knee joint. However, it remains doubtful if work with a model can really simulate operative conditions in patients, and many model knee joints are unsuited to this purpose. The Sommer company in Coburg has developed a model knee (Fig. 20) which is specially adapted to arthroscopic requirements; with the aid of this model the trainee can become familiar with the equipment and study the investigative

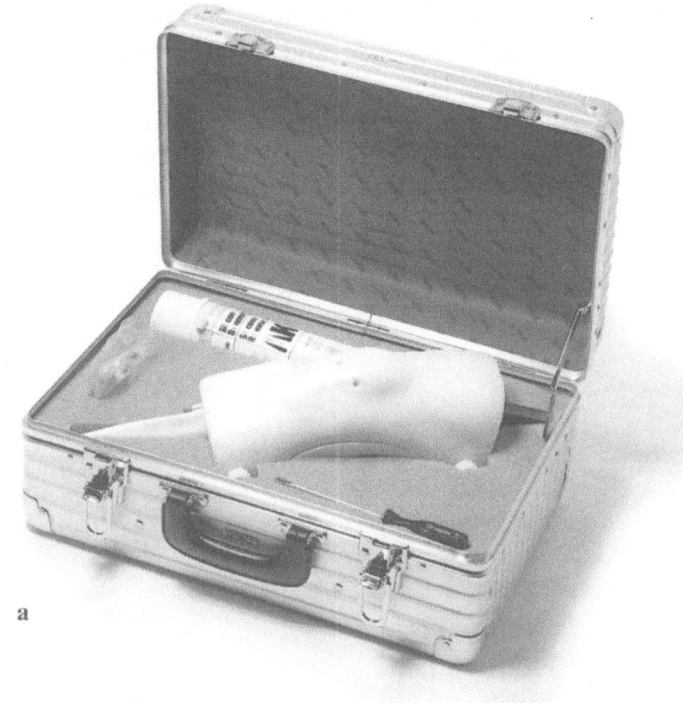

a

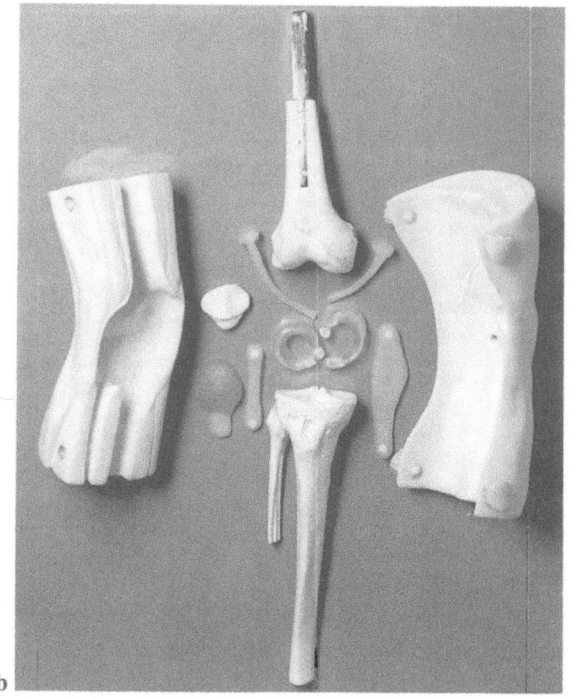

b

Fig. 20a, b. CLA model knee

18

procedure and manipulation of the various instruments. The student also learns to appreciate the magnification effect produced by very close approach of the optical system to the observed object. However, training in the investigative procedure is the most important; using the 30° optical system and, if possible, the video camera, particular approaches can be practiced.

An exercise on the right knee joint could be as follows. Lateral insertion in the typical anterolateral approach. Focusing on the medial condyle with the 30° viewer turned upwards. By moving the lower leg in different angles of flexion, the entire articular surface of the medial condyle is brought into the visual field. The medial condyle remains in focus in 30° flexion. If the light-cable attachment is rotated through 90° to the left (when the light cable is at 180° to the direction of view), the body and anterior horn of the medial meniscus come into view. If the light cable is rotated through 90° to the right from the initial positions, the lateral border of the medial condyle comes into view together with the entrance to the posterior recess and possibly even the posterior horn of the medial

meniscus. At this point it is usually necessary to advance the arthroscope slightly in order to see the posterior horn of the medial meniscus. Refocusing of the arthroscope on the medial condyle with upward line of sight. The tip of the arthroscope is moved to the intercondylar region and elevated above the infrapatellar synovial plica (not present in the model). Focusing of the anterior cruciate ligament. Focusing of the lateral condyle. The lateral meniscus is located merely by rotation of the arthroscope in a similar manner. Obviously, in the practice model exact "figure 4" positioning as in the patient's knee is not possible, so the complete investigative procedure is not reproducible. It is essential for the trainee, with the arthroscope in the patellofemoral joint, to bring first the back of the patella and then the trochlea into view merely by rotation of the optical system, just as was done for the menisci. The first 50 model studies serve mainly for the learning of this maneuver and the acquisition of a routine (Fig. 21).

Fig. 21. Practicing on the model knee

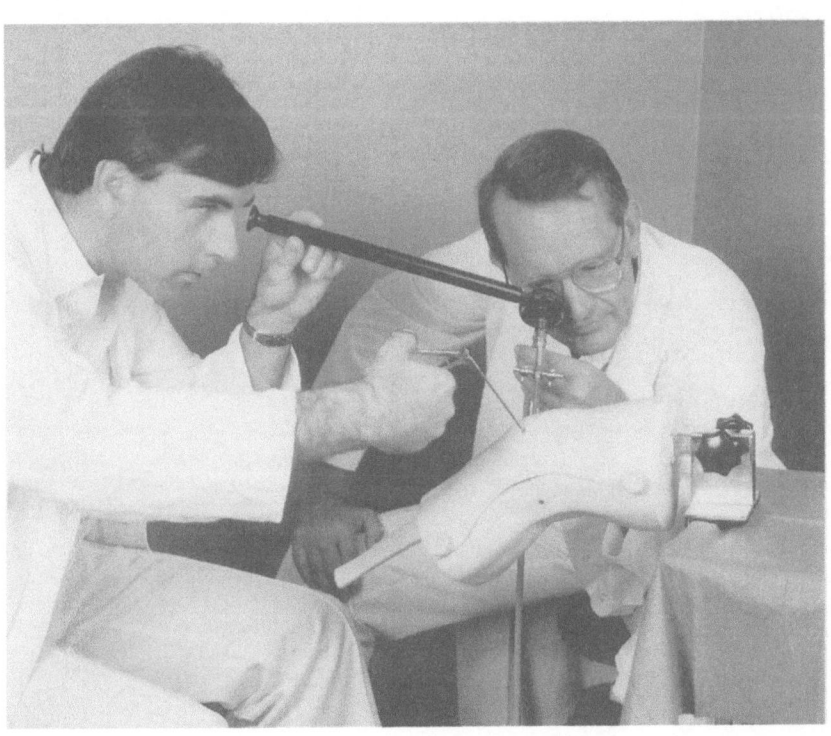

Once the trainee has developed an adequate routine with the equipment on the model, in vivo studies of patients under anesthesia can begin. Obviously, the initial work concerns only diagnostic arthroscopy. After the trainee's first experience and with the emergence of the initial problems, a second arthroscopy course or a visit to an experienced colleague is advisable as a refresh. Only then can any individual problems be discussed, mistakes eliminated, and new ways pointed out. The arthroscopist will realize, after a large number of diagnostic arthroscopies, that the skill required for arthroscopic operations is being acquired. A small palpation hook will nearly always have been used in diagnosis. The detection of the hook in the knee is not as simple as might be initially supposed. The instruments are very often held crosswise and it is not possible to bring the hook into the visual field. However, the surgeon will usually notice that the instruments come into contact within the knee. At first this is allowed to happen deliberately and then, by bringing the outer ends of the instruments closer together, their inner ends are separated, thus bringing the instrument automatically into the visual field. The intercondylar region is a suitable place for detecting the tip of the instrument, which can then be guided visually to the required site. The model knee is eminently suitable for practicing this maneuver.

CHAPTER 4
Documentation of Arthroscopic Investigation

Documentation is as important for this as for other procedures. Various methods are available, and can usually be combined.

4.1 Written Records

As always, written records of the findings of arthroscopy or arthroscopic operation remain the most important part of the procedure. Semischematic operation reports have proved most satisfactory. A short history and clinical findings should be appended at the top with the personal data. A schematic diagram enables the surgeon to record his findings very easily. It still seems indispensable at present to give a short personal operation report describing the overall arthroscopic situation. It is not possible, merely by completing a form, to give the reader a correct impression of the procedure (Fig. 22). Since the operation report may be destined for computer storage, it is important that it should, not accumulate so many data that they are not readily comprehensible; every scientific practitioner should, therefore, personally complete the operation sheet or supply the data. It is essential for the operation report to be dated; especially with arthroscopic operations, guesses are quite unreliable in practice. In the absence of an anesthetic report, the time should be stated.

4.2 Photographic Documentation

The written operation report is supplemented by photographic documentation. Towards the end of the arthroscopy, especially in diagnostic procedures, photographs can be taken even with an nonsterile camera. A Polaroid instrument is suitable for this. Using an enlargement attachment, Polaroid photographs with a diameter of 4 cm can be taken that are well-focused and adequate for immediate information.

Obviously, slides are most suitable for building a photographic record. It is certainly safer initially to record the main findings photographically, though, as experience increases, such records may be dispensed with in cases without pathologic findings. Whereas the beginner will be inclined to overdocumentation, the experienced practitioner will limit himself to a few pictures or to the main finding. To avoid confusion it is advisable to label the slides with the patient's number immediately; this is no longer a problem with the data screen of modern cameras. As the pictures often cannot be correctly arranged at a later date, it is advisable to refer to this documentation in the operation report itself as this considerably facilitates subsequent classification. Photographic documentation during arthroscopic operations is associated with problems of sterility, so that taking photographs from the television monitor is an excellent alternative. Also, electronic printouts of images on paper will certainly be possible in the near future and can be improved to such extent as to ensure that information can be given immediately to the physician who continues treatment.

4.3 Video Recording

A well-functioning television system is essential for recording a procedure on video tape. The professional U-matic tape system is the most suitable for this purpose. It satisfies the highest requirements for recording and reproduction. Transfer to simple video systems as well as rerecording onto the American video system (NTSC) is possible. Recording the entire operation is often too expensive, so the surgeon should be able to record the most important stages of the operation by means of a foot-switch.

Fig. 22. Sample operation report form   ▷

Orthopedic Department

Kreiskrankenhaus Rheinfelden

Medical Director Dr. H.R. Henche

Arthroscopy report

AS-No.:

Date:

Patient's name:

Date of birth:

☐ Knee joint
☐ Shoulder joint
☐ Other joints

☐ Right ☐ Left

Prearthroscopic diagnosis:

Arthroscopic diagnosis:

Arthroscopic treatment:

Treatment plan:

Approach:				
☐ Lateral	☐ Medial	☐ Suprapatellar		
☐ Ventral	☐ Dorsal			
☐ 2 Approaches	☐ 3 Approaches	☐ 4 Approaches		

Duration: _____ min   **Complications:**

Reason: **History:**

☐ Uncertain diagnosis   ☐ Trauma
☐ Inclusive assessment   ☐ Effusion   ☐ Serous ☐ bloody
   of anticipated lesion   ☐ Locking
☐ Progress monitoring   ☐ Giving way of knee
☐ OP   ☐ Feeling of instability

Knee joint – clinical findings:

☐ Joint-line tenderness   ☐ Medial   ☐ Lateral
☐ Patellofemoral tenderness   ☐ Swelling   ☐ Effusion
☐ Loss of extension   ☐ Loss of flexion

☐ Lateral instability   ☐ Medial   ☐ Lateral
☐ Anterior drawer sign   ☐ Lachmann   ☐ Pivot shift
☐ Anterior drawer sign

Arthrogram: ☐ Positive ☐ Negative ☐ Not done   Nature: _____

Previous operations: _____   Date: _____

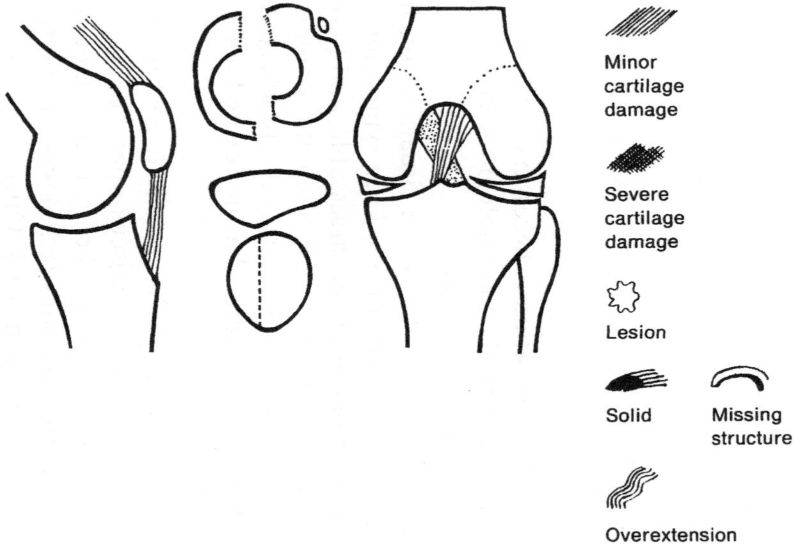

Anaesthesia: ☐ Local ☐ Spinal ☐ General

Documentation: ☐ Polaroid ☐ Transparency ☐ Video

Report:

Minor cartilage damage

Severe cartilage damage

Lesion

Solid

Overextension

Missing structure

23

CHAPTER 5
Indications for Arthroscopy

Arthroscopy is indicated when clinical and radiologic examinations of the knee joint do not allow definitive diagnosis. This applies just as much to chronic knee pain as to an acute injury. If a displacement within the knee joint is suspected as the cause of symptoms, arthroscopy will provide the most exact information. The uses of arthroscopy are:

1. To establish the diagnosis in knee pain or injury when clinical and radiologic assessment is unreliable.

2. To monitor the course of events precisely, as when assessing whether cartilage transplants are properly incorporated or whether cruciate ligament repairs or reconstructions are adequately functional.

3. To plan the operative procedure in recent injuries of the knee joint; also, to decide whether operation is necessary when there is definite clinical and radiologic evidence of articular cartilage damage.

4. To help clarify the situation conclusively in cases of chronic knee symptoms otherwise not objectively assessable, and to reassure the patients, and often the parents of young girls (who are frequently affected by obscure knee pain), that no severe knee joint disease exists.

5. To operate, especially to remove loose material and in meniscus operations; operative procedures are being used increasingly as instruments and techniques are perfected (see Chap. 18, p. 106). Operative procedures should only be carried out during arthroscopy when the operation will be at least as successful as arthrotomy.

CHAPTER 6
Preparation of the Patient for Arthroscopy

6.1 Explanation and Appointment

The indication for arthroscopy nearly always emerges during a consultation with an orthopedist or accident surgeon in the consulting room or casualty department. Even at this stage the patient should be informed of the nature of the anesthetic and the likely course of the procedure. Obviously, the possibility of complications such as infection should also be mentioned. In chronic complaints – though not in acute injuries – several days at least should elapse before the actual investigation, so that the patient may have the opportunity to reflect on whether he really wishes to undergo the procedure. The surgeon's position is more difficult in the case of referral investigations. If the decision has been made by the referring colleague, the patient is frequently admitted directly for arthroscopy and seen by the surgeon on this occasion for the first time. If the surgeon is not convinced that arthroscopy is the correct course of action, he should have the courage not to go ahead with the operative procedure.

As the availability of arthroscopic studies and operations is limited in clinics and practices, dates for these procedures in chronic cases are often fixed weeks in advance. This has the advantage that information on the procedure and possible complications can be sent to the patient with the written notification. The patient can then at home sign the informed consent form and thereby indicate that the operation is not being performed without due consideration. The patient brings this notification on the day set for the investigation. It also contains practical advice, e.g., that he should come for examination having not eaten, and should not drive himself (Fig. 23).

If arthroscopy is done on an outpatient basis, reception at the operating theater is carried out by appropriately trained staff. The patient is provided with theater garments and the knee joint is prepared by shaving and sterilization with an alcohol solution. It is very important to look after the patients from their entry into the (to them) strange changing-room next to the theater onwards, up to and including and during the operation. Shivering may be due not only to anxiety but to the thin operation garments and the normally cool operating theater conditions; here, reassurance and a warm covering during the often unavoidable waiting time work wonders.

Besides shaving and sterilization, a trial of the position on the operating table with the leg supports is sensible, particularly when the operation is to be performed under local anesthesia. As the patient cannot see the surgeon, a nurse should be in attendance at the head-end of the operating table throughout the entire procedure. When the proceedings can be viewed on the monitor, the patient's attention is diverted, leading to a significant improvement in leg muscle relaxation. This obviously makes the investigation easier.

Orthopedic Department

Kreiskrankenhaus Rheinfelden

Kinderklinik Lörrach

Leaflet for Patients

Nature and importance of knee joint imaging and its aftertreatment

Dear patient!

Imaging of the knee joint (arthroscopy) makes it possible to assess injuries and damage within the joint. Moreover, in recent years refined techniques and special intruments have made it possible to treat many lesions and injuries in the knee joint arthroscopically, thereby replacing conventional operative methods. For you, this method has the advantage that it can usually be carried out without admission to hospital and with relatively little risk.

Nature of the investigation:

Under local anesthesia an optical instrument (arthroscope), about the size of a pencil, is inserted into the knee through a small incision. The approach usually chosen is at the outer side below the knee cap. After inserting the instrument, gas or fluid is pumped in under regulated pressure. Every structure in the knee can now be precisely inspected; the image is transmitted directly via a video camera to a television set and you will be able to follow the procedure too.

If you wish, you can obtain a VHS video copy: the charge to cover our expenses is about 60 DM

It is often necessary to check the joint structures with a probe; this instrument is inserted into the joint through a second small incision.

After conclusion of the study the air or fluid is sucked out, the instrument removed, and the small incision closed with a stitch.

Certain injuries and lesions can be operated on arthroscopically at the same session, e.g., meniscus tears or loose bodies.

No further anesthesia is usually required for this.

The aftertreatment will then depend upon the procedure carried out.

Procedure after diagnostic arthroscopy

You will have had a bandage applied after the procedure. This must not be too tight and you should loosen it if necessary. You can remove it yourself after 48 hours and cover the wound with an ordinary adhesive plaster.

You should limit your activities for the first 2 days. Please do not walk about more than necessary, although full weight can be taken on the knee for a few steps. If there is pain or a tight feeling, an ice pack should be applied and the limb kept elevated. Pain-killers can be taken as required.

"Gurgling" and "splashing" sounds in the knee are normal and are due to small amounts of residual fluid or gas; these will be completely absorbed. However, should the feeling of tightness in the joint increase you should consult your doctor, who may have to put a needle into the knee.

The stitch or stitches will be removed after 8–10 days. Washing and showering are allowed after 2 days, but baths should be avoided for 2 weeks.

Procedure after arthroscopic operations

Similar instructions apply as above, except that you should limit your activities for a longer period. Exactly how long will vary, depending on the type of procedure, but you will be informed by us about this. The use of two elbow-crutches is generally necessary to take the weight off the leg that has been operated on. Please begin muscle-tightening exercises (at the front of the thigh) at the 2nd day and do these 3 times a day for at least 10 minutes. A short check-up by your doctor or by us will be necessary to monitor your condition. Please bear in mind that, despite the small incision, an operative procedure has taken place in your joint and that this calls for a longe recovery period.

If there is unexpect edly severe pain, redness, swelling of the lower leg, and fever, please report immediately to your doctor or to us.

Telephone Kreiskrankenhaus Rheinfelden: 07623 94371

PD Dr. Henche
Senior Surgeon

Fig. 23. Explanatory leaflet for arthroscopy patients

6.2 Positioning

We prefer the patient to be placed on the operating table in a supine position, with the knee in a support designed especially for arthroscopy. The lateral supports should allow the exertion of powerful varus or valgus stress. The leg holder itself is covered with a specially designed sterile towel (Fig. 24).

After preparation of the entire limb by disinfection with a suitable solution, as for arthrotomy, the foot and lower leg are enclosed in a sterile stocking. The thigh is placed in the leg holder with its sterile covering. Large operation towels are then applied, as is customary for arthrotomy. We have abandoned the practice of covering the knee with an adhesive drape, as parts of the drape may be torn off by the trocar and be transferred into the knee joint.

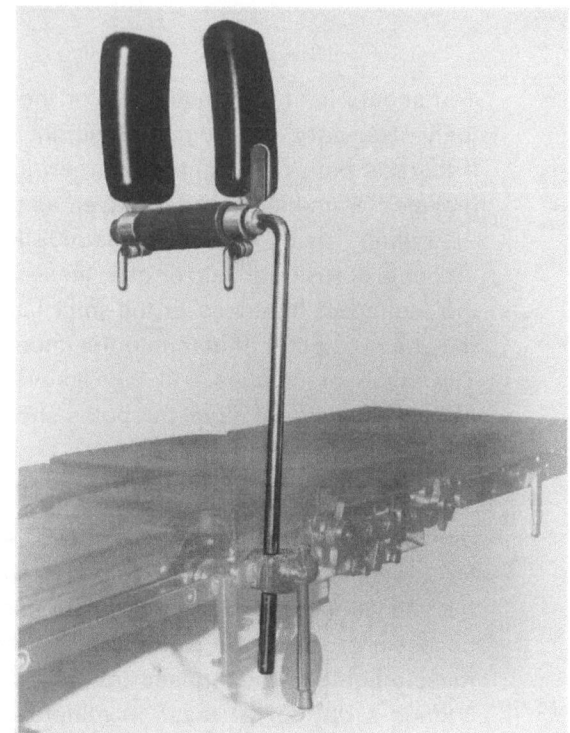

Fig. 24. Leg holder (Maquet)

CHAPTER 7
Theater Nurse's Preparations for Arthroscopy

The preparations for arthroscopy are not limited to correct positioning of the patient on the operating table and draping. The requisite nonsterile accessory equipment as well as the actual arthroscopy instruments with the attachments to the nonsterile parts are arranged around the operating table. The prepared sterile table for the arthroscopy equipment is placed on the side of the knee to be operated on. Those instruments that may be required for the particular type of investigation and operation are placed here ready for use, always including the outer tube with its obturator and the arthroscope. Sterile hoses for filling the joint with gas or fluid are attached to the appropriate accessory apparatus. Likewise, after attachment to the arthroscope, the light cable is connected to the light source, which is located behind the surgeon. The surgeon now has the knee to be investigated in front of him, his assistant on one side to move the knee appropriately, and on the other side the small sterile table with the operation instruments. Behind the surgeon are the nonsterile accessory items of equipment such as the gas or fluid supply, suction pump, and light source. The television system with the video recorder is placed appropriately at the other side of the operating table. The cable to the camera must be carried across the patient to the surgeon's side, most suitably by a suspension-pulley system. The camera itself and at least 1 meter of the camera cable towards the monitor are enclosed in sterile wrapping. This wrapping also surrounds the eyepiece of the arthroscope, so no nonsterile part of the equipment becomes involved during arthroscopy using a video camera. With the surgeon viewing directly through the arthroscope, the black portion (eyepiece) must be regarded as nonsterile.

CHAPTER 8
Care of Equipment

All parts of the arthroscopic equipment are cleaned and autoclave sterilized just like all operation instruments. Special attention is given to the optical system, for which gas sterilization with acetylene is undoubtebly the best method. This sterilization facility is not universally available and there is also the disadvantage that after sterilization the equipment must be aired for 24 h in a so-called airing conduit, i.e., the eyepieces can only be used once every 24 h. The same applies to sterilization in formalin vapor, where reinsertion of the optical system also has to wait for 24 h. Rapid disinfection is possible with Cydex solution, reuse of the arthroscope being possible 20–30 min after immersion in the bactericidal solution. The disadvantage is that the Cydex solution cannot kill spores, although there is no evidence that the infection rate with this type of sterilization is higher than with gas sterilization.

Apart from sterilization, care of the delicate instruments and testing of their functional performance is of the greatest importance. The quality of the optical system must be assessed after every investigation. Bending leads to failure of the light-conducting system and therefore to loss of illumination during the investigation, which will be revealed first by the quality of the photographs. The performance of the light cable must also be checked. Deposits on the glass fiber bundles at the ends of the cable lead to very great loss of light. Fusing of the ends of the glass fibers with consequent rapid loss of illumination occurs particularly with very powerful light sources, such as the xenon lamp.

As regards the equipment, special attention must be given to ensure that the blades of forceps and scissors have not suffered fatigue fractures. Good care and supervision of the instruments reduces the risk of instrument breakage in the knee joint during the operation. Special attention must also be paid to the sealing of the tubing used in filling the knee joint with gas. As the tubing deteriorates the system can lose pressure and clarity of viewing within the knee may become impaired. Pressure loss in the knee is frequently an indication of inadequate attention to the attached system.

If the gas insufflator is connected to a bacterial filter, this too must be regularly inspected or the filter changed at the prescribed intervals.

CHAPTER 9
Anesthesia for Arthroscopy

Basically, three different types of anesthesia can be used for arthroscopy and arthroscopic operations, the type used depending on external circumstances and constraints. On the one hand, the experience and reliability of the surgeon play a decisive part; on the other, the policy of the hospital administration or of the medical insurance fund have to be taken into account. As any form of anesthesia involves risk, the surgeon must be familiar with all the advantages and disadvantages of the various techniques and reach his decision in conjunction with the external circumstances and the patient's wishes. Reliance on a single type of anesthesia is undesirable.

9.1 General Anesthesia

General anesthesia has considerable advantages and will be employed particularly by surgeons who are still gaining experience and have not yet developed a long-standing routine for diagnostic arthroscopy or operative procedures. The patient is completely relaxed and a tourniquet is easily applied. The surgeon is unhurried in the investigation and operation. A further advantage is that the patient can move his legs as soon as he regains consciousness.

However, the disadvantages of general anesthesia are not insignificant. In particular, the patient has to grant the surgeon a sort of general "power of attorney" before the operation so that diagnostic and operative procedures may be decided on during the operation. For many patients this is a disagreeable situation, especially if the procedures to be carried out have only moderate success rates. A further disadvantage is that the use of leg holders may damage the lateral ligaments of the knee. With a powerful assistant,

the varus or valgus strain from pressure or traction on the lateral ligament may be great enough to cause partial or even complete rupture of the ligamentous apparatus. Even fractures of the femur may occur; some have been reported in the literature (Saillant et al. 1986). Again, the patient will not notice if fluid or gas under excess pressure is forced into the musculature above or below the knee in recent injuries. Thereby, general anesthesia incurs an increased risk of thrombosis, especially as a tourniquet is often employed. Another disadvantage to be considered is that general anesthesia relieves the surgeon from pressure of time, which for many surgeons is unfortunate as they may persist with operations that have been started but which prove impracticable to complete. Operation times then arise that can be harmful for the patient. Of course, this disadvantage should not be attributed to the general anesthesia in itself; it is for the surgeon to decide on his own time limit, especially where operative procedures are concerned.

9.2 Regional Anesthesia

The only form of regional anesthesia to be considered here is spinal anesthesia, whose main advantage, as opposed to epidural anesthesia, is that it produces complete muscle relaxation. Unlike general anesthesia, it is possible to talk with the patient who can even watch the findings on the television monitor and can participate in discussion of further procedure. This type of anesthesia lasts long enough to relieve the surgeon from time constraints but, as the patient is usually conscious throughout the operation, the surgeon cannot extend the procedure indefinitely as under general anesthesia. However, spinal anesthesia also has its disadvantages, such as the well-known long and unpredictable recovery phase. The patient must be kept under observation and cared for in hospital for several hours. The legs cannot be moved very well right away, and this leads to an increased risk of thrombosis if a tourniquet has been used. Just as with general anesthesia, the patient cannot feel pain if fluid or gas under increased pressure is forced into the tissues around the knee joint. A further undesirable consequence of spinal anesthesia, especially in young people, is the frequent development of headaches which may persist for several days, preventing the patient from resuming work even when the after effects of the arthroscopy have long subsided. Moreover, one disadvantage of general anesthesia that has already been mentioned also applies to spinal anesthesia: a powerful assistant may produce injuries to the knee joint or thigh during the investigation.

9.3 Local Anesthesia

Indisputably, the most refined form of anesthesia is local anesthesia, especially for diagnostic arthroscopy. This has the advantage that it is not absolutely necessary to have an anesthetist, though of course the patient should be requested to fast before attending for examination, not on account of the local anesthesia itself but because of the possibility of one of the exceedingly rare complications of this type of anesthesia developing. An excess of local anesthetic agent may lead to a fall in blood pressure and, in rare cases, to convulsions of the petit mal type. The patient must fast before local anesthesia so that, the anesthetist can undertake intubation should such complications arise. It is highly advisable, therefore, that the anesthetist should stand by during arthroscopy under local anesthesia. However, in none of 4000 arthroscopies under local anesthesia has this precaution proved necessary so we have dispensed with the insertion of an intravenous line during local anesthesia. Often, a patient undergoing arthroscopy after a light breakfast

gives the impression of better toleration of this procedure than one who has fasted for several hours and is therefore hungry. However, for legal reasons we think it better to require the patient to fast before the investigation, although we do not insert an intravenous line preoperatively despite similar legal considerations.

9.4 Technique of Local Anesthesia (Fig. 25)

The knee joint is shaved after application of soap solution. Sterilization is then carried out with an alcoholic solution or with the sterilizing agent customary for the operation. Injection of local anesthetic is performed under sterile conditions as for any puncture of the knee joint. At the desired site a skin wheal is raised with a 2% local anesthetic solution (mepivacaine) mixed with a small amount of a vasoconstrictor agent. The deeper layers are likewise anesthetized with this solution. Not more than 2 ml is used at any one site. When the synovium has been infiltrated the tip of the needle enters the joint cavity and it suddenly becomes very much easier to inject the anesthetic solution. This is an infallible sign of correct positioning of the needle tip. The knee joint is now filled with a 0.25% anesthetic solution. It is reasonable to use a long-acting agent; filling with 20 ml bupivacaine suffices. However, it is perfectly reasonable to inject up to 40 ml, in which case the dilution of the anesthetic agent should be 0.125%. With proper instillation, it has been shown that even greatly diluted anesthetic solutions produce the same effect and that circulatory and central complications are reduced to a minimum in this way.

An important test as to whether it is the knee joint cavity rather than the infrapatellar fat pad that has been distended is to observe what happens when the needle is removed from the cannula. Slow dripping from the end of the cannula of the artificially produced effusion shows that all is well. If, however, there is a jet of anesthetic solution from the cannula, it means that the fat pad or other structure in the knee joint has been in-

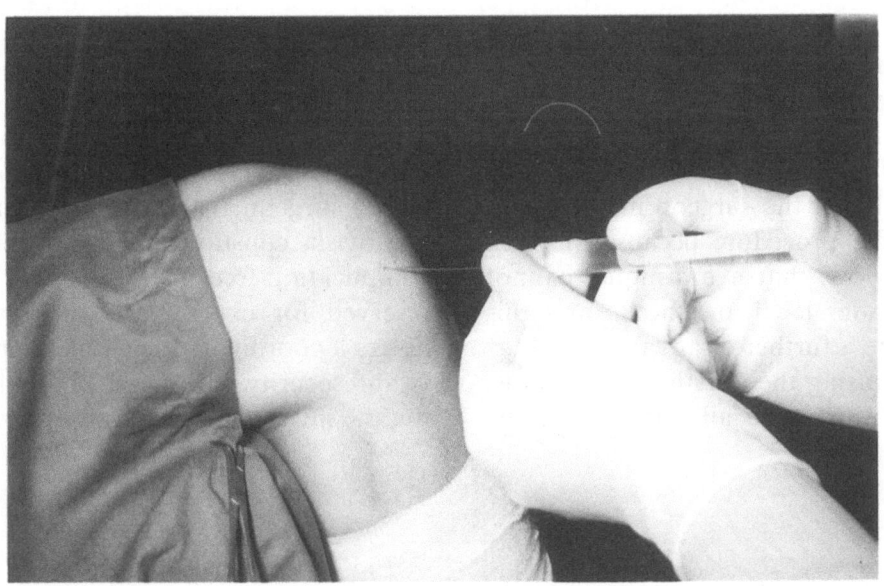

Fig. 25. Local anesthesia of the knee cavity and incisions

filtrated. In addition the patient has probably mentioned a feeling of pressure during the injection. With correct instillation of the local anesthetic solution the patient expresses no pain, or at most only a slight sensation of pressure or feeling of coldness. In any case, when one is uncertain whether the needle tip is within the joint it is advisable to change the site of injection, possibly choosing suprapatellar infiltration of the local anesthetic as the conventional insertion site. Distension of the fat pad from the anterolateral approach customary for arthroscopy may make the investigation impossible or at least very difficult. Nevertheless, if the fat pad is distended and the surgeon and patient are disinclined to dispense with arthroscopy on that day, it has been found useful to move the knee vigorously and then to wait at least 30–60 min, when it is usually possible to carry out the procedure without marked disadvantages.

There should be a pause of at least 10–15 min after injection of the local anesthetic. Even then, in rare cases, the patient experiences brief pain during the stab incision and insertion of the trocar into the knee joint cavity. However, with proper anesthesia the actual investigation is always painless. The duration of anesthesia depends on the agent employed – between 60 and 120 min with long-acting anesthetic solutions. Advantages of local anesthesia are that it can be used rapidly and without complications, and that premedication is not necessary. The patient can move the knee immediately after the investigation or operation and, depending on the procedure, may be able to bear weight on the leg. The time restriction inevitably resulting from the use of regional or local anesthesia counts as an advantage, as it protects the patient in many cases from very long and therefore strenuous procedures.

However, the disadvantages of local anesthesia should not be overlooked. It does not produce complete muscular relaxation – many patients find it extraordinarily difficult, for instance, to relax the quadriceps in order to permit inspection of the patellofemoral joint and the superior recess. Of course, with increased surgical experience and routine and with proper mental conditioning of the patient the number of those unable to relax during the procedure becomes insignificant. However, a certain degree of muscle tone is always present and therefore it is more difficult to perform arthroscopic operations under local anesthesia with full confidence. To this is added the time restriction on the surgeon. It is safe to assume that, under local anesthesia, an arthroscopic operation with both gas distension of the knee and continuous saline irrigation will be unacceptable to the patient after some 60 min. In contrast to general anesthesia, the surgeon may have to discontinue the procedure because of pain. It is also obvious that a tourniquet cannot be applied under local anesthesia, and this may constitute a further disadvantage.

When choosing the anesthetic technique, the surgeon must take all relevant factors into account: the patient's wishes, local conditions, the surgeon's routine, type of procedure and any other constraints. Usually, it may be said that general anesthesia is the most reasonable method for the inexperienced surgeon. There is no doubt that local anesthesia constitutes the most refined and complication-free method, but it should be reserved for experienced surgeons and requires a coordinated team to ensure the safety and security of the patient at all times during the investigation or operation.

CHAPTER 10
Approaches to the Knee Joint

The lateral approach, close to the knee joint cavity, has proved most satisfactory. With the knee bent at a right angle, the lateral joint space is easily found anteriorly. The thumb is used to palpate an anterolateral depression bounded medially by the patellar ligament, proximally by the lower border of the patella, and distally by the edge of the head of the tibia. The incision is made approximately in the center of this lateral depression (Fig. 26). It is important that the incision should lie directly over the joint space, and if there is any doubt it is preferable to choose a more proximal approach. From the lateral approach it is possible to inspect nearly all the important parts of the joint. However, the general rule to apply in the choice of approach is that the region opposite the skin incision is the easiest to inspect. It must be stated that, with experience, even the lateral joint region can be completely and thor-

oughly inspected from a lateral incision. As already mentioned, the figure 4 position of the knee is important here as it best opens up the lateral joint cleft. The patellofemoral joint and the suprapatellar recess are likewise open to inspection. The intercondylar region is usually best inspected from the lateral approach and the inner aspect of the medial femoral condyle is almost completely exposed. The anterior attachment of the posterior cruciate ligament is clearly seen, provided it is not obscured by fatty tissue and synovial membrane. The anterior cruciate ligament can be fully inspected with the 30° optical system. To reach the attachment of the anterior cruciate ligament to the lateral condyle, it is advisable to carry out the approach close to the patellar ligament.

The inner aspect of the lateral condyle can also be fully inspected, and intubation of the dorsolateral recess is likewise possible in this manner. In about half the cases, with the arthroscope below the anterior cruciate ligament and above the posterior horn of the

Fig. 26. Lateral approach

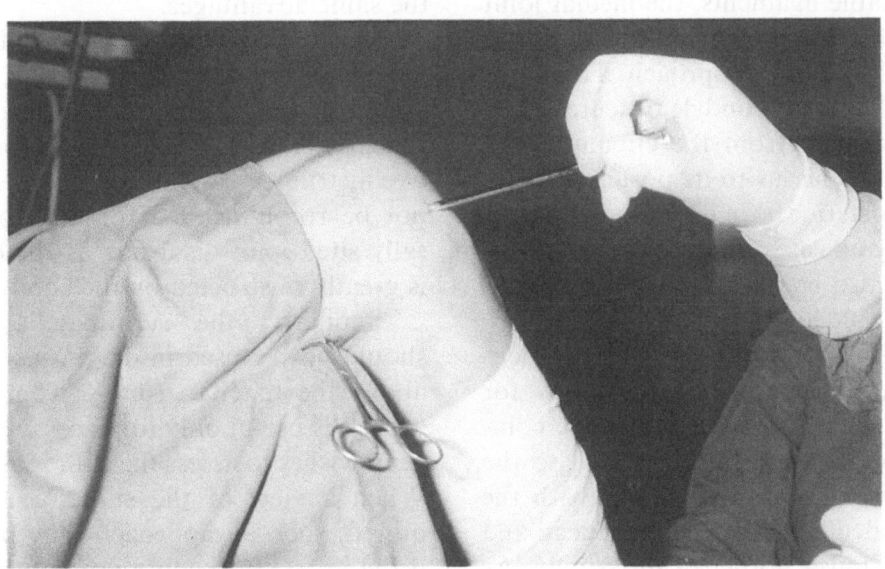

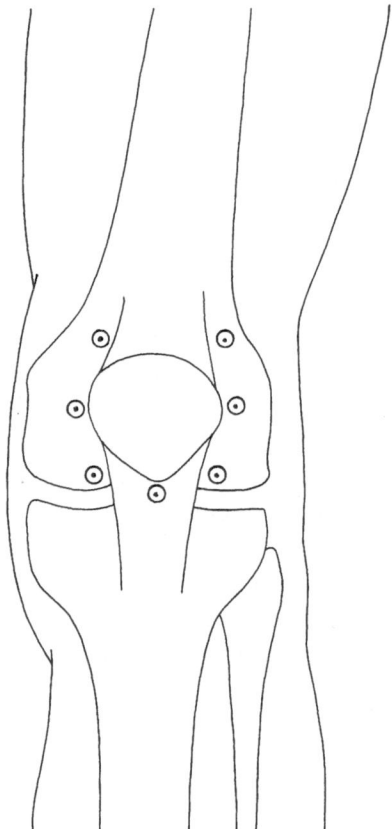

Fig. 27. Anterior approaches to the knee joint

lateral meniscus, it is possible to view the dorsolateral recess. Exchanging the 30° optical system for a 70° system makes it possible to view the posterior tibial margin with the origin of the posterior cruciate ligament. In knee joints with stable ligaments, the medial joint compartment cannot always be completely viewed from the lateral approach. The bulge of the medial femoral condyle obscures from view the transition from the circumference of the medial meniscus to its posterior horn, though the posterior horn itself can be clearly seen in nearly all cases. The edge of the meniscus should also be visible in nearly all knee joints with stable ligaments.

The medial approach (Fig. 27) is particularly suitable in diagnostic arthroscopy for precise assessment of the lateral joint compartment. Here too, the fossa medial to the patellar ligament is easily palpable with the thumb, bounded below by the tibial head and above by the lower border of the patella. As with the lateral approach, the incision is made at the center or upper half of this depression. At the medial aspect it seems particularly important for the approach to be directly over the joint cleft in order to avoid damaging the meniscus, and also not to be too greatly hampered by the fat pad during the inspection. The medial approach is not often chosen for diagnostic purposes and usually serves for insertion of the small hook used for probing structures within the joint cavity. In particular, the medial meniscus can be palpated from here for tears and flap formation. In operative procedures on the lateral meniscus it may be helpful to insert the arthroscope from the medial side of the knee.

Variants of these two anterior approaches include Gillquist's approach through the patellar ligament and Patel's approach at the mid-patellar level. The transligamentous approach introduced in Sweden has the advantage, compared with an extreme lateral or medial approach, of allowing significantly better instrumentation of the posterior recess while the lateral and medial views remain satisfactory. Its disadvantage is that it damages such an important structure as the patellar ligament, which means that the central portion of the ligament cannot be employed immediately for replacement of the anterior cruciate ligament. This approach is not absolutely necessary since lateral and medial approaches sited very close to the patella have the same advantages.

The approach recommended by Patel, very high above the joint space, is perhaps due to finding that a higher approach is particularly suitable for manipulation of operative instruments within the knee joint. It cannot be recommended for diagnosis of dorsally sited joint disorders as the dorsal view is greatly obstructed by the condyles.

Similarly, the suprapatellar approach should not be used in diagnosis. An incision above the patella, usually from the lateral aspect, is useful only for cases where the surgeon wishes to assess the suprapatellar recess. When a view of the superior recess is required, such an approach may be necessary if the usual approaches are not good enough

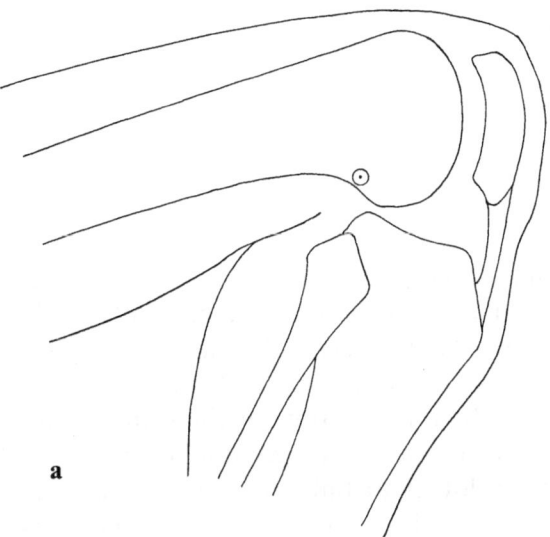

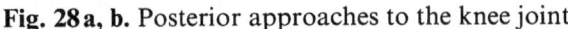

a

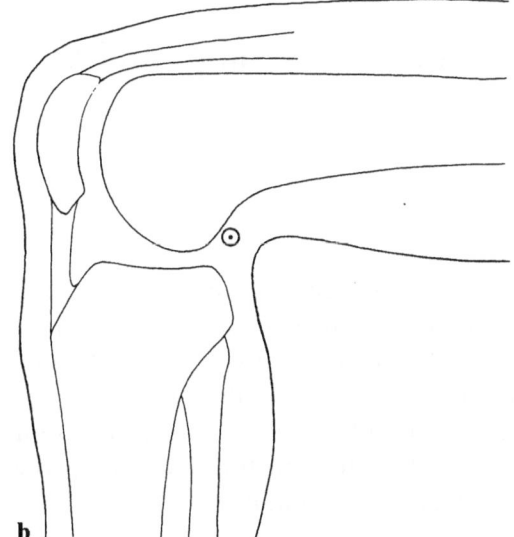

b

Fig. 28 a, b. Posterior approaches to the knee joint

due to scarring from numerous previous operations. The suprapatellar approach also serves for the insertion of operation instruments, and the removal of loose bodies is best carried out by this route.

For certain problems it is necessary to inspect the dorsal recesses (Fig. 28). One of the most important indications is the presence of large free loose bodies which are mobile in the posterior recess on one or other side and cause frequent pain within the joint and sometimes also in the popliteal fossa. Under these circumstances, no locking occurrs at all. These recesses are very difficult to inspect from in front and it is impossible to displace the loose bodies forwards, even with irrigation. In such cases, dorsolateral in-

sertion of the arthroscope is advisable, most suitably above the head of the fibula, anterior to the biceps tendon, and behind the popliteus tendon. Here, the incision is made about 1 cm above the palpated joint space.

The same applies to the dorsomedial approach, where the incision is made close above the pes anserinus tendon with the knee flexed at 60°–90°. Inspection of this recess also allows the posterior horn of the medial meniscus to be seen. It must be left to the surgeon to decide whether this justifies such an approach. This approach is also important when looking for loose bodies and lost portions of menisci or foreign bodies, such as parts of the operative equipment.

To sum up, it can be said that the anterolateral approach combined with a medial approach for the probe hook is adequate for 95% of diagnostic arthroscopic examinations.

CHAPTER 11
Examination Using Fluid or Gas Media

Basically, illumination of the knee joint can be performed in two different media. Normally, the investigation is carried out with the joint cavity distended with fluid; gas is less commonly used to expose the joint. It is possible, and sometimes advantageous, to combine both techniques.

11.1 Filling the Knee Joint with Fluid

The knee joint can be distended with Ringer solution or normal saline. Disadvantages such as synovial irritation by saline have not been demonstrated with certainty. It is advantageous to perform the first filling of the joint via a 2- to 3-mm needle in the suprapatellar recess. This is followed by insertion of the arthroscope which is more easily done in tightly distended joints and with less risk of damage to the articular cartilage (see p. 46). At this point it is sensible to introduce the fluid via the arthroscope. It is usually satisfactory to use infusion bottles, which should be suspended at least 1 m above the knee. The thick needle originally placed in the suprapatellar recess then acts as an overflow system. For practical purposes, the greater the through-flow of fluid, the clearer the view. However, too great a flow also produces a lot of turbulence and, especially in severe synovitis, the view within the joint may be repeatedly obscured by synovial fragments. Therefore, the flow should be so regulated that the fluid remains clear while turbulence is restricted to a minimum. The advantages of this type of joint distension are obvious. No expensive equipment is required. The pressure in the joint cavity is regulated by the height of the infusion bottle and possibly by control of the overflow. Those who prefer a more precise method may use the pumps supplied by various firms for fluid filling of the knee joint. These permit choice and adjustment of pressure within the knee, as necessary. The biggest disadvantage of fluid distension of the knee joint is the so-called "aquarium effect" (Fig. 29), when the syno-

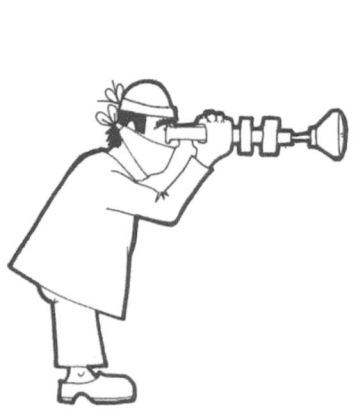

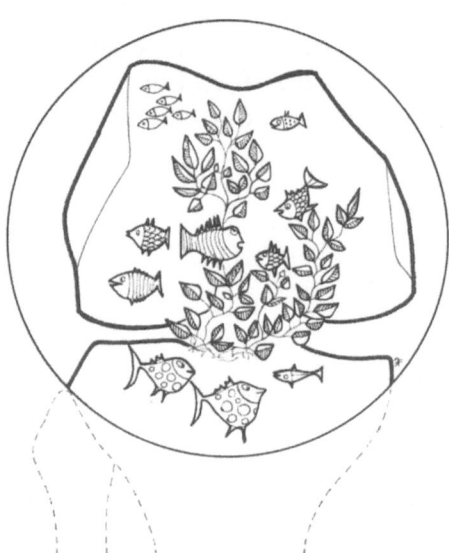

Fig. 29. "Aquarium effect"

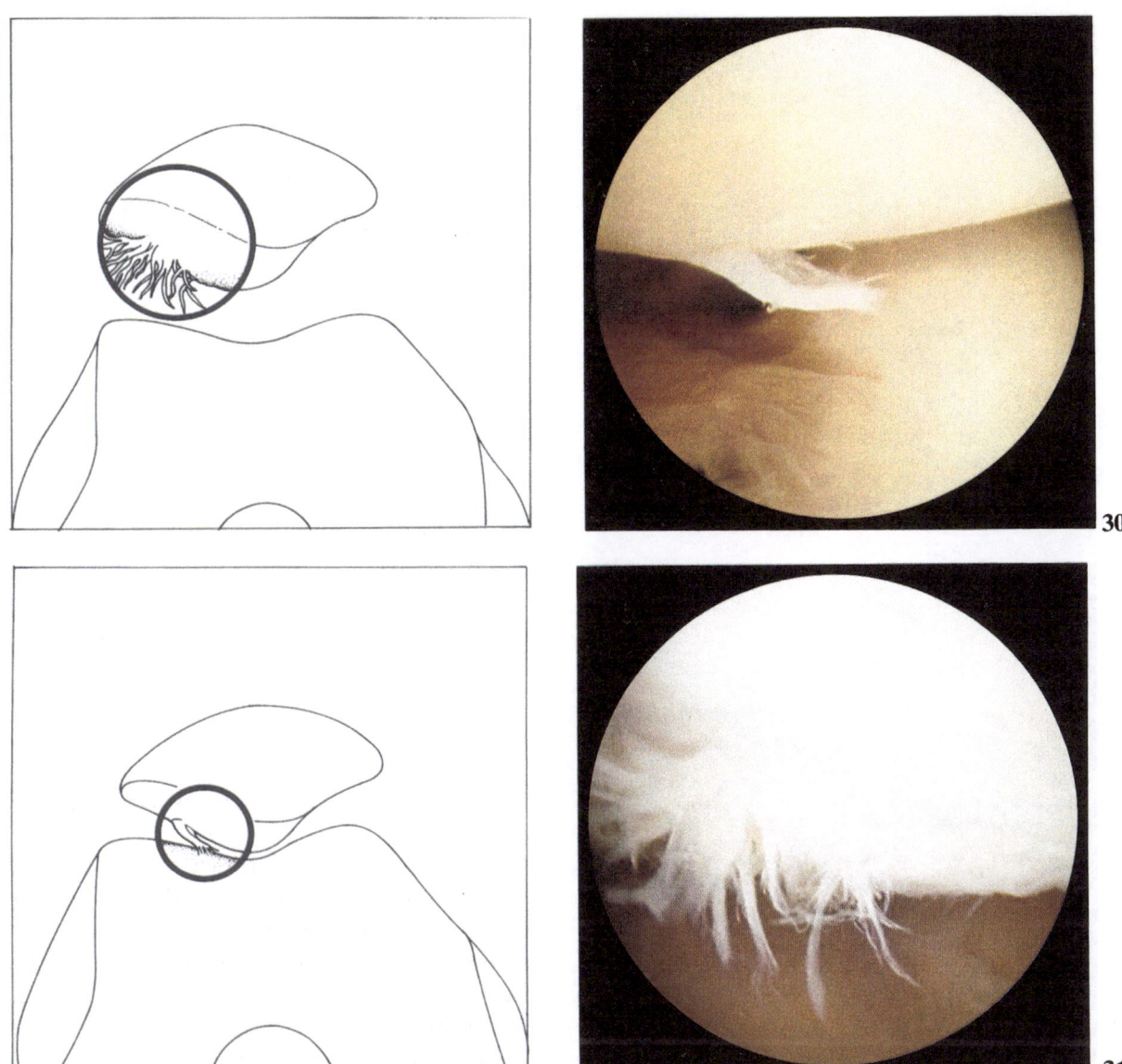

vial villi behave like water plants in an aquarium, moving with the turbulence of irrigation in the direction of the flow. Cartilage shreds and fraying of the articular cartilage surface are in this case very readily (too readily?) detectable and may lead the surgeon, especially if inexperienced in arthroscopy, to diagnose severe cartilage damage (Figs. 30–32). Hence the maxim of the experienced: "The knee joint distended with fluid appears more diseased than it really is." The insertion of a small hook under water greatly helps to clarify the picture and suspected ruptures or partial ruptures of the cruciate ligaments can be assessed more realistically.

Fig. 30. Image of a minimal cartilage defect at the back of the patella using a fluid medium

Fig. 31. Low-grade chondromalacia patellae. The aquarium effect makes it appear very large and deep

39

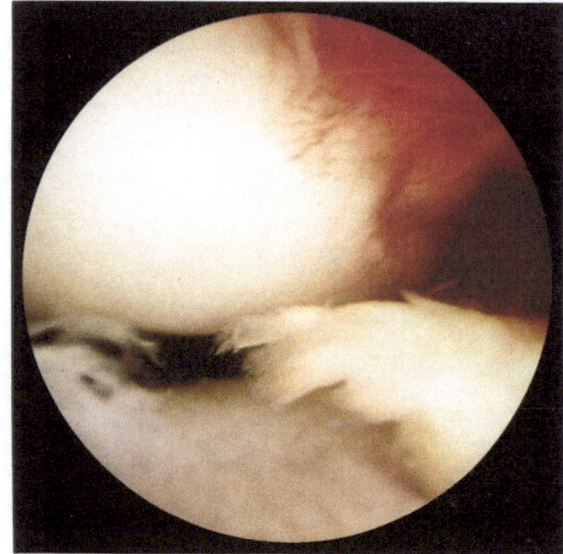

a

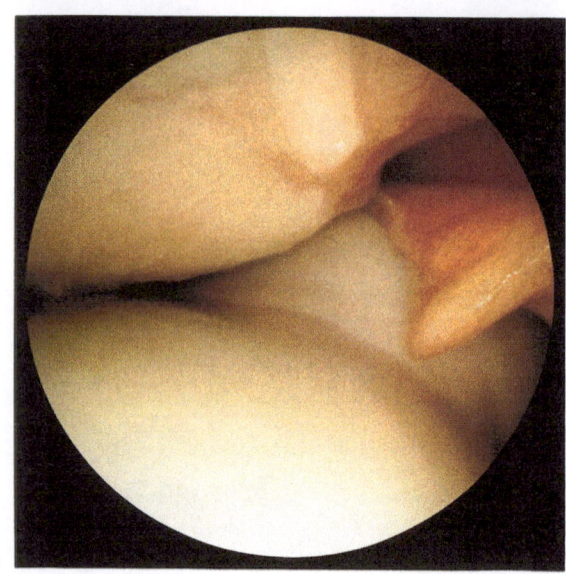

b

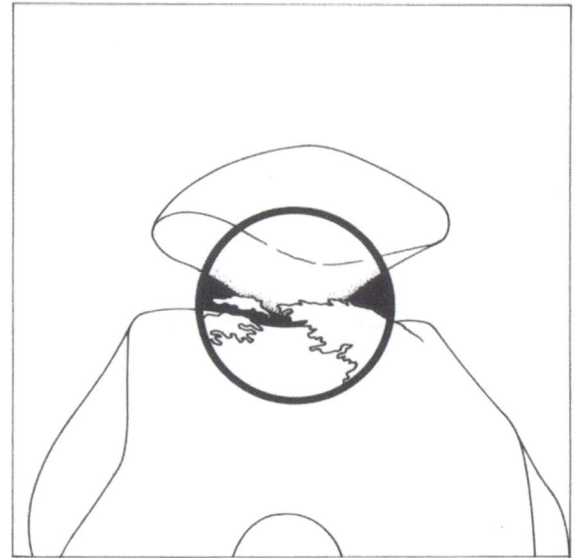

Fig. 32a, b. The appearance of the inflammatory synovial changes and of the tip of the infrapatellar fat pad vary according to the medium used to fill the joint

11.2 Filling the Joint Cavity with Gas

In principle, the knee joint cavity can be filled with various gases and also with air (Fig. 33); CO_2 and N_2O are most often used. CO_2 seems to be the most risk-free as it is very rapidly absorbed by the body, transported by the bloodstream within minutes, and expired. Under local anesthesia it has the additional advantage (or disadvantage) of causing a burning feeling as soon as subcutaneous emphysema begins to develop. This is the most important difference from N_2O, where the absence of pain sensation during emphysema formation under local anesthesia may be considered a disadvantage. If the knee is distended at a pressure not exceeding 60 mmHg, there is virtually no risk of emphysema within the first 30 min. The gas to be used should be passed through a bacterial filter to ensure sterile filling of the joint. The outstanding advantage of gas distension is the natural appearance of the knee joint cavity. It has already been stated that one of the preconditions for successful arthroscopy is the best possible view, and this is better guar-

A second, controllable, disadvantage of fluid filling, as with gas filling, is that it may lead to fluid, or gas, entering damaged structures between the thigh or lower leg musculature, and in a few cases even under the skin. If the fluid pressure in the knee is uncontrolled and excessive, fluid and air may even be expressed into the scrotum (Henderson et al. 1982). Obviously, this can happen only under general or regional anesthesia, for the patient under local anesthesia will be able to warn the surgeon immediately.

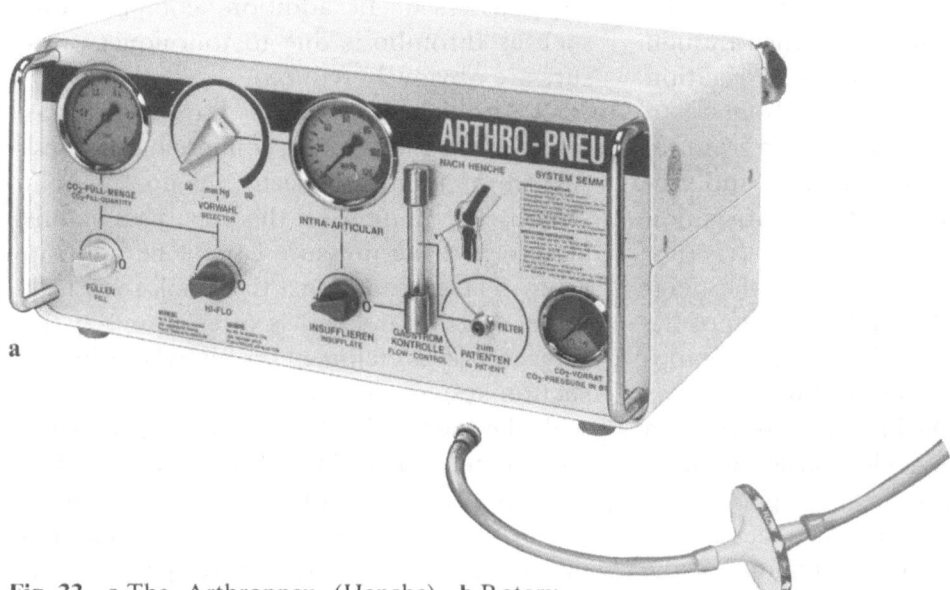

Fig. 33. a The Arthropneu (Henche). b Rotary pump (Storz)

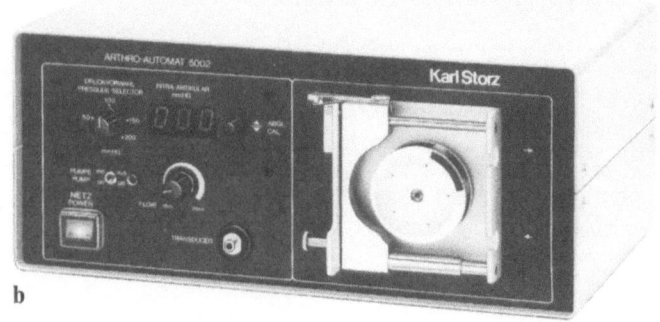

anteed by gas than by fluid. The knee structures retain their natural shape and the customary appearance as seen in arthrotomy. In contrast to fluid distension, possible bleeding, such as may well occur with a very inflamed synovium, does not obstruct the view with gas filling.

However, straightforward gas filling of the knee without previous irrigation with a fluid medium is not practicable. Even the healthy knee joint contains small amounts of synovial fluid which, by wetting the optical system, gives rise to a distorted image. Furthermore, contact of the optical system with the mucosa sometimes obscures the view. Therefore, the combined use of irrigation and subsequent gas filling is the best method for diagnosis.

11.3 Alternate Filling of the Joint Cavity with Fluid and Gas

As already mentioned, it is advantageous to combine both techniques. The cavity should first be distended with fluid in order not to damage the articular cartilage of the knee joint during insertion of the arthroscope. When local anesthesia is used, the anesthetic agent is introduced with the irrigation fluid. Under general anesthesia it has proved satisfactory to puncture and distend the knee from the superior synovial recess, the surgeon aspirating the irrigation fluid or local anesthetic before introducing the gas. If synovial fluid persists in the knee the problem of foam formation often arises; this may be a nuisance where vision is concerned though it is rapidly improved by repeated irrigation and suction. However, further obstacles to vision may develop such as bleeding from recent injuries. In this case, irrigation and suction must be continued until the irrigation fluid becomes clear. Subsequently, the knee can be filled with filtered gas and the diagnostic procedure can begin. Reduction of the gas pressure using specially designed equipment is absolutely essential; Fig. 33 shows a system (called the Arthro-pneu) developed by the Wisap company. The considerable reduction in gas pressure makes it possible to work without a tourniquet, which means that it is easier to detect inflamed regions of the synovium and localization of synovial disease within the knee joint cavity can be more pre- cisely assessed. In addition, complications such as thrombosis due to tourniquet pressure are obviously reduced.

A problem occasionally arises with gas filling of the knee joint – collapse of the pressure in the joint may occur, for no apparent reason. The pointer on the apparatus stands at zero and the pressure cannot be built up again. The surgeon must then look for a leak in the system, and this is often found at the arthroscope attachment or elsewhere in the suction system, frequently at the connection with the bacterial filter. With an established routine, neither the changeover from fluid to gas nor the solving of such minor technical problems need cause undue delay. To sum up, this combined method gives perfect visualization and outstanding photographic and video documentation.

CHAPTER 12
Anatomic Considerations

Clearly, nobody is likely to undertake arthroscopy if he is not thoroughly familiar with the anatomy of the knee joint. However, the anatomy of the knee joint as seen through the arthroscope is in no way comparable with that seen by the anatomist. It is extremely difficult to find one's way about the knee joint with the thin instrument. The conventional concepts presented in anatomy textbooks cannot be directly utilized during arthroscopy.

Under normal circumstances the closed knee joint contains neither air nor large quantities of fluid. The arthroscopist must therefore clearly understand that the synovial membrane is in direct contact with an opposing synovial membrane or with the surface of the articular cartilage; the empty spaces which are sometimes portrayed in anatomy textbooks do not exist in the knee joint. By filling the joint with fluid or gas the situation is radically altered. It will help the arthroscopist to find his way about the joint if he remembers that the cartilage and menisci remain in their original places, whereas the synovial membrane and joint capsule are lifted away from the joint itself by the increase in intraarticular volume. It is clear that the patella, for example, is not displaced to the same degree as parts of the suprapatellar recess.

Certain anatomic structures are easily confused and are therefore given special mention in this chapter. The investigator should pay particular attention to the infrapatellar fat pad and its attachment, the intrapatellar synovial fold. The intrapatellar fold is inserted below the trochlea and tautens when the knee joint is inflated. If the fold is particularly thick an inexperienced arthroscopist may take it to be the anterior cruciate ligament. However, it cannot be confused with the latter structure if the investigator remembers its origin and insertion. The identification of the alar folds presents similar problems. These are lateral prolongations of the infrapatellar fat pad in the anterior joint capsule. These capsular folds, parts of which contain thick fibrous tissue are situated in the lower part of the patellofemoral joint to the right and left sides of the infrapatellar fat pad when the knee joint is completely extended. With increasing flexion they are pulled distally together with the infrapatellar fat pad, giving the appearance of the wings of a big bird, the body of which is the fat pad. These alar folds can look like menisci to the inexperienced arthroscopist and, indeed, their shape, color and consistency sometimes resemble those of the meniscus (Fig. 34). Another particularly striking anatomic feature seen during arthroscopy is the transverse ligament which joins the two anterior horns of the menisci. In the vicinity of the site of insertion between the transverse ligament and the anterior horn of a meniscus one sometimes sees a fold which may appear to the inexperienced arthroscopist to be a tear in the anterior horn of the meniscus. One should beware of being misled by this structure (Fig. 34).

The lateral contours of the femoral condyles are particularly clearly displayed during arthroscopy. The anatomist distinguishes the articular surface of the patellofemoral joint (the trochlea) and the articular surface of the femorotibial joint (the condyles). The two articular surfaces are separated by the linea terminalis (trochlear-condylar line). In the course of careful lateral inspection during arthroscopy this slight ridge at the junction of the patellofemoral and femorotibial joint surfaces is almost always easily recognizable. Proximal to this line (at the distal end of the

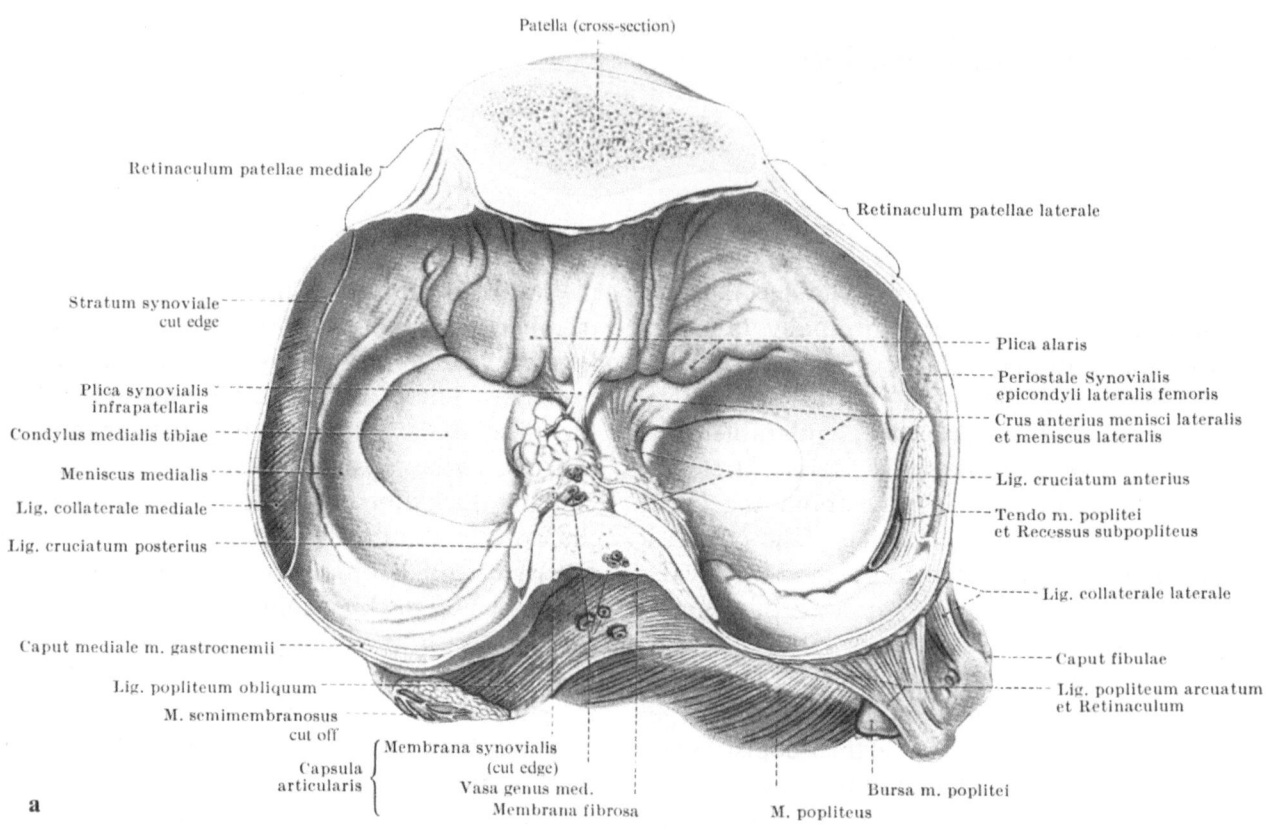

Patella (cross-section)

Retinaculum patellae mediale

Retinaculum patellae laterale

Stratum synoviale
cut edge

Plica alaris

Periostale Synovialis
epicondyli lateralis femoris

Plica synovialis
infrapatellaris

Crus anterius menisci lateralis
et meniscus lateralis

Condylus medialis tibiae

Lig. cruciatum anterius

Meniscus medialis

Tendo m. poplitei
et Recessus subpopliteus

Lig. collaterale mediale

Lig. cruciatum posterius

Lig. collaterale laterale

Caput mediale m. gastrocnemii

Caput fibulae

Lig. popliteum obliquum

Lig. popliteum arcuatum
et Retinaculum

M. semimembranosus
cut off

Capsula
articularis
{ Membrana synovialis
(cut edge).

Vasa genus med.

Membrana fibrosa

Bursa m. poplitei

M. popliteus

a

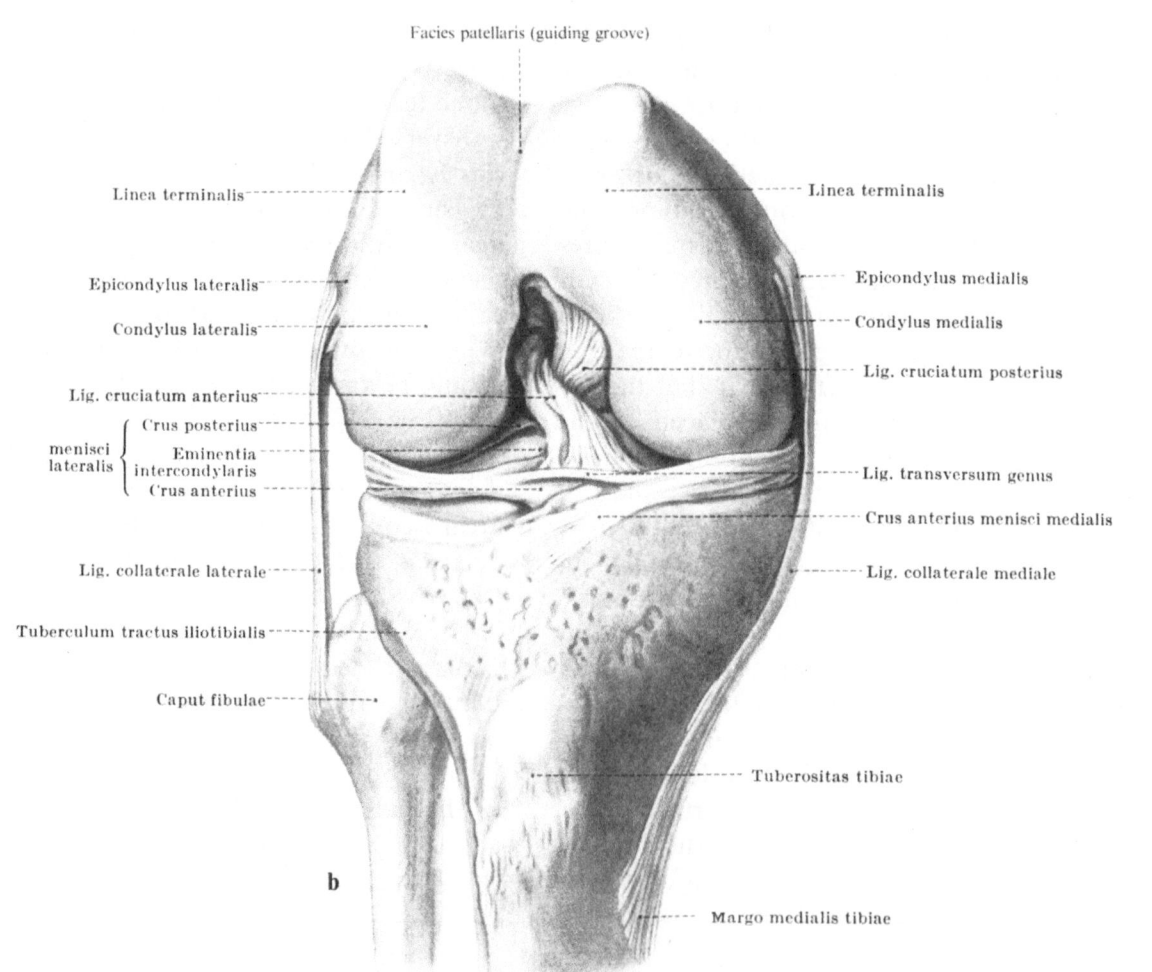

Facies patellaris (guiding groove)

Linea terminalis

Linea terminalis

Epicondylus lateralis

Epicondylus medialis

Condylus lateralis

Condylus medialis

Lig. cruciatum anterius

Lig. cruciatum posterius

menisci
lateralis
{ Crus posterius

Eminentia
intercondylaris

Crus anterius

Lig. transversum genus

Crus anterius menisci medialis

Lig. collaterale laterale

Lig. collaterale mediale

Tuberculum tractus iliotibialis

Caput fibulae

Tuberositas tibiae

b

Margo medialis tibiae

44

⊲ **Fig. 34a, b.** Anatomy of the knee joint (from Lanz and Wachsmuth 1972)

trochlea, so to speak) there may be shallow impressions. These are mainly caused by the lower border of the patella. Impressions, some of them very deep, are more frequently seen distal to the trochlear-condylar line. Not uncommonly they have the appearance of gaps in the cartilage. These depressions are caused by abutment of the anterior horn of the medial meniscus and the edge of the tibia against the proximal end of the condyle when the knee joint is completely extended. It is difficult to draw a line between physiologic impression and pathologic damage, especially in the region of the medial condyle.

The arthroscopist is therefore advised to revise carefully his knowledge of the anatomy of the knee joint before proceeding to examine a patient. There is, in all probability, no beginner who has not made an incorrect diagnosis or wrongly identified an anatomically normal structure.

CHAPTER 13

Arthroscopic Procedure

13.1 Insertion of the Arthroscope into the Knee Joint

Once the surgeon has decided on the site of approach, the skin incision is made with a pointed scalpel. This incision should always be slightly too small; if it is too large in relation to the outer tube gas may escape from the knee during insufflation of the joint. This hampers the investigation as no pressure can then be built up in the joint. With fluid distension, fluid escapes through the overlarge incision and causes undesirable "flooding." After making the relatively undersized incision, the pointed trocar is inserted into its sheath. These components must be interlocked.

With the lateral approach, the surgeon now introduces the instrument parallel to the articular surface of the tibia and radially towards the center of the joint, aiming somewhat towards the anterior attachment of the posterior cruciate ligament. With continuous

rotation, the outer tube is advanced toward the center of the joint. Penetration of the joint capsule by the trocar point is clearly felt, but on no account must the pointed trocar be allowed to penetrate the joint completely. Should this nevertheless occur, the surgeon will often detect a minor injury at the attachment of the posterior cruciate ligament to the inner aspect of the medial femoral condyle. Aiming in this direction will in any case prevent damage to the articular cartilage. Once the surgeon feels that the joint capsule has been pierced, the pointed trocar is exchanged for the blunt one. At the same time the position of the knee joint is changed from a right-angled or at least 60° position to full extension. With the blunt trocar, the outer tube is now pushed into the patellofemoral joint (Fig. 35). After some practice the

Fig. 35. Direction of insertion of the instrument into the patellofemoral joint in extension

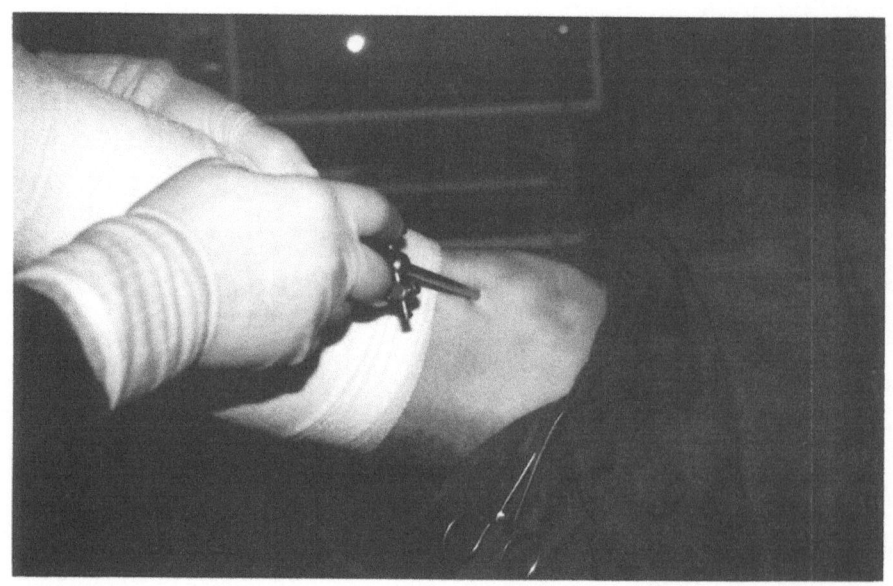

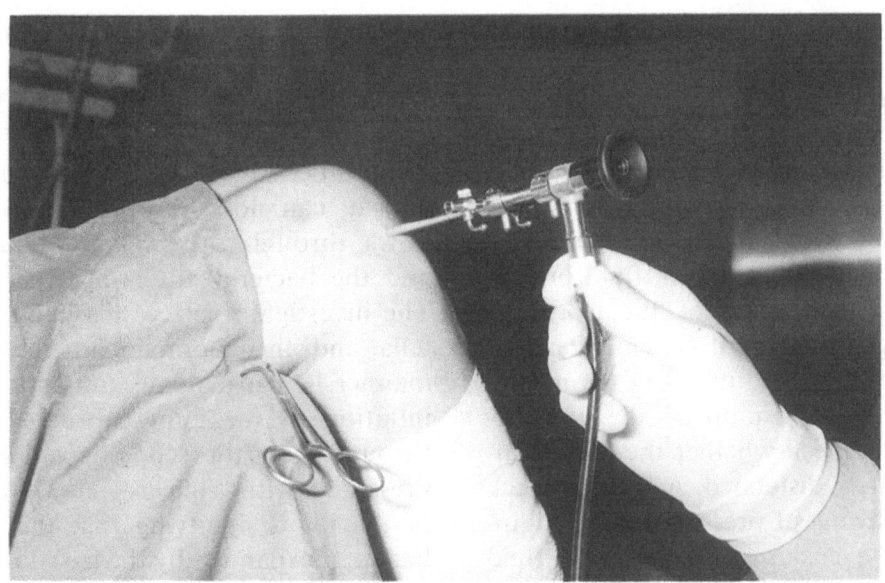

Fig. 36. Position of the inserted arthroscope parallel to the condylar axis with the knee flexed at right angles

surgeon will know whether the instrument is really in the knee joint, as the trochlea and its shape can be accurately traced with the outer tube. If the trocar sheath is still covered with a synovial layer the trochlear margin cannot be clearly palpated by the trocar with the knee in extension. Once the knee capsule has been definitely punctured, the surgeon positions the outer tube parallel to the condylar axis and the knee joint is simultaneously flexed (Fig. 36). A characteristic snapping movement indicates that the instrument is correctly placed. This procedure can be repeated in the reverse direction with the tube reintroduced into the patellofemoral joint with the knee extended. This reintroduction of the instrument parallel to the condylar axis results in anterior displacement of the infrapatellar fat pad by the outer tube. The insertion of the trocar sheath into the joint cannot be practiced and verified often enough. If the surgeon is not convinced that the tip of the outer tube is actually within the knee joint cavity, under no circumstances should fluid or gas be pumped into the joint, since if the tube is outside the synovial sac the introduc-

tion of gas or fluid will make the investigation impossible. Every surgeon has probably on at least one occasion distended the fat pad with fluid to such an extent as to prevent further investigation, without having had even a glimpse of the articular surface.

Let us assume that the trocar sheath now lies exactly in the joint cavity, displacing the fat pad anteriorly with its broad side. The blunt trocar can now be removed. Any fluid in the joint can be emptied via the trocar sheath – a sure sign that this is correctly placed. It is advisable either to attach the suction system to the outer tube immediately or to collect the effusion in a kidney dish, but complete evacuation of the joint, entailing blind manipulation of the tube, should be avoided. The optical system with its attached light cable is carefully inserted into the outer tube, the theater nurse having already prepared the ancillary attachments to the trocar sheath. The attachments for suction and for gas or fluid introduction can be fixed quickly and easily with maintenance of complete sterility, having first ensured that all the taps on the outer tube are closed. If no fluid has so far been discharged the suction system is connected, and any effusion or previously introduced local anesthetic should now be aspirated. If this does not occur, the correct positioning of the tube in the knee joint is in doubt and the introduction of gas or fluid should be postponed. The optical system should be withdrawn, the trocar reinserted and a further attempt made to puncture the superior recess with the knee extended. This should be continued until it is possible to suck out at least some fluid.

The joint is now filled with fluid or gas. With correct positioning of the trocar, a glance through the optical system often immediately reveals the contours of the medial condyle. The surgeon palpates the suprapatellar recess to check whether the joint is already adequately distended. A further check is from monitoring of pressure by the equipment. Initially, sucking the irrigation fluid out of the knee is difficult and demands some practice. The fluid is removed from the knee under visual control, and it is therefore advisable to place the end of the optical system in a part of the joint where suction is unhampered by synovial membrane. In most cases the medial compartment is suitable, the arthroscope being advanced here so that the end of the optical system comes to lie on the anterior horn of the medial meniscus, and can then be guided backward to intubate the dorsal recess. However, complete evacuation is frequently achieved only if the lateral joint compartment is located and the joint space opened up dorsally in the figure 4 position, allowing the fluid to be sucked out. At the same time the suprapatellar recess can be emptied by manual pressure. Pressure on the popliteal fossa can also massage the fluid forward and facilitate its suction.

Almost all the irrigation fluid can be evacuated from the knee joint in this manner. Small "puddles" do not compromise the investigation to any serious degree. If there was joint effusion prior to the investigation or if the fluid from the first irrigation was particularly cloudy, the washout procedure is repeated two or three times in the manner described above.

Once the joint has been satisfactorily irrigated the corresponding main tap on the side of the instrument tube is closed. The second main tap on the opposite side of the instrument tube, to which the CO_2 supply is attached, can now be opened. The CO_2 gas flows through the pressure-reducing valve and the bacterial filter into the knee joint. The investigator places his hand on the patella and the suprapatellar recess. In this manner he can palpate and assess the rapid inflation of the joint capsule. On looking through the arthroscope he will suddenly be presented with a clear view of the interior of the joint, signifying that the joint space has been expanded by the gas. The knee joint is now ready for arthroscopic inspection.

If the investigator has succeeded in filling the joint satisfactorily with CO_2 gas following the irrigation procedure he can be said to have the most difficult part of the investigation behind him. The irrigation of the joint with Ringer solution and the removal of the liquid by suction are procedures which, in many cases, are less simple than they appear to be. The points at which mistakes are especially likely to occur are the following:

1. The worst mistake which one can make is to fill the suprapatellar fat pad with Ringer solution or to allow infiltration of liquid or gas between the synovial membrane and the joint capsule. A knee joint which has been "filled" in this manner can no longer be inspected with the arthroscope and the investigation therefore has to be abandoned. One should always bear this in mind when infiltrating the joint with local anesthetic.

2. Leakage in the afferent or efferent tubing is another frequent cause of problems during arthroscopy. Whereas the flow of Ringer solution to the arthroscope and its infusion into the joint are relatively easily monitored, it is sometimes difficult to obtain the correct degree of suction for evacuation of fluid from the joint. If the vacuum is excessive, synovial tags are immediately sucked into the gaps between the optical system and the outer tube of the instrument and prevent the evacuation of further fluid from the joint.

At the same time there is characteristic reddening and blurring of the arthroscopic image. Inadequacy of suction is usually caused by leakage at one of the couplings and makes sucking out of the joint slow and laborious. If the arthroscopist has a clear view of the joint but the instrument fails to suck up the fluid he should not lose patience but should check the tubes which are attached to the instrument; the site of leakage is frequently revealed by a stream of air bubbles.

Another cause of difficulty in sucking out the knee joint is an excessively large skin incision, which allows air to enter the joint along the outside of the arthroscope. Here too, the subsequent stages of the arthroscopy are made more difficult and the result is, in some cases, not completely satisfactory.

3. A further complication (the one which is most easily avoided) is incorrect operation of the small afferent and efferent taps. Whenever opening or closing the main taps attached to the outlet tube of the instrument or the accessory three-way tap, the less-experienced arthroscopist should check carefully that he is opening the correct channel. One of the commonest mistakes is to leave the gas supply tap open. This error may be made at the beginning of the investigation and allows the infused Ringer solution to flow in the direction of the CO_2 cylinder and pass into the bacterial filter, which then ceases to function. If the arthroscopist has not already realized his mistake he will be made aware of it as soon as he attempts to fill the knee joint with CO_2. A less harmful combination of tap positions is that which results when one attempts to irrigate the knee joint with Ringer solution and simultaneously forgets to close the suction tap. The Ringer solution then takes the short route through the three-way tap attached to the outer tube of the instrument and does not flow into the joint. On glancing through the arthroscope in such a case the investigator will be momentarily puzzled by the lack of turbulence (since no fluid is flowing into the joint) but should have little difficulty in identifying and correcting his error. It cannot be overemphasized that closure of the main taps on the outside of the instrument is one of the most important manual operations during arthroscopy.

N.B.: Throughout arthroscopy at least one of the two main taps should be in the closed position.

A further problem which may complicate arthroscopy, and which may even arise during the initial stages, is bleeding. The skin incision is usually followed by slight external bleeding. If a small artery has been transected it is usually compressed by the outer tube of the arthroscope, which has a relatively large diameter, and this prevents further bleeding. Bleeding from the synovial membrane is frequently associated with inflammation of the latter tissue. It is advisable to irrigate the joint two or three times. The bleeding from the synovial membrane does not always stop and the advantage of subsequent filling of the joint with CO_2 gas is that bleeding does not compromise the examination, since the resulting pressure inside the joint also compresses the synovial vessels. Even if slight bleeding continues, gas inflation has the advantage over liquid filling that it maintains a clear view of the inside of the joint. The liquid-filled joint has to be continuously perfused in order to keep the irrigation fluid even relatively clear. The arthroscopic examination may be regarded as a sterile operation up to the point at which the operator's eye comes close to or accidentally touches the eyepiece of the arthroscope. Any aids such as the use of a sterile mask, sterilization of spectacles, and similar maneuvers cannot overcome the fact that direct viewing through the arthroscope means that the operation is not sterile. An important advange of using a video system is that this shortcoming can be overcome.

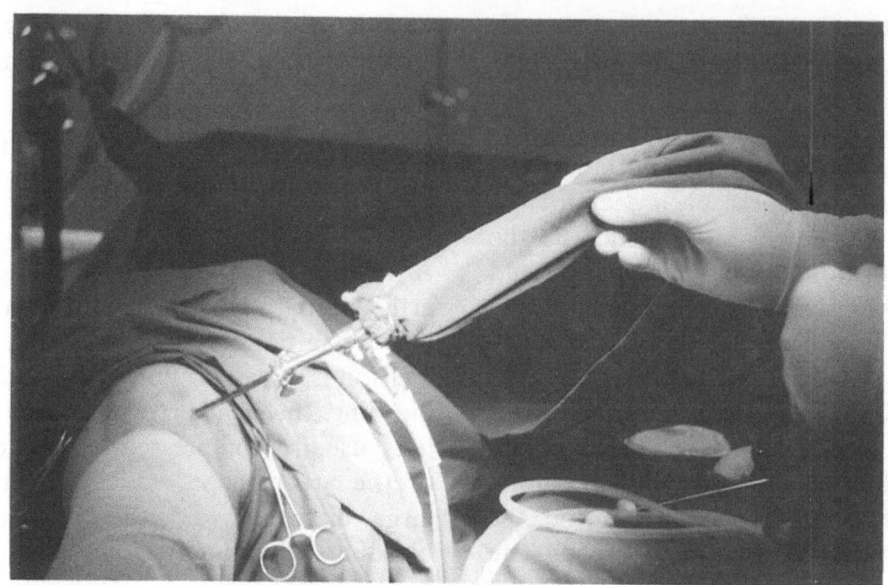

Fig. 37. Video camera in sterile sheath

The small portable television cameras (see p. 14) can be either sterilized themselves or more simply wrapped in sterile bags (Fig. 37). Arthroscopy employing video techniques can be undertaken therefore as a completely sterile procedure. This is also an important consideration in operative procedures. It is strongly recommended that the operative technique be made completely sterile by using a television camera and monitor screen. Disposable plastic sheets can be used for sterile wrapping of the video camera. We have found useful strong tubular drapes of at least 1–1.5 m in length, connectable at both ends, that are tied by the surgeon in the sterile area over the still sterile arthroscope eyepiece and are tied up to the camera cable away from the operating table by the nonsterile theater orderly (see Sect. 2.). Impermeable, disposable plastic tubing is also available.

13.2 Systematic Inspection of the Knee Joint Using the Lateral Approach

13.2.1 Initial Situation

The knee is flexed to about 60°–70° and positioned on the knee holder. The outer tube lies obliquely in front of the femoral condyles, displacing the infrapatellar fat pad forward. The connectors are attached and the optical system inserted into the outer tube. The video camera is attached to the optical system under sterile conditions. The surgeon holds the camera in its sterile sheath in his right hand, the left hand is placed on the knee for additional orientation, and his eye is fixed on the monitor which stands on the opposite side. It is assumed that some local anesthetic and irrigation fluid remain in the knee and the outlines of structures now appear in the fluid. The camera is carefully moved to and fro until the uniform reddish or white "curtain" on the monitor screen is resolved into definite outlines. First to be recognized is the sharp outline of the medial femoral condyle. The surgeon must continually check the direction in which he is guiding his arthroscope. Aids to orientation on the camera and eyepiece must be so coordinated that, at any given moment, he can say what is visible on each section of the televi-

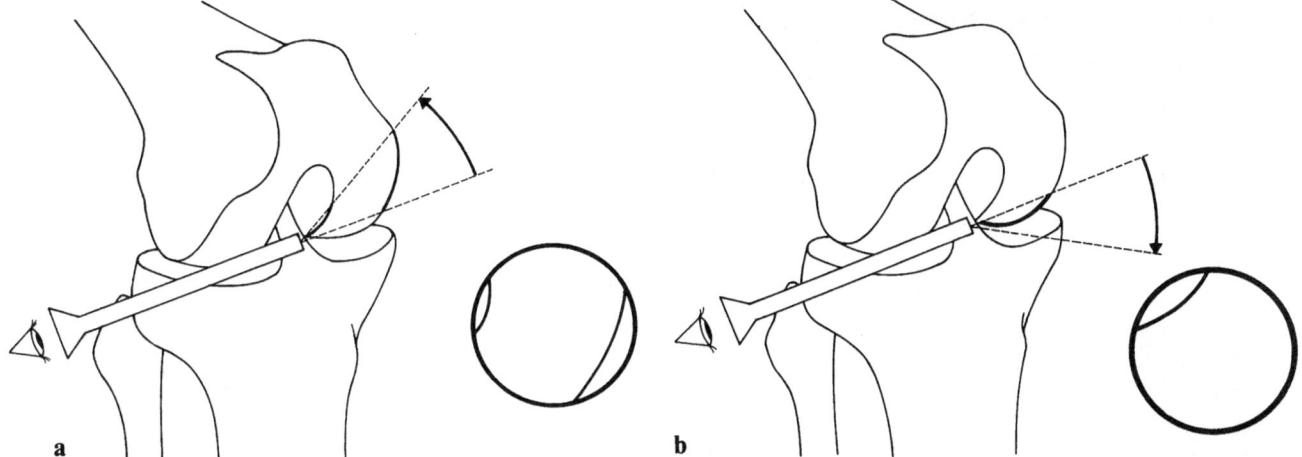

a   b

sion image (above, below, right, or left). Only in this way can the arthroscope be guided from the emerging contour in the right direction. Once the outline of the condyle is recognized on the monitor, gas can be introduced. Frequently, a clear view with the gas bubble appears in the upper half, while the residual fluid can be seen in the lower half. As previously described, the fluid is now sucked away, beginning in the region with the least synovial membrane. The surgeon fixes the inner border of the medial femoral condyle as a landmark and a starting-point for inspection of the knee joint. The arthroscope is guided along the margin of the medial femoral condyle in the direction of the medial joint space, the knee now being flexed at about 30°, while the assistant is instructed to hold the joint in the valgus position. By rotation at the light cable the arthroscope can now be focused on the condylar surface and the medial condyle can be completely inspected by alternate flexion and extension of the knee. It should be remembered, however, that rotation of the camera itself is undesirable and that only the arthroscope should be moved to gain an upward view of the condyle. On the other hand, the monitor image must remain upright (Fig. 38). Once the surgeon has visually "probed" the medial femoral condyle, slight elevation of the camera and approximately 90° rotation of the optical system bring the anterior horn and periphery of the medial meniscus into the visual field

Fig. 38. a Correct and **b** incorrect viewing of the medial femoral condyle

(Fig. 39). The medial meniscus is easily recognizable, almost always standing out in contrast to the tibial plateau and the adjacent synovium. Inspection of the meniscus begins at the anterior horn region and the surgeon must be aware that the fibers of the transverse ligament converge towards the site of attachment on the anterior horn (Fig. 40). The inexperienced arthroscopist may misinterpret this normal finding as a tear in the region of the anterior horn. If the surrounding synovial membrane appears normal, i.e., uninflamed, it may be assumed that what is seen is a strong transverse ligament, especially as a tear in the anterior part of the meniscus is extremely rare. More often, especially with unstable knee joints, the anterior horn of the medial meniscus droops forward over the tibial margin, completely exposing the anterior margin of the tibial head. This "instability" of the anterior horn of the meniscus probably has little pathologic significance; it appears to be just a feature of typical anteromedial instability. The arthroscope is now introduced further toward the medial joint space, following the course of the meniscus over half its periphery. At this point it is advisable to combine a valgus position of the knee with outward rotation of the lower leg (Fig. 41) since this, together

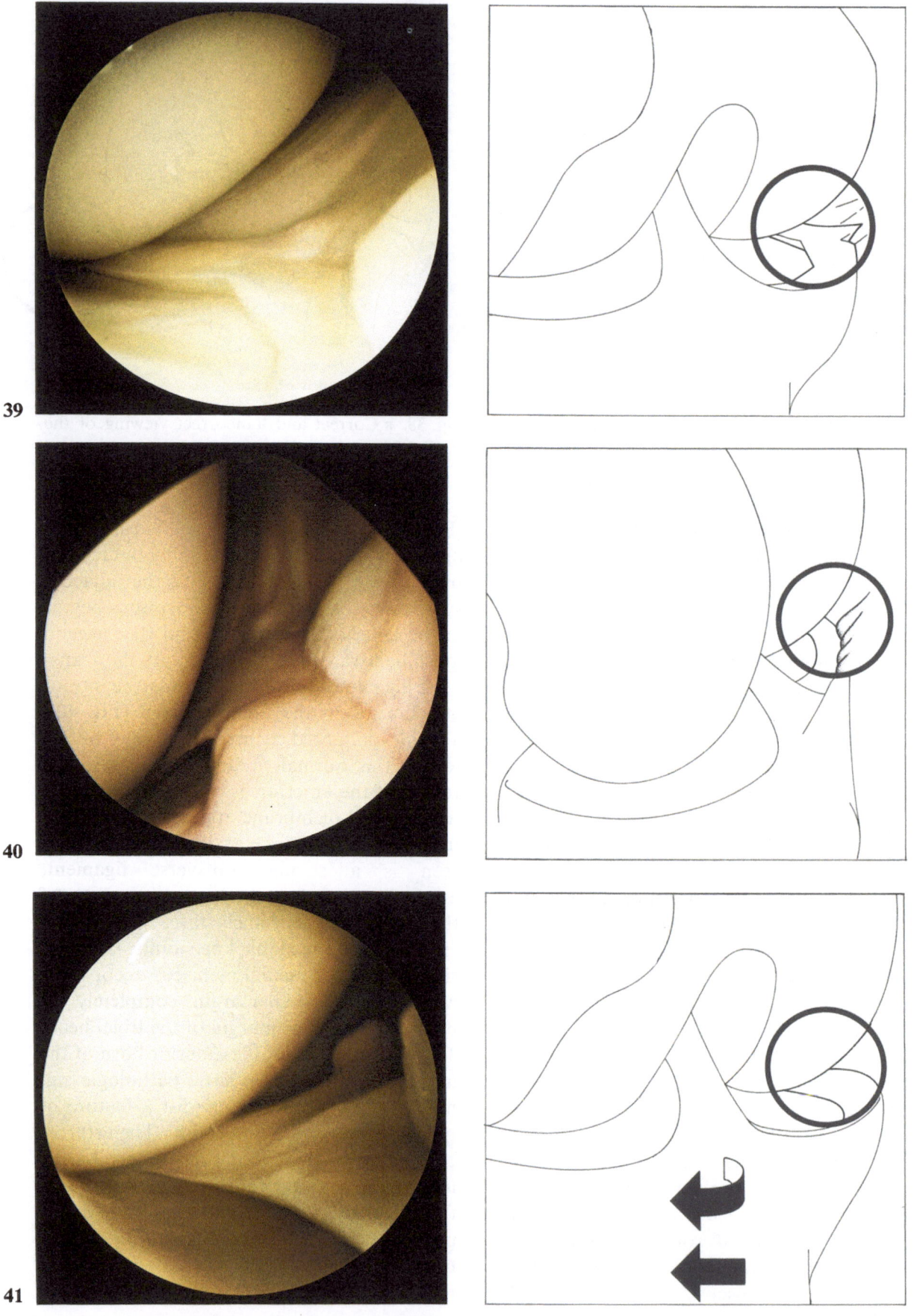

39

40

41

52

with appropriate tentative rotation of the arthroscope, helps to bring the instrument beneath the periphery of the meniscus, so that the underside of the meniscus can be checked for possible tears. The tibial plateau can be inspected from almost the same position, the arthroscope (without camera) being rotated somewhat more to give a view of the plateau from above. It is interesting that that portion of the articular cartilage of the plateau covered by the meniscus is often more yellow in color than the uncovered portion. The arthroscope is now withdrawn from where it bridges the periphery of the medial meniscus and is directed more toward the intercondylar region. It is apparent that the meniscus disappears behind the medial condyle and can no longer be seen as far as the posterior horn region. This is always the case when the arthroscope is directed outward from the middle of the knee towards the meniscus. If the arthroscope is rotated through 180° the anterior horn and periphery of the meniscus disappear and the surgeon's view moves from the body of the medial meniscus towards he middle of the joint. In nearly every case, beginning at the transition from the periphery to the posterior horn, it suddenly becomes possible to follow the free edge of the meniscus in its entirety to the end of the posterior horn. If the knee joint is somewhat unstable, the whole of the posterior horn is thus brought into the visual field. From this position one may see the so-called "rucked carpet" appearance of the medial meniscus, which should not be regarded as abnormal, especially after 30 years of age (Fig. 42). In this situation the probe hook can be inserted from the medial aspect and the base of the meniscus palpated from the periphery right round to the posterior horn. Frequently, this can be optically displayed by applying pressure on the body of the meniscus from underneath (Fig. 43).

The medial condyle, the tibial plateau, two-thirds of the medial meniscus, and the free margin of the meniscus in the posterior horn region are now inspected. The inner aspect of the medial femoral condyle is again used as a guideline, and the knee is extended with the arthroscope alongside this. The transition between condyle and trochlea is often quite apparent and the trochlear-condylar line is seen as a smooth ridge. The view is then suddenly blocked by a "yellow curtain" – part of the infrapatellar fat pad which prevents uninterrupted field of vision into the patellofemoral joint. With further swinging of the optical system and the knee in about 20° flexion, the lower point of the patella and the beginning of the trochlea often enter the visual field.

13.2.2 Inspection of the Patellofemoral Joint

As the arthroscope is swung around in the direction of the patellofemoral joint it is essential that the instrument is not withdrawn too far from the knee. It is often better to insert the arthroscope rather deeper at the outset. The arthroscope is then removed in precisely the opposite direction to that used during its introduction. The view of the lower end of the patella is abandoned, and the arthroscope is brought over the medial trochlear margin with a slight jolt as the knee is extended. If the surgeon is unsure whether the arthroscope has been placed too deeply,

---

◁ **Fig. 39.** Normal medial meniscus in flexion of the knee without rotation of the lower leg

Fig. 40. Attachment of the anterior horn of the medial meniscus with converging fibers of transverse ligament (normal appearance)

Fig. 41. Medial meniscus with lower leg in maximum outward rotation and valgus. When the collateral and cruciate ligaments are intact the medial femoral condyle may obscure the transition from the periphery to the posterior horn

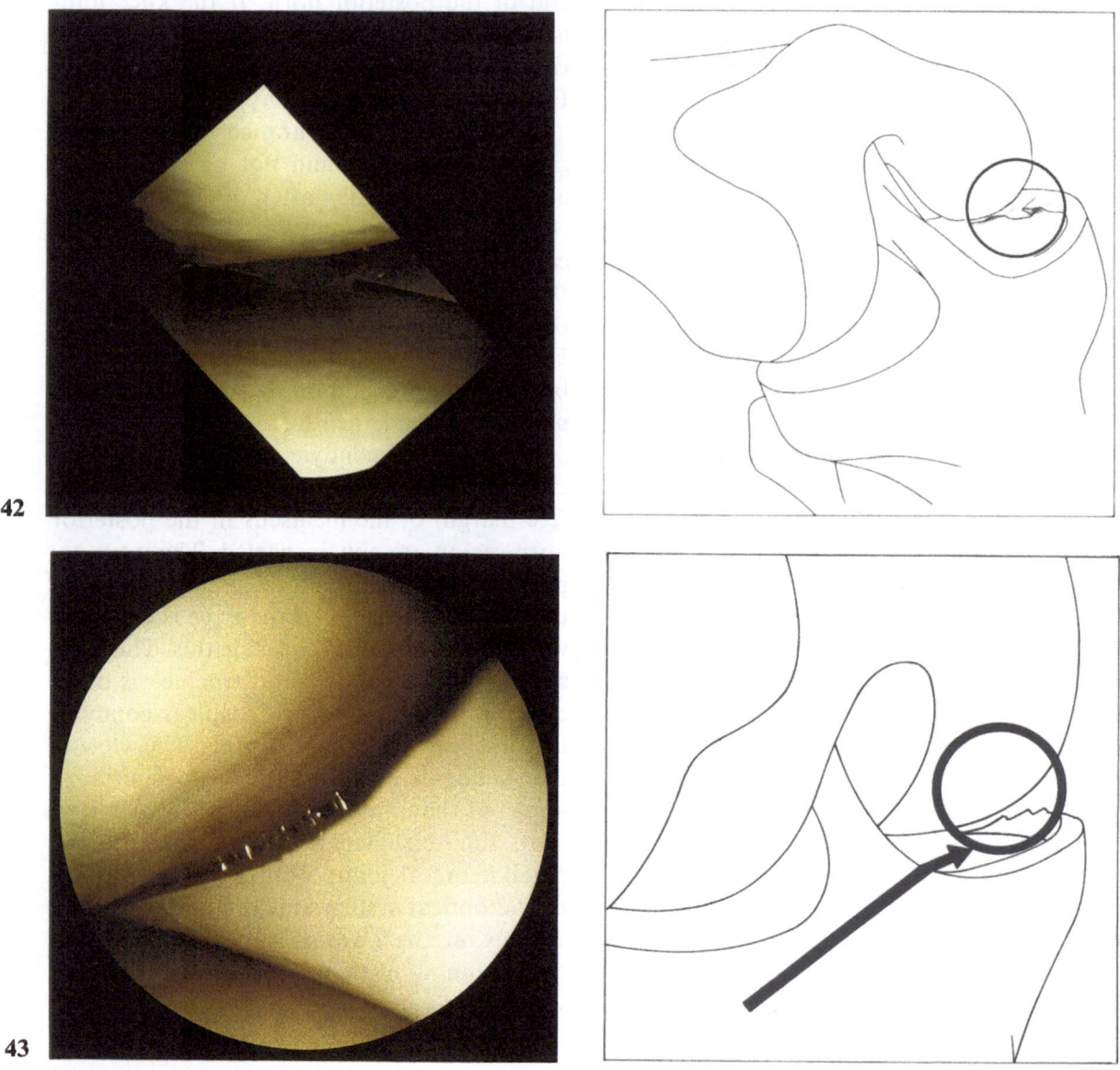

Fig. 42. "Rucked carpet" appearance at the posterior horn of the medial meniscus

Fig. 43. The underside of the meniscus; the lens is directed obliquely upwards

or not deeply enough, in the knee joint he must inspect the joint from outside. If the inner side of the patellofemoral joint or the superior recess is strongly illuminated (this translucency phenomenon can be made use of when looking for foreign bodies), the surgeon may be fairly sure that he is deep enough, or possibly even too deep in the recess. If the light begins to shine through the skin at the apex of the patellofemoral joint, or even laterally, the greatest care should be taken not to withdraw the trocar prematurely. It is always advisable in such cases to discontinue the introduction of fluid or gas

54

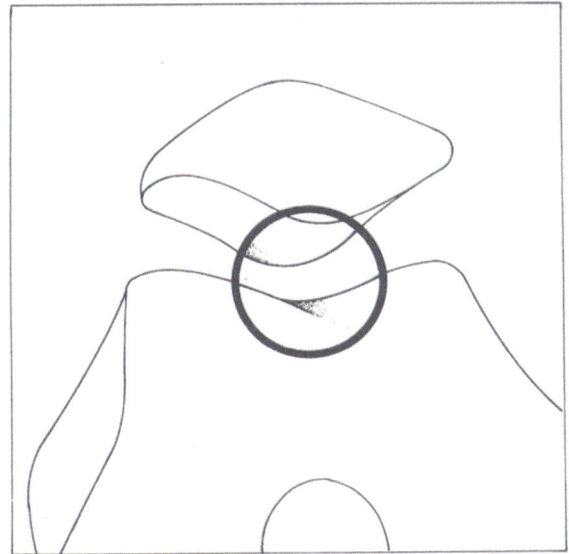
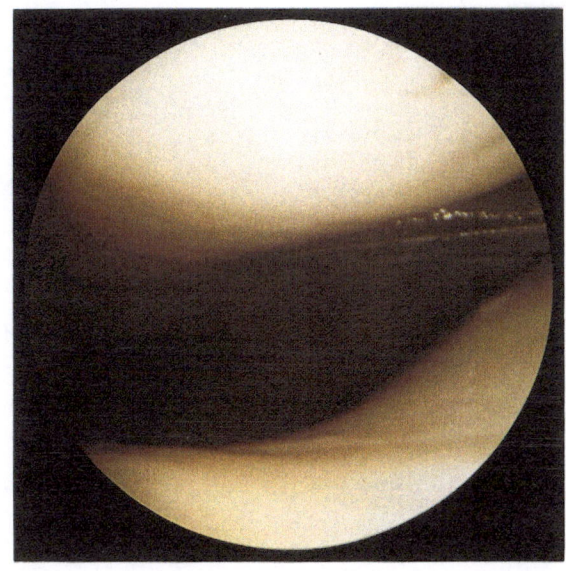

Fig. 44. View of the normal patellar undersurface with the knee fully extended

until the correct position of the arthroscope can be reconfirmed. No light spot is visible when the end of the optical system is exactly beneath the patella. It is advisable, therefore, to insert the arthroscope deeply into the joint and to visually locate the medial border of the patella as it is gradually withdrawn. This is usually successful. At this stage the surgeon must ensure that the optical system is aimed directly upwards. This is essential for a complete inspection of the often steeply angled medial facet of the patella. Here, complete extension or, if possible, hyperextension of the knee joint is necessary. The patella normally stands off some 1–1.5 cm from the trochlea, and inspection of its entire undersurface is therefore a simple and rapidly learned step in arthroscopy of the knee (Fig. 44). Patients under local anesthesia are often not completely relaxed and a reminder to relax from time to time is useful. Inspection can easily be made by to-and-fro displacement of the patella medially and laterally. In this way the surgeon can also move the patella across the optical system and simultaneously assess the joint closure between the patellofemoral articular surfaces.

After inspection of the patella the optical system is rotated through 180° and the whole of the trochlea studied. This is done with the knee fully extended, moving from the medial to the lateral side. Special attention should be paid to the trochlear margins (Fig. 45) for evidence of shearing fractures of the articular cartilage. Here, too, movement of the patella by the surgeon's hand may provide information. At the proximal medial end of the trochlea, the level of the ridge at the junction of articular cartilage and bone (Outerbridge's ridge) can also be readily assessed (Fig. 46). Special attention should be paid to the midline of the trochlea, where cartilage defects are often found after contusion of the patella.

Assessment of the function of the patellar articular surface is further aided by positioning the arthroscope at the distal pole of the patella. This requires it to be withdrawn by some 1–1.5 cm, which can be done even with the joint still extended, though it is advisable to flex the joint gradually while this is being done to about 30° (Fig. 47). The surgeon can now observe the greater part of the patellofemoral joint from a relatively remote position (as in axial X-ray views) and can also see how the joint space gradually closes. Normally, the first cartilaginous contact begins at the lateral side of the joint (Fig. 48), and with increasing flexion it is often noted that

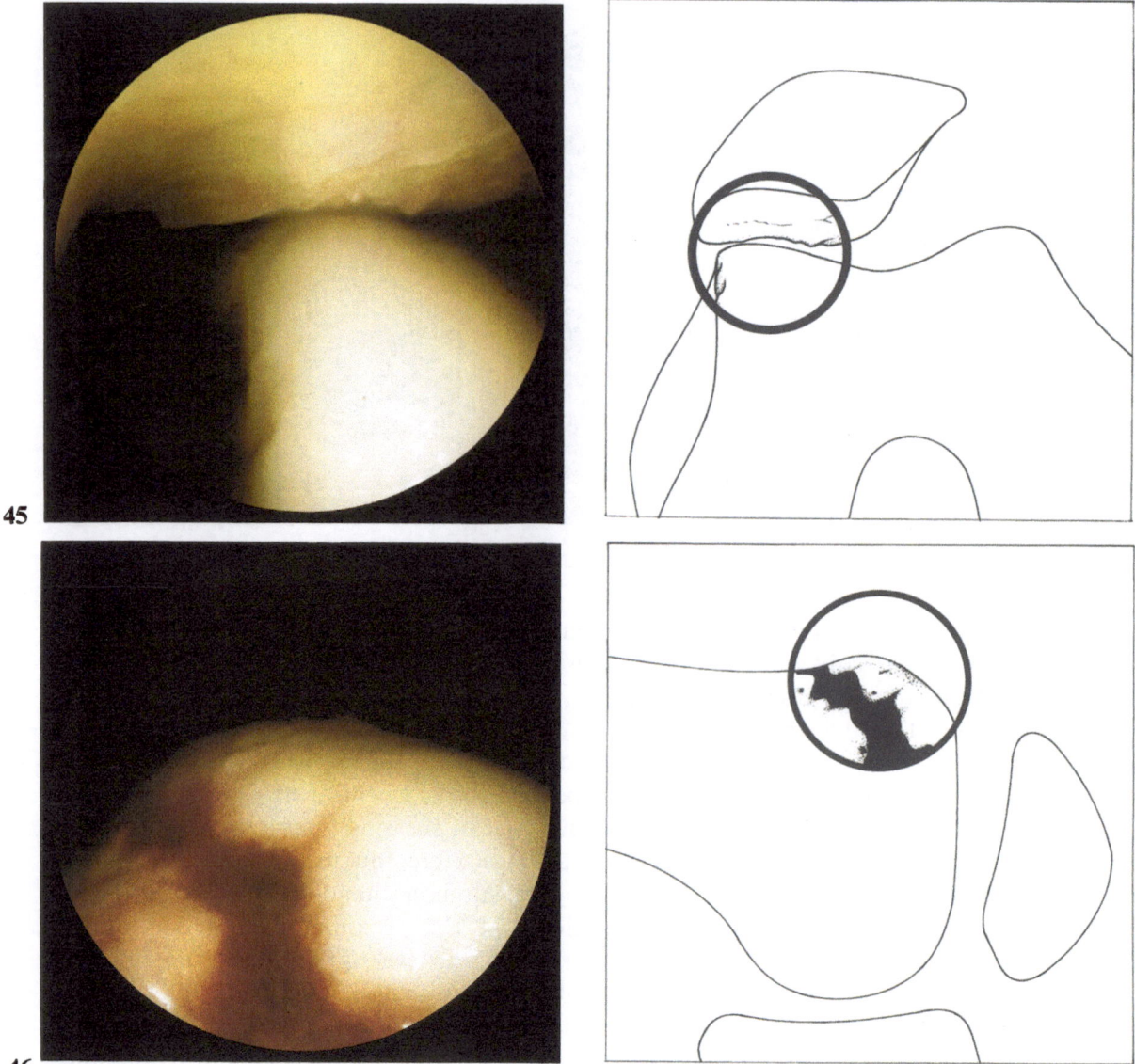

Fig. 45. Normal lateral trochlear margin with lateralized patella and moderate patellar chondromalacia

Fig. 46. Outerbridge's ridge with recent hemorrhage at the osteocartilaginous junction after contusion of the patellofemoral joint

Fig. 47. Normal patellofemoral joint with lateral ▷ contact at about 30° of flexion

Fig. 48. Early medial contact in the patellofemoral joint with unusual lateral widening

Fig. 49. Normal medial plica with minor chondromalacia at the medial patellar facet (patella omitted from diagram)

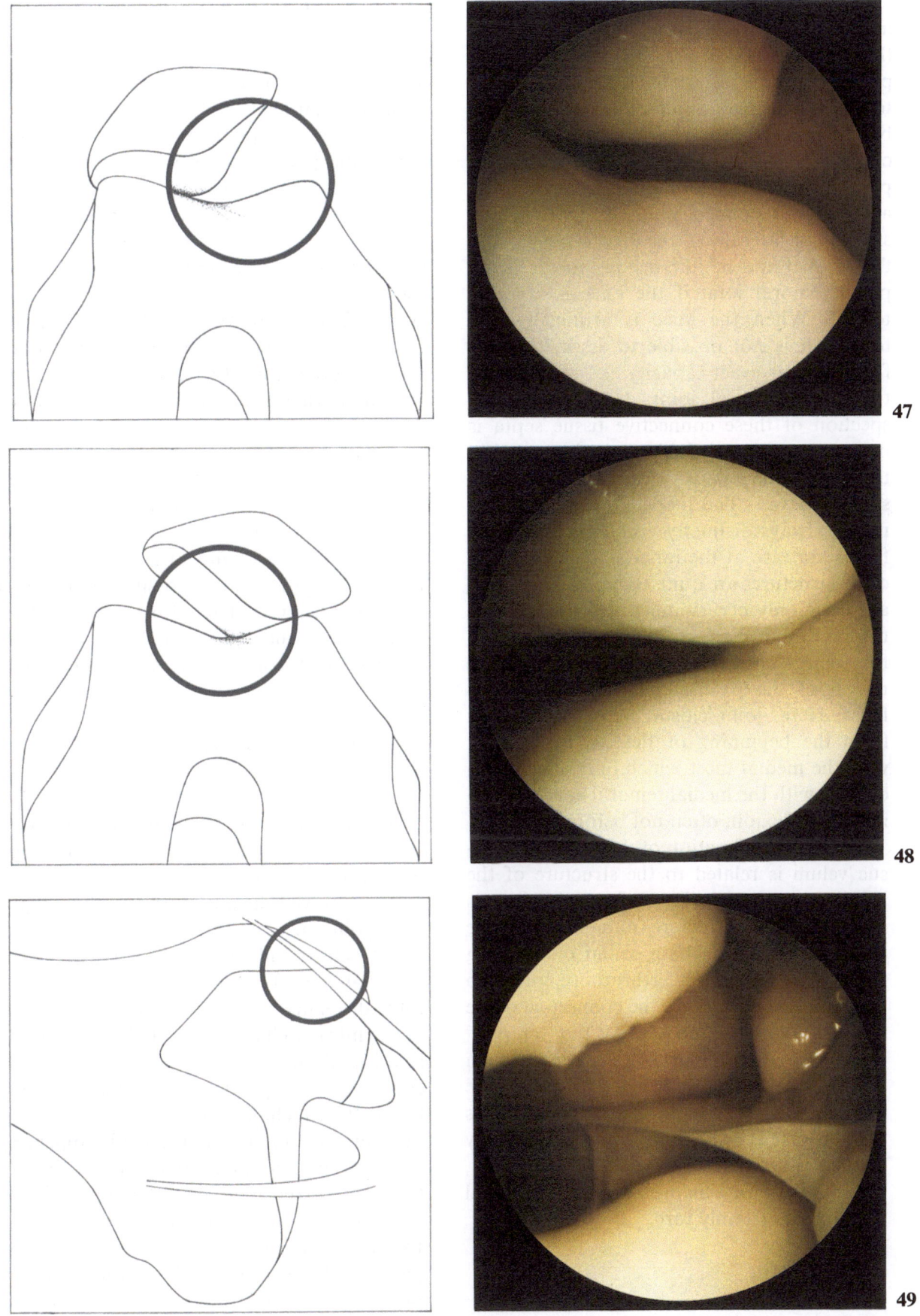

47

48

49

57

part of the medial facet of the patella comes into contact with the trochlea. Inspection of the joint beyond 50°–60° of flexion is seldom possible as the infrapatellar fat pad begins to obscure the image and it is no longer possible to bring the optical system sufficiently close to the joint. The alar folds also form part of the patellofemoral joint system. These are adjacent connective tissue septa which spread out laterally in the joint capsule from the fat pad and lie like menisci in the distal patellofemoral joint if the knee is not distended. When the knee is artificially distended, it is not possible to assess the alar folds in their exact capacity as "menisci" of the patellofemoral joint. Nevertheless, inspection of these connective tissue septa is important and each fold can be inspected in turn from the opposite side with the joint slightly flexed. The medial fold (Fig. 49) is nearly always distinctly visible; rudimentary forms are rare at the inner side while duplicated structures are quite common. The lateral fold is only occasionally as distinct as the medial due to the fact that there is no room for such a connective tissue septum in the region of the patellofemoral articular surfaces. Here, joint closure is complete even from the beginning of flexion, in contrast with the medial facet which only comes into contact with the medial femoral condyle with increased flexion, often not before 90°.

Thus, the formation of the connective tissue velum is related to the structure of the patellofemoral articular surfaces. As there is a slight negative pressure in the healthy knee joint, (the slight sucking sound on opening the synovial cavity at arthrotomy comes to mind), it is obvious that the connective tissue septa extend into and occupy the "empty" joint space. Hence, marked formation of such a fold is linked with the negative pressure between the patellofemoral articular surfaces only in extension. When the folds are very distinct they are possibly subject to trauma, but inflammatory changes due to mechanical factors are certainly rare.

13.2.3 Inspection of the Suprapatellar Recess

The suprapatellar recess is completely lined with synovial membrane, the color of which varies with the pressure within the knee. When the joint capsule is very greatly distended the lining mucosa becomes pale and judging whether inflammation is present or not therefore calls for some experience. The application of a tourniquet further hinders the assessment of synovial inflammation and should therefore be avoided. The prerequisite for this assessment is the precise control of the pressure within the knee.

The normal suprapatellar recess contains folds of a septal nature which project into the recess (Fig. 50). Sometimes the upper recess can be completely divided by such a septum into two halves, though this is unusual. More often the recess is visible through a round or oval aperture in a transverse septum. A classification is possible, but not of great importance (Hempfling 1987). These connective tissue septa are delicate and easily distinguished from postoperative adhesions.

13.2.4 Inspection of the Intercondylar Region

After inspection of the suprapatellar recess – again with complete extension or hyperextension of the knee – the tip of the arthroscope is moved distally in the midline of the knee joint, i.e., in the intercondylar fossa. The trochlea ends at the attachment of the synovial fold. This tautens markedly in the fully distended knee and ends at the apex of the infrapatellar fat pad. The synovial fold is normally easily recognizable and usually consists of a single delicate connective tissue band. Its attachment to the fat pad is easily recognizable, the latter frequently appearing in the visual field like a thick yellow tongue. Changes in the region of the synovial fold are rare, apart from inflammatory reddening. Every beginner runs the risk of mistaking a particularly thick synovial fold for the anterior cruciate ligament, but identification of its

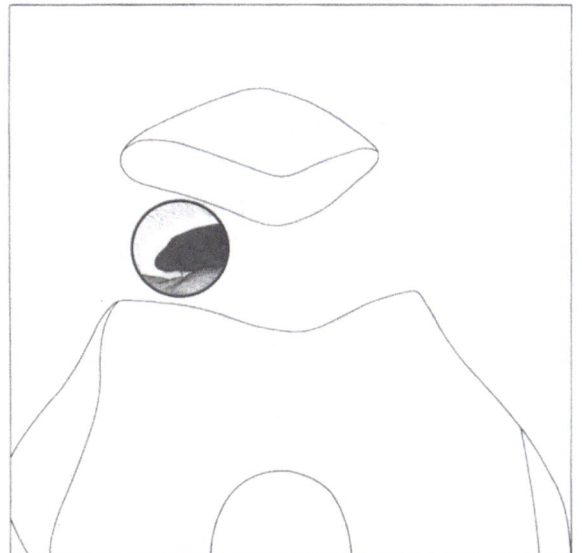 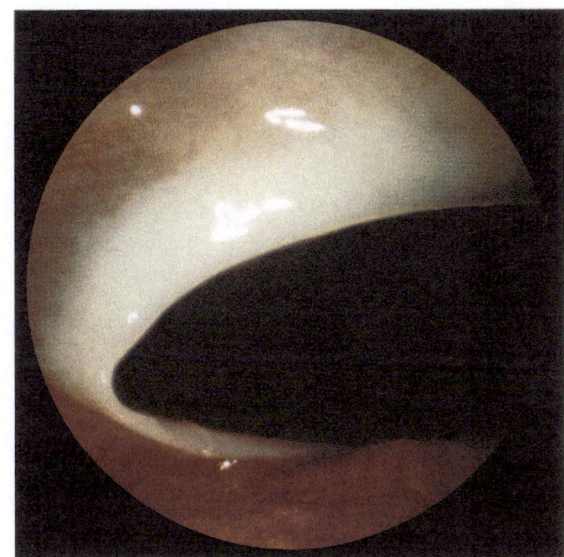

Fig. 50. Normal connective tissue septum in the suprapatellar recess

attachment to the end of the trochlea makes it clear that the structure concerned is the synovial fold (Fig. 51).

To ensure optimal identification of the anterior cruciate ligament the optical system is depressed and simultaneously rotated by some 90°. The ligament runs more or less parallel to the synovial fold and is easily recognized where it fans out to its broad-based attachment in the anterior tibial region. The individual sinewy fibers of a healthy anterior cruciate ligament can easily be made out. Fine vessels are often visible on the surface of the ligament (Fig. 52). The anterior cruciate ligament is visible along its whole length. Although with normal positioning only the lower third can be seen, the attachment to the femoral condyle is identified by rotation of the optical system and viewing towards the lateral femoral condyle. At this time parts of the posterior horn of the lateral meniscus often come into the visual field. This positioning is usually conducive to an attempt by the assistant to elicit the anterior drawer sign at about 40°–60° of flexion. The structure and function of the anterior cruciate ligament can be assessed in this manner,

especially its often defective and avulsed attachment to the lateral femoral condyle. If the lateral condyle presents a large free surface and allows direct viewing into the posterior recess, it is likely that the anterior cruciate ligament has been avulsed.

After inspection of the anterior cruciate ligament the inner aspect of the medial femoral condyle is examined. It is often covered with a thin fatty layer and sometimes also lined with synovial membrane. However, the attachment of the posterior cruciate ligament is easily identified in half the cases examined (Fig. 53). The inferior extension of the posterior cruciate ligament is best displayed when the anterior ligament is absent. Complete exposure of the posterior ligament from the lateral approach is virtually never possible. In a few cases it is possible to intubate the posterior and medial recess medial to and somewhat above the anterior cruciate ligament, and then to identify the attachment of the posterior cruciate ligament to the back of the tibia with a 70° optical system. It is more convenient to intubate the dorsolateral recess, and here too the 70° system can give information on the course of the posterior cruciate ligament.

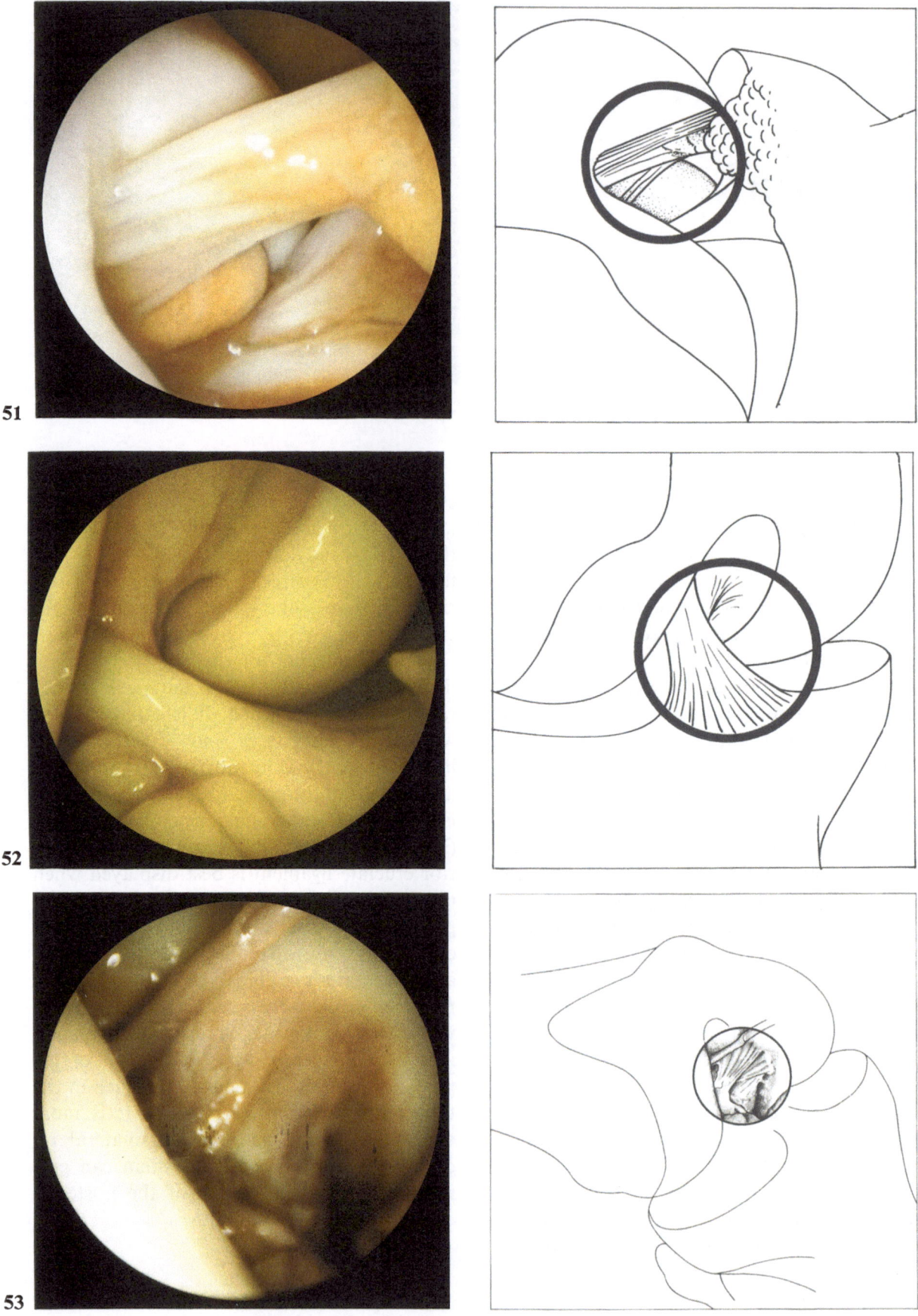

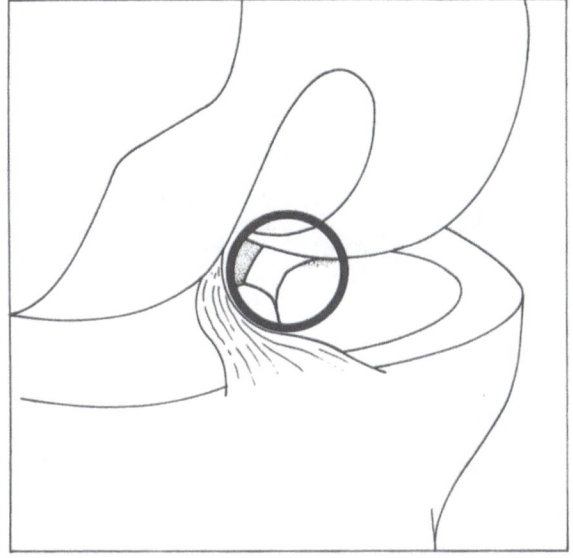

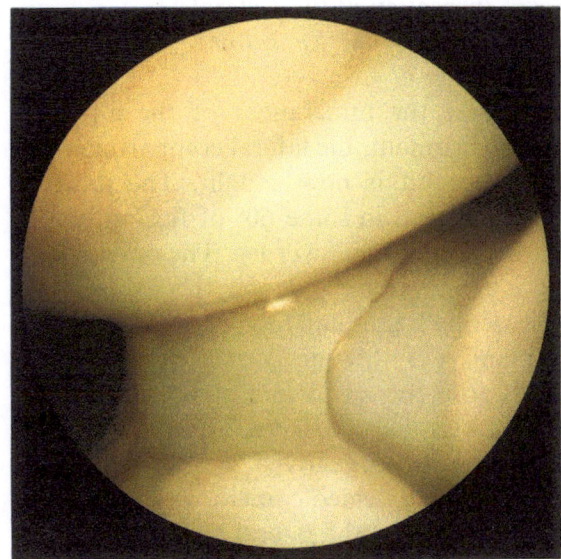

13.2.5 Inspection of the Posterior Horn of the Medial Meniscus

The posterior horn of the medial meniscus can be identified and fairly well inspected from the intercondylar region. With the 30° viewing system the course of the anterior cruciate ligament is crossed almost at a right angle and the attachment of the posterior cruciate ligament comes into view. Now an attempt is made to advance the arthroscope under gentle pressure in the direction of the dorsomedial recess, the direction of viewing being maintained medially and slightly distally with the 30° optical system. It is nearly always possible to identify the attachment of the medial meniscus in the region of the posterior horn in this way and to look for tears (Fig. 54). Here, too, insertion of the probe

Fig. 54. Normal posterior horn of medial meniscus

hook to pull on the posterior horn of the meniscus is essential. This positioning is extremely important for operative procedures. Severely inflamed knee joints obviously make this course of investigation difficult.

If, using a dorsolateral approach, it is impossible to move the arthroscope medially to the posterior horn of the medial meniscus because of lack of space, the arthroscope should be withdrawn somewhat and an anterolateral approach to the posterior horn chosen. Apart from withdrawal of the arthroscope, only 180° rotation of the instrument is necessary (see Chap. 3). As well as these standard positions for inspection of the posterior horn, it may be necessary in certain cases to view more from above or below (by rotation of the arthroscope) depending on the choice of approach and especially on the level of puncture. It is often helpful, at the same time, to rotate the lower leg laterally while maintaining its routine valgus position. Precise location of the posterior horn of the medial meniscus is the most important and most difficult task in the investigative procedure, and must be fully mastered by every arthroscopist before performing arthroscopic operations.

◁ **Fig. 51.** Normal medial synovial plica

Fig. 52. Normal anterior cruciate ligament

Fig. 53. Proximal half of the posterior cruciate ligament with attachment to the medial femoral condyle

13.2.6 Inspection of the Lateral Compartment of the Knee Joint

Starting at the attachment of the anterior cruciate ligament, the lateral compartment of the knee joint is now sought. The joint is best positioned in some 60° of flexion, without rotation of the lower leg. The optical system is slowly retracted and the axis of the arthroscope is gradually swung into the sagittal plane. As the surgeon is now looking downward, the operating table should be lowered by some 20–30 cm. The operating table will need to be moved to and fro during studies with the video camera.

Inspection of the lateral compartment of the joint from the lateral approach is technically rather difficult. The arthroscopist should always be aware of the exact position of the end of the instrument, as there is always a risk of it slipping out of the knee joint.

By carefully extending the knee to about 30° of flexion and with the assistant producing maximum varus, it is possible to survey the entire lateral joint space. Here again, the surgeon should rotate the angled optical system so as to obtain a good view of the lateral meniscus and the underlying tibial plateau. The exposed portion of the tibial plateau is normally very small; cartilage defects are often found at this site. The color of the lateral meniscus contrasts only slightly with that of the articular cartilage layer. Its characteristic feature is its sharp medial border which is nearly always plainly visible. In the maximal varus position, at various degrees of flexion between 30° and 60°, the sharp edge of the posterior horn of the lateral meniscus comes into view and thorough examination of the body of the posterior horn is usually possible.

The assistant should be instructed to perform all manipulations of the joint slowly and steadily throughout the examination. Here, the video system affords real help, as the assistant can see the effects of his manipulations on the screen. During the study of the lateral compartment, use of the so-called figure 4 position should not be omitted (Fig. 55), as this position permits optimal

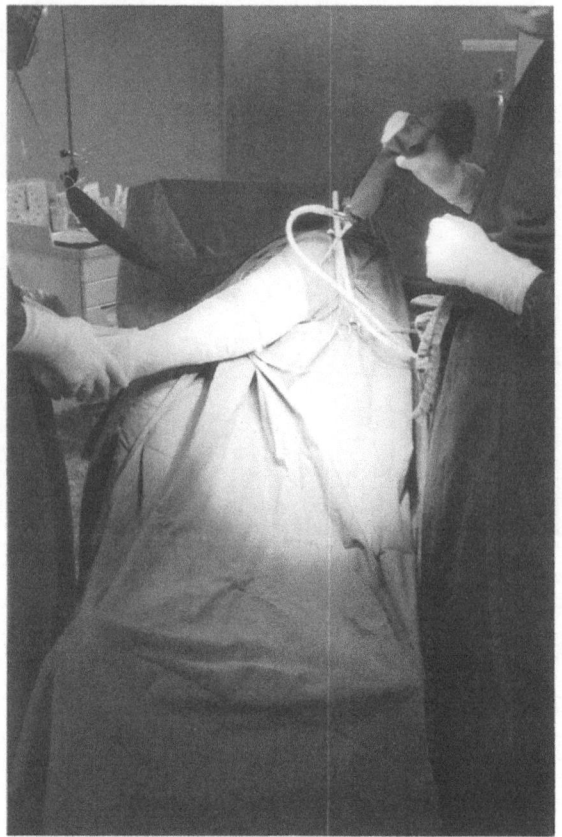

Fig. 55. Figure 4 position for examination of lateral joint space

closure of the lateral joint space. Both the upper and lower surfaces of the lateral meniscus should be completely visible. It is nearly always possible to display the popliteal hiatus and to bring the popliteus tendon into the visual field. The probe hook should be introduced from the medial aspect and the lateral meniscus palpated (Fig. 56). By extending and stretching the knee joint and looking towards the lateral femoral condyle, this can be completely illuminated and examined. Using the figure 4 position already mentioned, it is often possible to introduce the arthroscope fairly easily over the posterior horn of the lateral meniscus into the posterolateral recess. The fibers of the posterior cruciate ligament are seen medially, the instrument passing beneath them. A 70°-angled optical system can be used in the posterior recess for backward viewing and to give a better

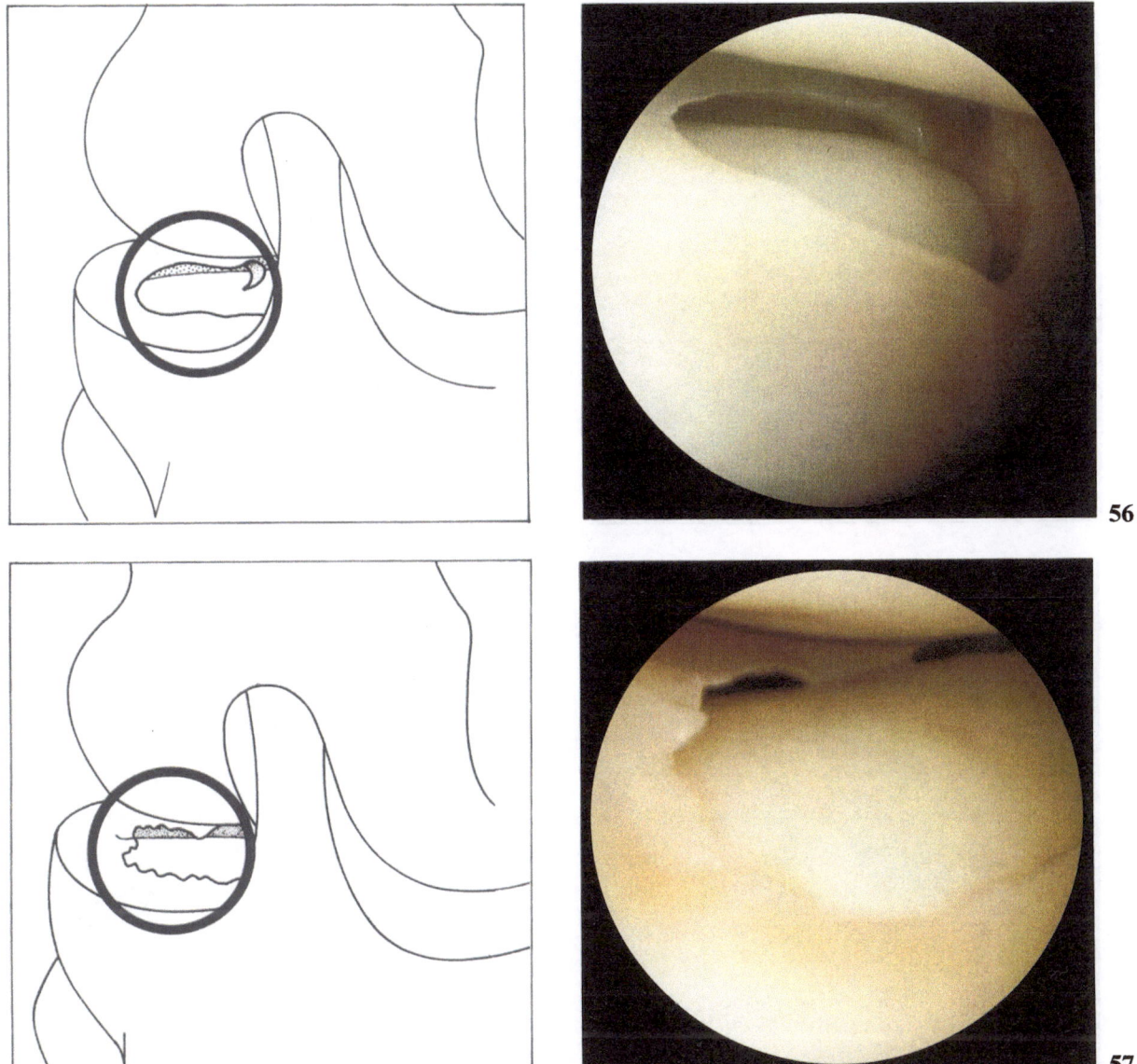

Fig. 56. Normal lateral meniscus

Fig. 57. A wavy-bordered but perfectly normal lateral meniscus in a 40-year-old patient

side view when searching for possible loose bodies (Figs. 57–60).

By retraction of the optical system followed by further movement laterally into the lateral recess, it is possible to display this recess directly. However, this route is somewhat risky as incautious movement may result in rapid extrusion of the instrument from the knee. In such a case it is advisable to discontinue the introduction of fluid and gas through the arthroscope. It is often possible, however, to demonstrate the lateral recess with its capsular folds and numerous plicae by slightly withdrawing and swiveling the in-

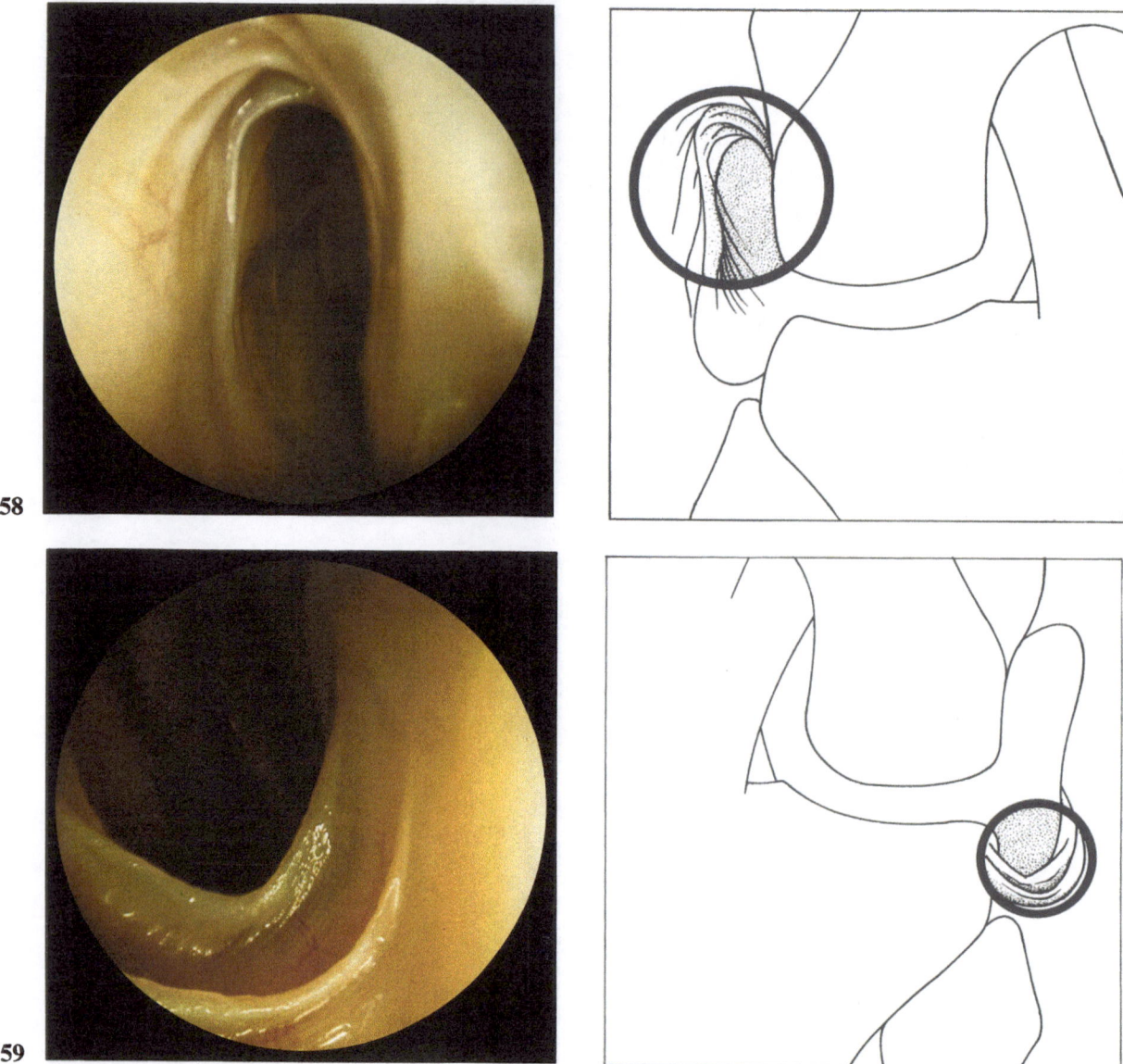

Fig. 58. Upper reflection of capsule and ligament at lateral femoral condyle

Fig. 59. Lower reflection of the capsule and ligament at the lateral femoral condyle, a common location for loose bodies

strument. Loose bodies or foreign bodies are most often found here in the lower part of the lateral recess, so that it may be helpful to position the arthroscope primarily in this position via the superior recess. As the knee is extended the optical system can be directed medially, when the patellofemoral joint together with the condylar or trochlear margin enter the side of the visual field. Withdrawal of the arthroscope anteriorly in full extension via the patellofemoral joint and over the condyles is easily performed. This concludes the tour of inspection from the lateral approach.

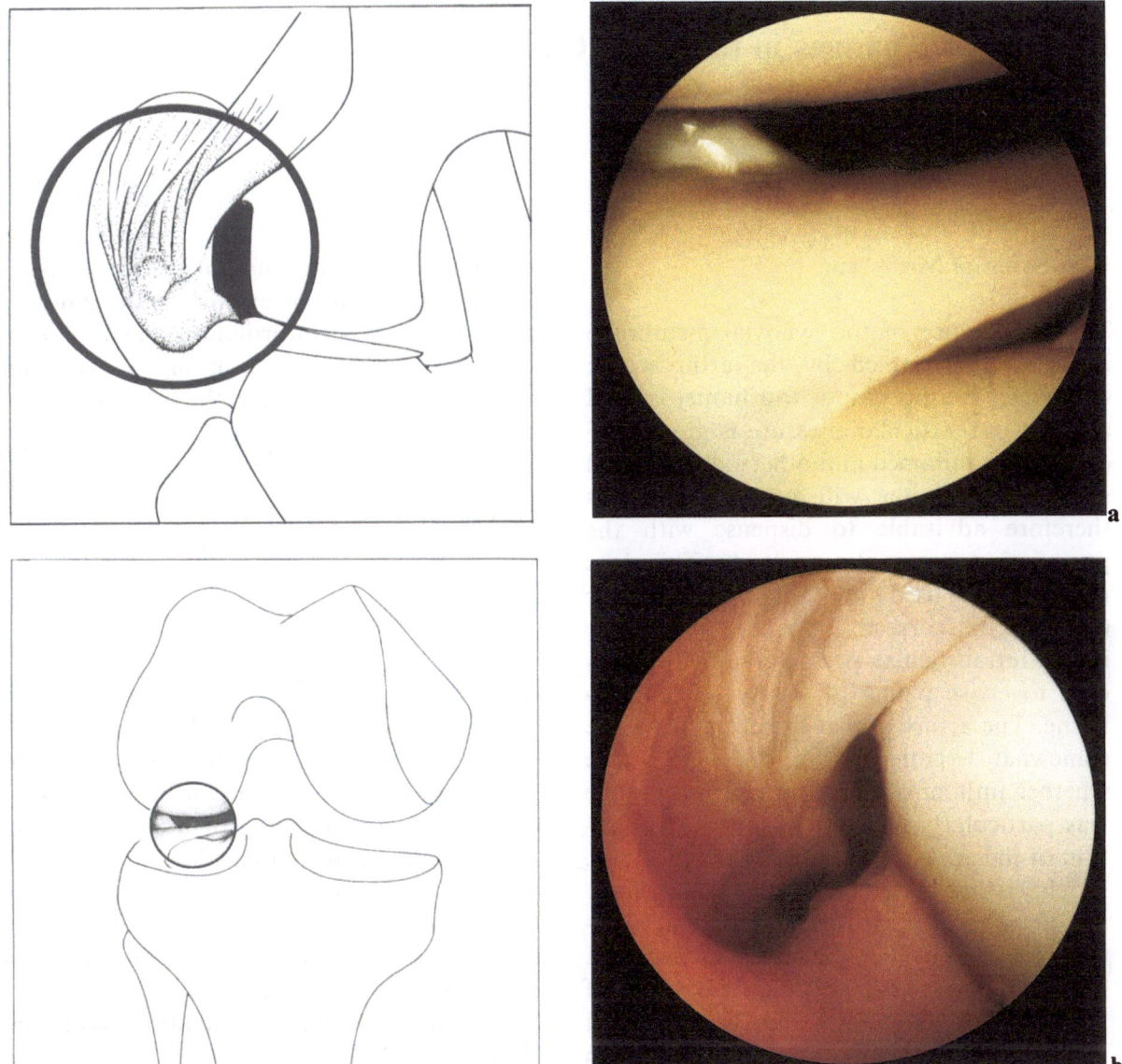

This procedure is only one of many possibilities and obviously a quite different inspection sequence is possible. However, at the end of the arthroscopy every observer must ask himself whether he has really displayed the entire knee joint. Thus, even definite findings of pathologic changes in the medial meniscus do not imply that complete and precise inspection (e.g., of the lateral folds in the superior recess) can be dispensed with.

Fig. 60. a Popliteus tendon in the popliteal hiatus of the lateral meniscus. **b** Popliteus tendon and outer border of lateral meniscus

CHAPTER 14

Pathologic Changes in the Joint Cavity

14.1 Synovial Membrane

The appearance of the synovial membrane is largely determined by the arthroscopic technique. If a pneumatic tourniquet is used and the intraarticular pressure is greatly increased, an inflamed and otherwise reddened synovial membrane will appear pale. It is therefore advisable to dispense with the pneumatic tourniquet completely. This does not need to be used if the combined technique (see p. 42) is correctly applied. An increase in the intraarticular pressure suffices on its own to cause paling of the synovial membrane. The arthroscopist therefore has to be somewhat experienced in order to judge whether inflammation is present. Watanabe was particularly interested in the interpretation of the appearance of the synovial types. By classifying them according to their shape and arrangement he tried to derive information relevant to the diagnosis of arthritis. There are, indeed, many different types of synovial folds. Their size and shape are best determined when the joint is filled with Ringer solution. With the slightest degree of turbulence the synovial folds then begin to move like seaweed and the "aquarium effect" becomes apparent. The tufts vary in shape from small and delicate synovial "trees" to thick polyplike structures. It can be said with some degree of certainty that the presence of delicate, florid and finely branched tufts is indicative of acute inflammation which has only been present for a short time. On the other hand, thickening of the branches of the synovial "trees"can be assumed to be a sign of chronic synovial irritation. Further differentiation of the synovial tufts by correlation of their appearance with different disease patterns is not possible. The arthroscopist cannot differentiate between chronic polyarthritis and nonspecific synovitis of the knee joint by examining the synovial membranes. The information which can be derived from examination of the synovial membrane is restricted to the following:

1. Inflammation is suggested by increased vascularity and the resulting reddening of the synovial membrane.
2. The presence of acute or chronic inflammation may be deduced from the shape of the synovial villi.
3. The thickness and arrangement of the villi indicate whether synovectomy or synoviorthesis should be carried out.

The success of the chemical synoviorthesis with osmium or yttrium can be assessed by arthroscopy. Blackening of the whole joint, including the articular cartilage, is known to occur following injection of osmium (Fig. 61). Follow-up investigation of a joint which has been successfully treated with yttrium or osmium reveals atrophy of the synovial membrane. The investigation should include a biopsy.

14.2 Pathologic Changes in the Medial Meniscus

As many previous studies have shown, the medial meniscus is most often affected by traumatic lesions around the age of 25 years. If the medial meniscus is not immediately torn by flexion-rotation and valgus strain of the knee, a tear usually occurs 1–2 years later secondary to persistent instability. The commonest type of tear is longitudinal, the extreme example of which is the bucket-handle tear. In a high proportion of cases a presumptive diagnosis can be made on the basis of the previous history and the clinical find-

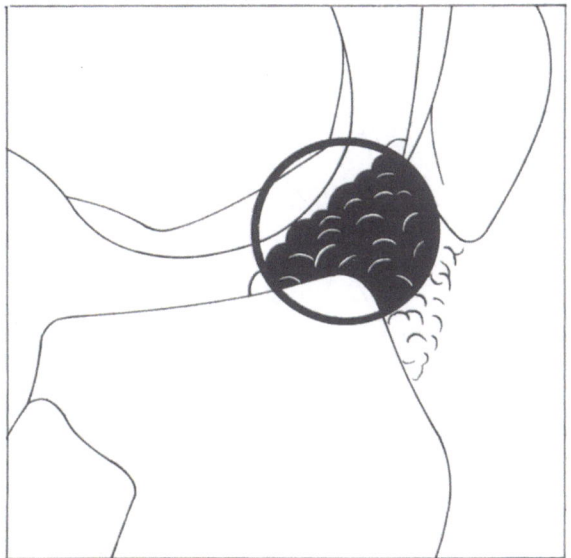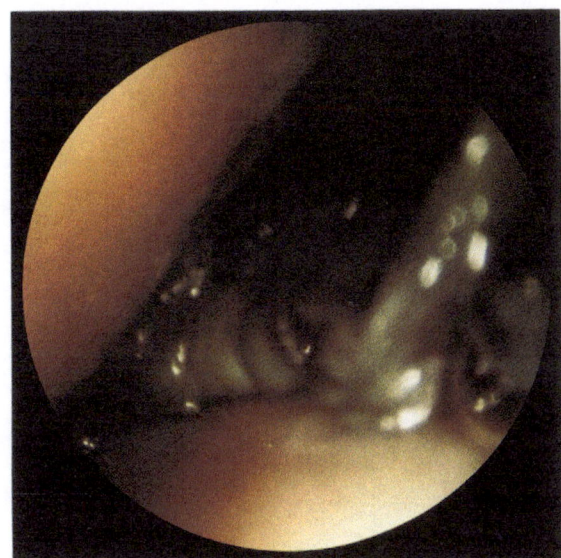

Fig. 61. Synovial membrane 8 days after injection of osmium

ings. Medial meniscus tears, which are not definitely traumatic in origin and are often purely degenerative, occur most commonly around the age of 40 and are a more difficult problem. Very often there is no simultaneous ligamentous lesion. Coarse longitudinal tears are manifested by sudden pain and a snapping sound when adopting the squatting position. Unfolding of the posterior horn, often a sequel to the "rucked carpet" formation in this region mentioned previously, may lead to flap tears. Horizontal tears, which are fairly common, may also exhibit significant degenerative components. Transverse tears of the medial meniscus are relatively rare and are frequently of no mechanical significance (Fig. 62). If a medial meniscus lesion is clinically suspected but cannot be confirmed immediately and reliably, it is essential to insert a diagnostic probe hook into the knee, usually from the medial side. It is possible with this hook to palpate the upper and lower surfaces of the meniscus, including the entire posterior horn, and to check for any flap formation. It is difficult to judge whether degenerative changes in the posterior horn are responsible for knee pain in a 50-year-old; ob-

viously, this depends on the general condition of the knee and the articular surfaces. Here again, the excellent view of the meniscus and the demonstration of very fine tears with the hook may automatically lead one to assume that the pathology found is responsible for the pain. It is essential that such inferences should not be carried too far, especially to the extent of operating on posterior horns with only minor degenerative changes. Such

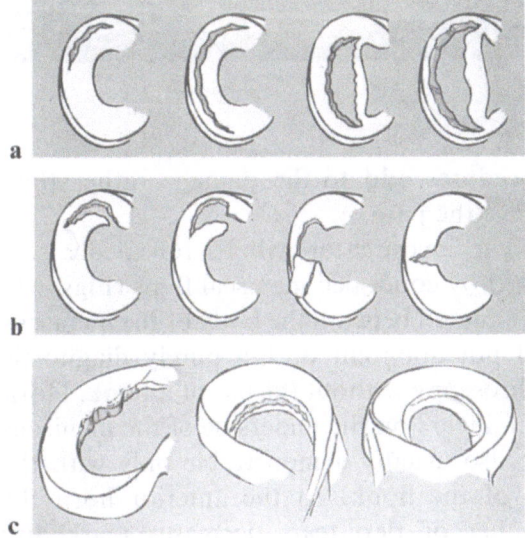

Fig. 62a–c. Types of meniscus tears. a Longitudinal tears, b flap and transverse tears, c degenerative changes and horizontal tears

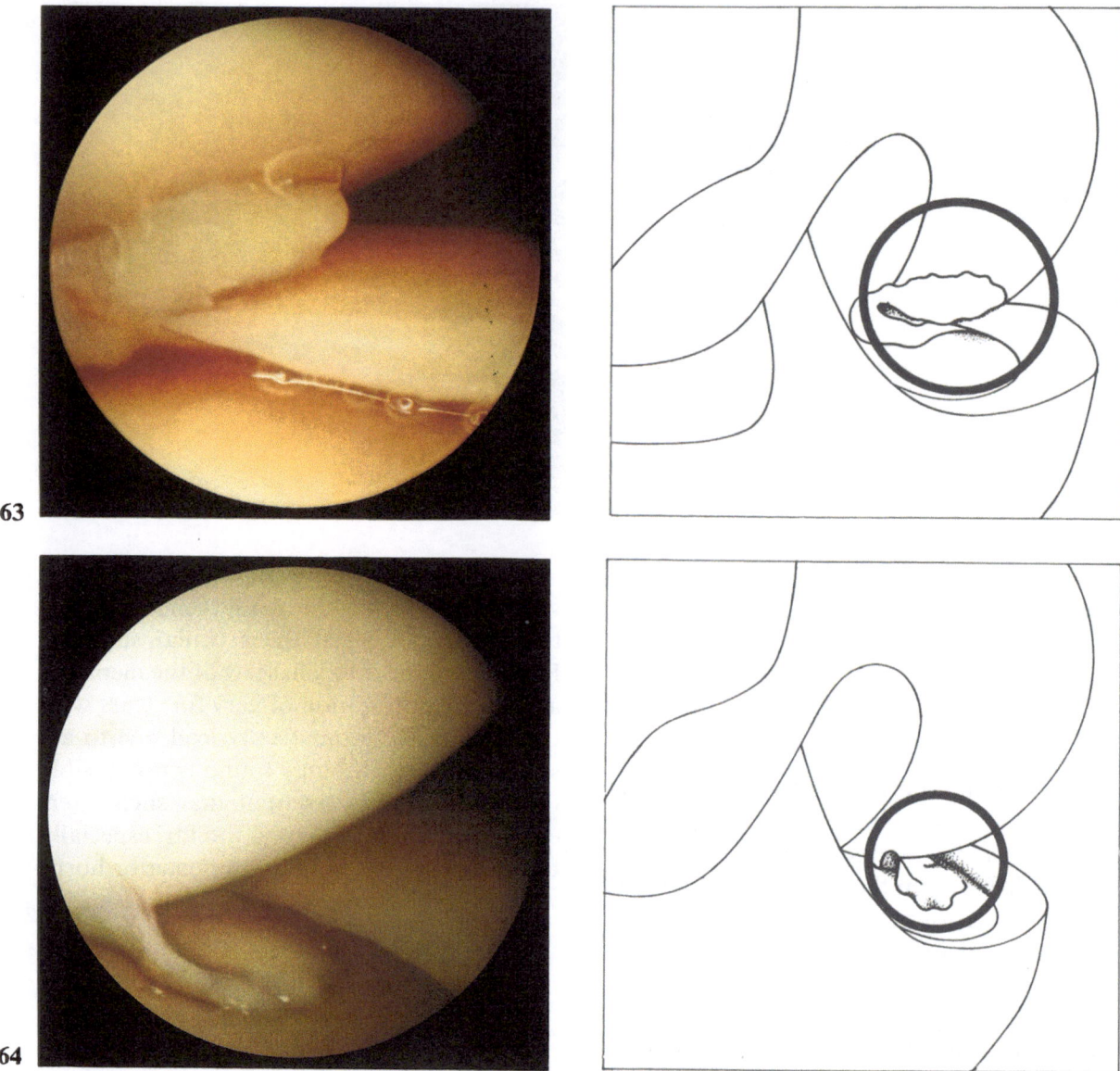

63

64

procedures add to the damage rather than relieve the pain.

The investigator will be repeatedly surprised by concealed meniscal flaps (Figs. 63–66) situated beneath the body of the meniscus and not apparent during purely diagnostic arthroscopy without the use of a hook. Horizontal tears on the underside of the meniscus are also usually demonstrable only with the aid of the hook. At the anterior horn the number of flap tears decreases markedly; here there is a marked transition to the bucket-handle tear. In the presence of a large bucket-handle tear, usually displaced inward,

Fig. 63. Flap tear of the medical meniscus lying above the body of the meniscus

Fig. 64. Flap tear of the medial meniscus arising from the posterior horn

---

Fig. 65. Small, clinically unimportant, transverse ▷ tear of the medial meniscus

Fig. 66. Large flap tear of the medial meniscus

Fig. 67. Inturned bucket-handle tear of the medial meniscus

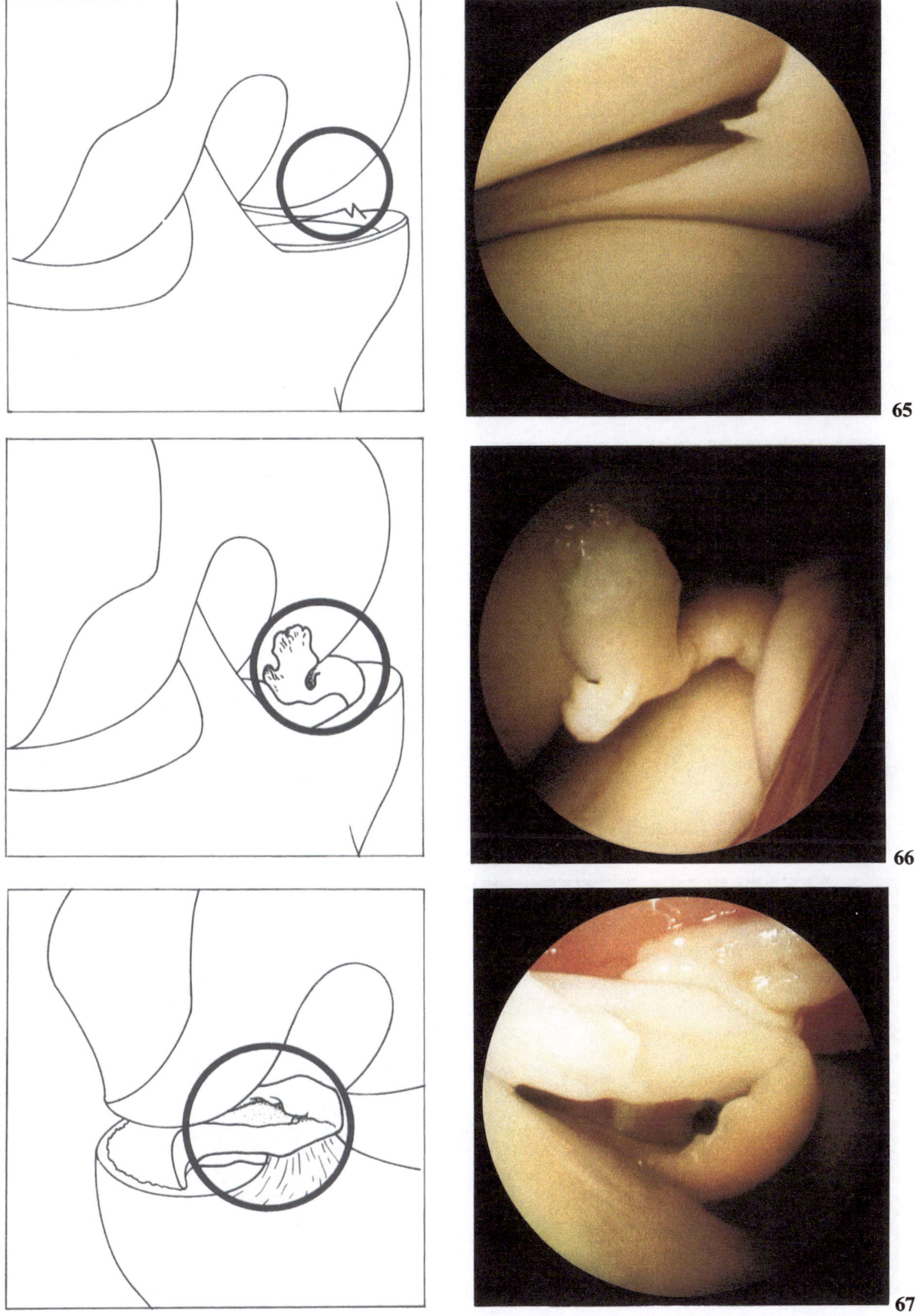

65

66

67

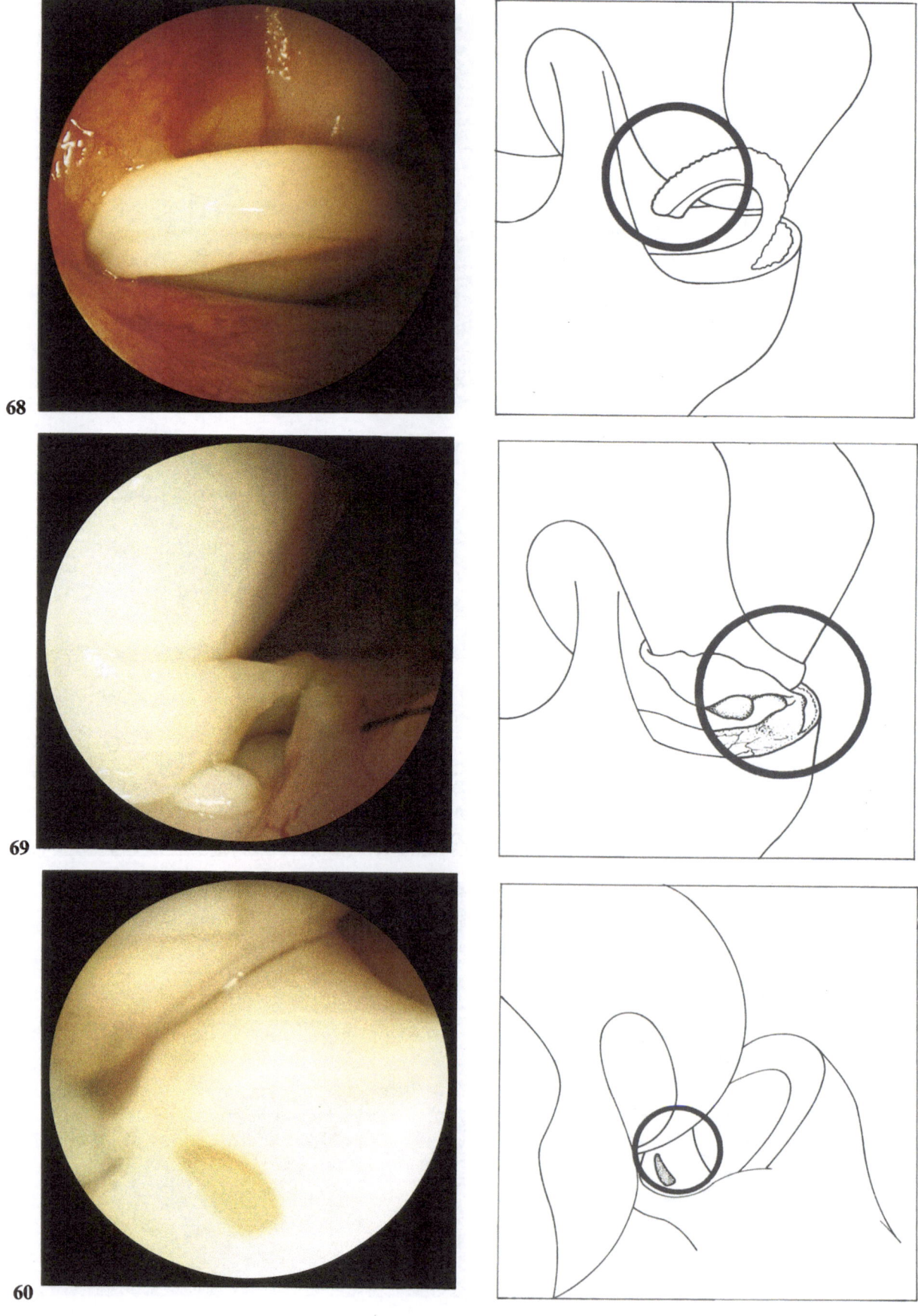

68

69

60

70

it becomes very difficult to inspect the intercondylar region and often it is only when the arthroscope is being withdrawn that the annular structure around the condyle is detected (Figs. 67–70). The transition zone in the region of the posterior horn should then be sought by appropriate rotation of the optical system towards the inner side of the knee and the bucket-handle tear subsequently followed up between the condyles as far as possible. It is only rarely that the surgeon has the good fortune to find that one end of the bucket-handle tear is already avulsed, with a large flap blocking the knee joint. The diagnosis is simpler when there is a traumatic meniscus lesion with anterior and often medial instability, as it is then easy to inspect the medial joint space. Obviously, in such a case it is easier to carry out operative procedures than in the stable knee joint.

◁ **Fig. 68.** Inturned, rounded-off bucket-handle tear of the medial meniscus with inflammation of the intercondylar synovium

Fig. 69. Anterior site of medial reflection of bucket-handle tear

Fig. 70. Small longitudinal tear in the base of the posterior horn of the medial meniscus

---

Fig. 71 a, b. Discoid lateral meniscus **a** before and **b** after tear

14.3 Pathologic Changes in the Lateral Meniscus

Exposure of the lateral meniscus is effected in the manner previously described. The pathologic changes in the meniscus are many and various. Transverse tears of the body of the meniscus are very common, but often of no clinical relevance. Marked spreading and instability of the body of the meniscus in the region of the popliteus tendon is not uncommon. Here, it is difficult to distinguish between the normal and the pathologic and an operation should not be undertaken if there is any doubt. Congenital discoid meniscus,

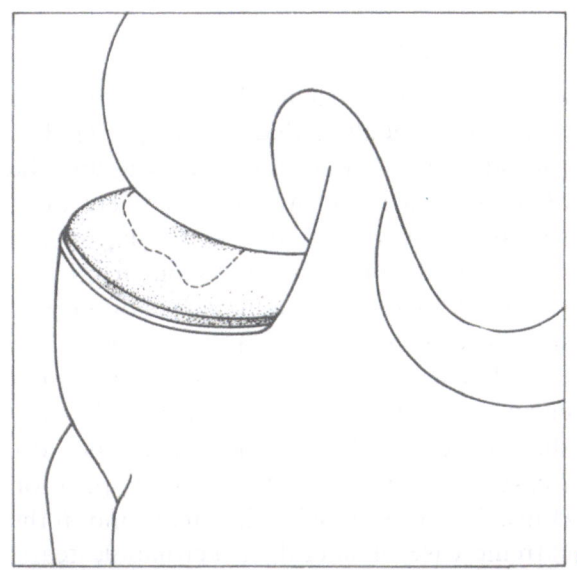

a

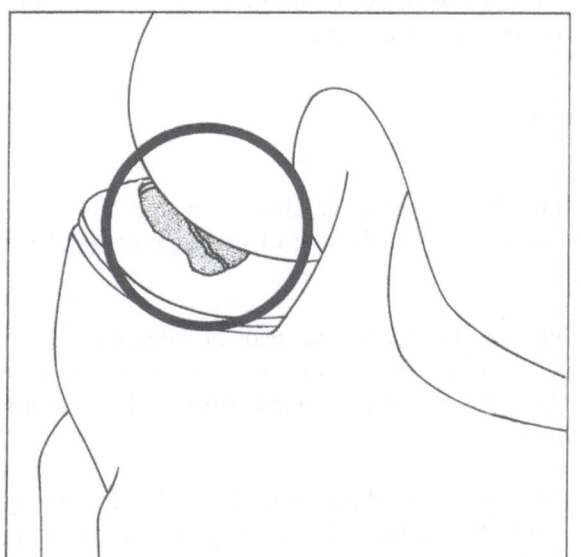

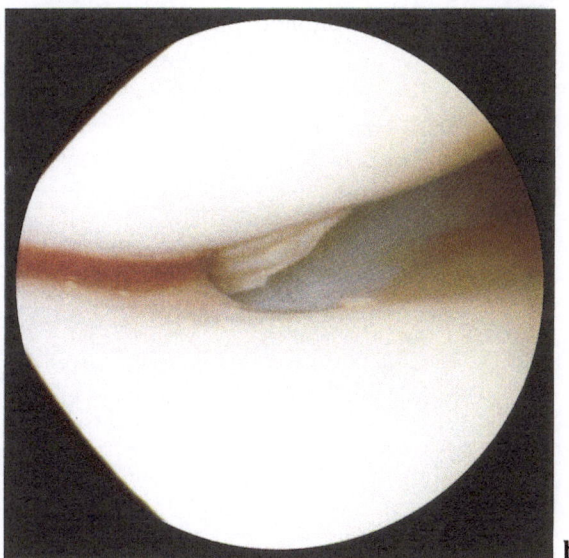

b

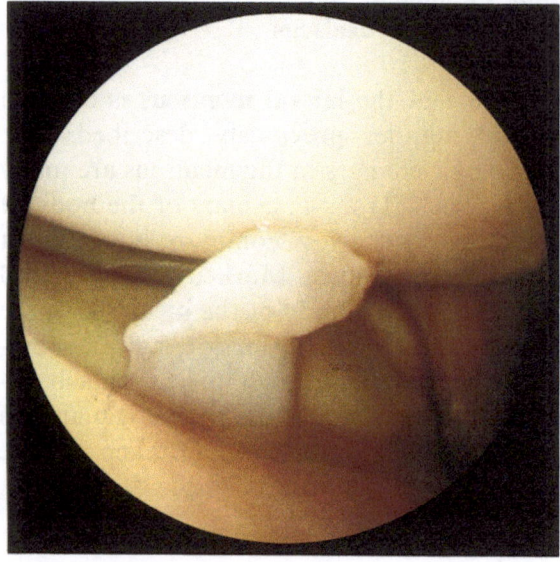 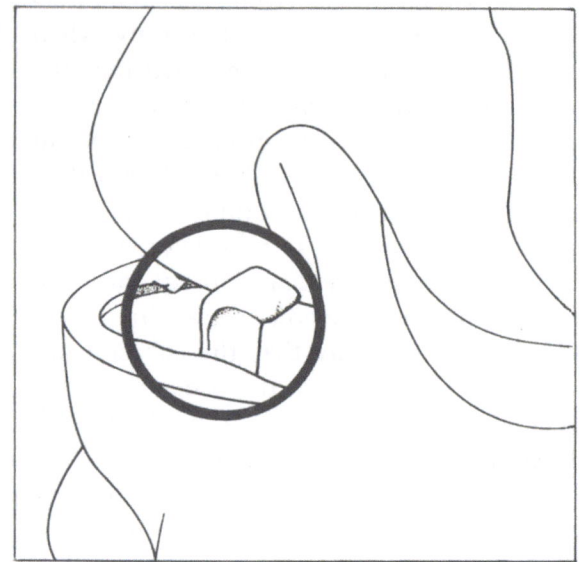

Fig. 72. Flap tear in lateral part of anterior horn

which is found particularly in the young, is especially difficult to diagnose (Fig. 71). The contrast between the lateral meniscus and the tibial plateau is in any case relatively poor and the observer often has the impression that he is dealing with a discoid meniscus. However, by inserting a hook it is often possible to elevate the delicate free edge of the lateral meniscus with its relatively small inner curve. A further guide is the usually very sharp border of the posterior horn, especially well-demonstrated in the figure 4 position (Figs. 72–75). In longitudinal tears and in the extreme case of lateral bucket-handle tears, pathologic evidence has often already been provided by the clinical picture. In terms of size and thickness, lateral bucket-handle segments are often twice as large as in the medial meniscus, so that the intercondylar region is then entirely occupied by the large bucket-handle flap. A certain degree of visualization and experience is required to make out the transition zone of the bucket-handle tear distinctly. Because of the size of the avulsed portion in longitudinal or bucket-handle tears of the lateral meniscus operation is not too easy, despite good opening-up of the lateral joint space (see Chap. 20).

Fig. 73. Degenerative changes in the lateral me- ▷ niscus with roughening of cartilage of tibial plateau

Fig. 74. Bucket-handle tear of lateral meniscus. The bucket-handle portion is not in the intercondylar space but is trapped between the tibia and femur

Fig. 75. Minor damage to the articular cartilage over the lateral tibial condyle following lateral meniscectomy

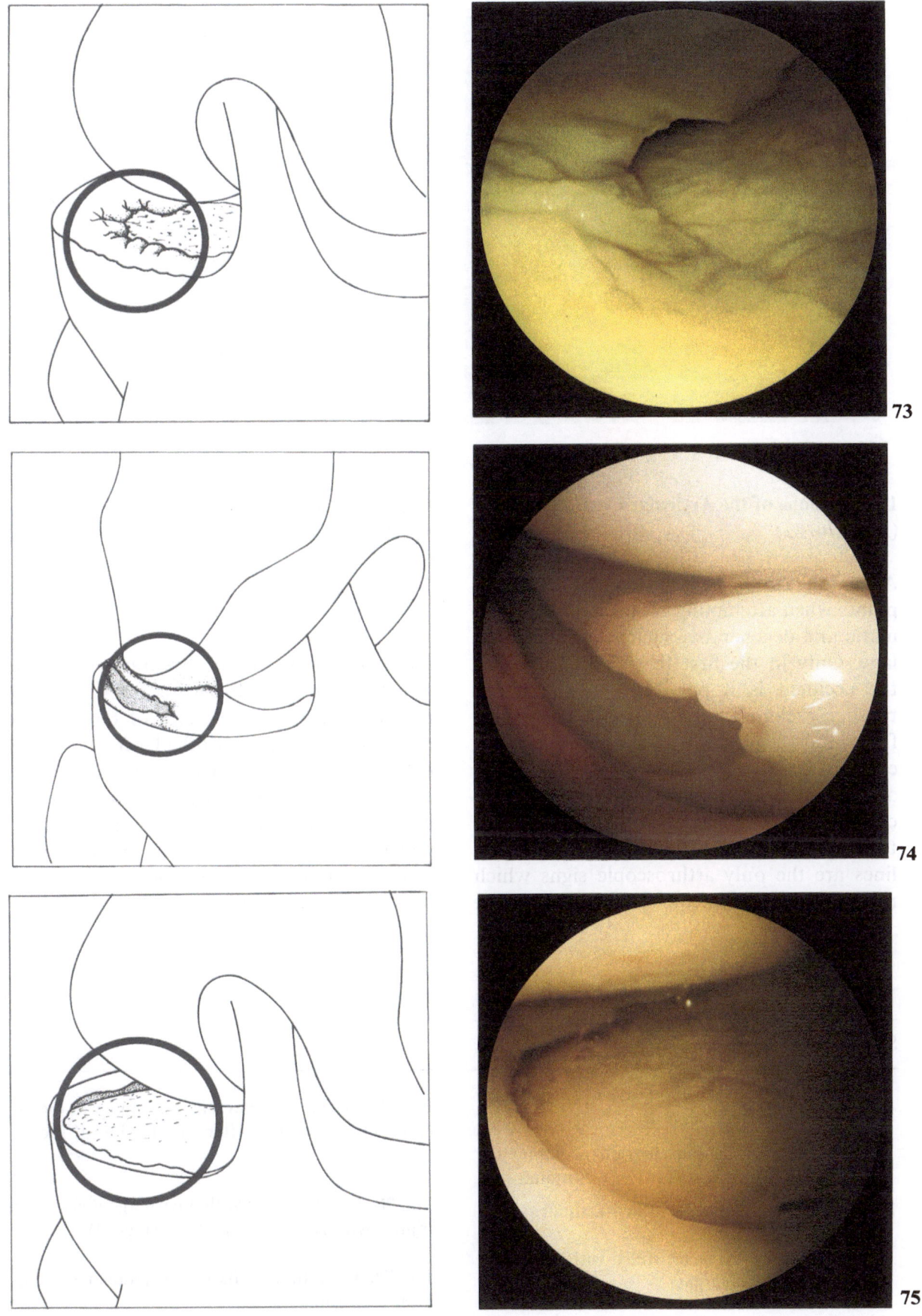

73

74

75

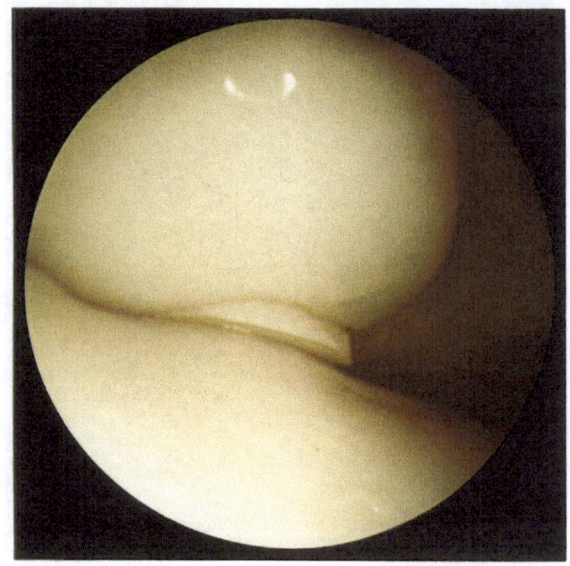

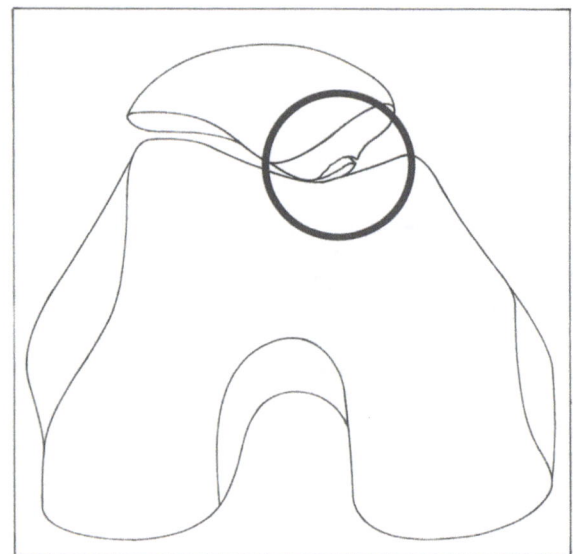

14.4 Lesions of the Articular Cartilage
(Figs. 76–83)

Attention should be paid to the following points when attempting to differentiate traumatic and degenerative changes in the cartilage. Only in the first few weeks following the accident is it possible to differentiate traumatic changes in the articular cartilage from those caused by degeneration. The edges of freshly fractured cartilage are sharp and clear cut and their appearance provides characteristic evidence that the lesion is post-traumatic in origin. These clear-cut fracture lines are the only arthroscopic signs which may be taken as unequivocal evidence that

Fig. 76. Recent traumatic articular cartilage damage due to shearing strain acting on the patella (stage I)

the lesion was caused by trauma. In the weeks and months following fracture of the articular cartilage the edges of the fracture gradually become smoothed off and it becomes increasingly difficult to decide whether the lesion was caused by trauma or by degeneration of the cartilage. A gap in the cartilage which has been present for more than 6 months cannot be ascribed with certainty to an accident (Table 1).

Table 1. Traumatic cartilage lesions

Stage	Age	Appearance	
I	Up to 6 weeks	Clear-cut fracture margin	Contusion, shear force,
II	6–24 weeks	Fracture margin rounded off	combined trauma
III	More than 24 weeks	a) Defect filled without raised margins b) Defect filled with raised margins	

Fig. 77. Recent articular cartilage injury at the lateral femoral condyle after subluxation of the patella ▷

Fig. 78. Older (3–6 months) cartilage defect after injury, with rounded-off edges (stage II)

Fig. 79. Longitudinal fissure in patellar cartilage after contusion

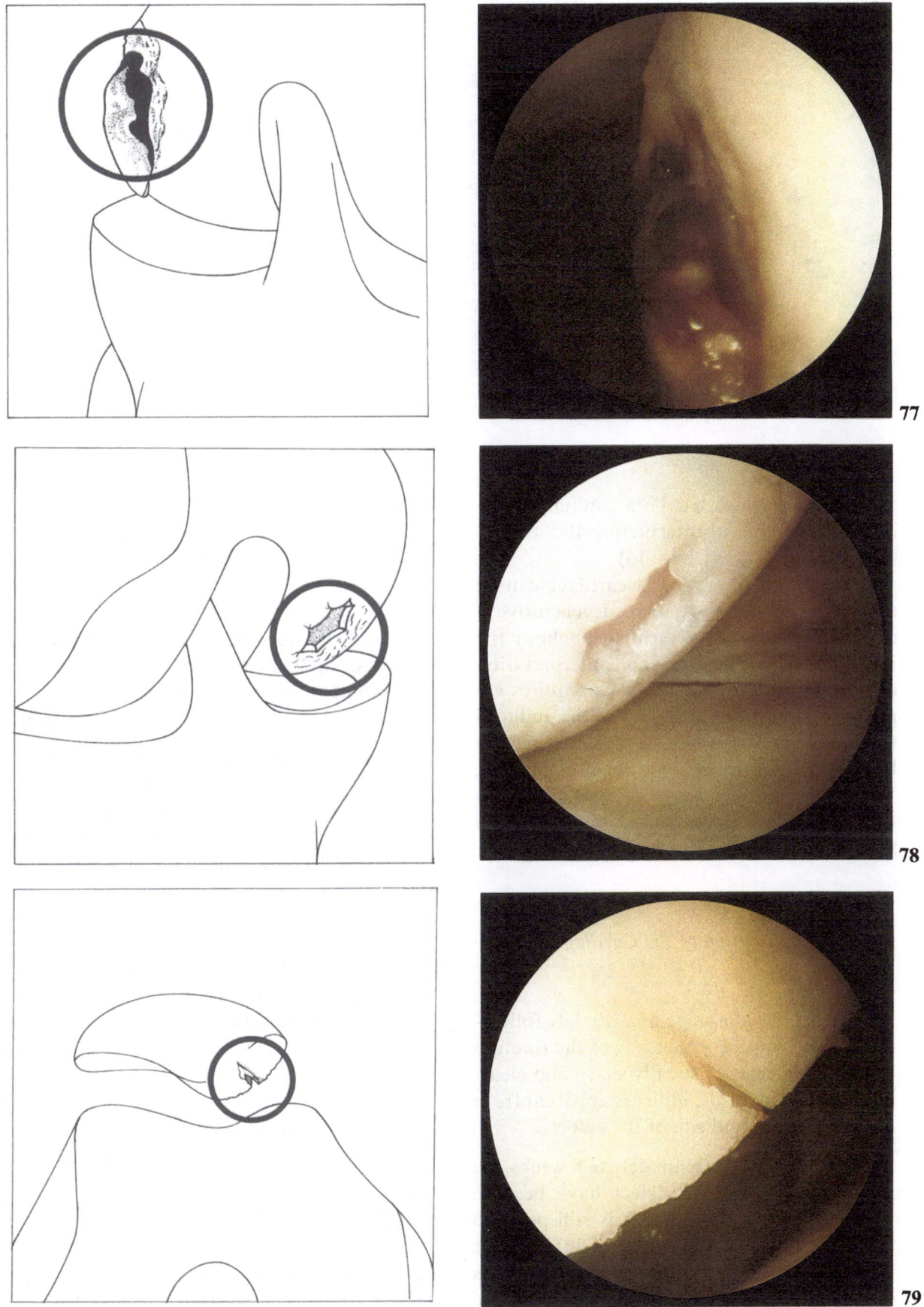

77

78

79

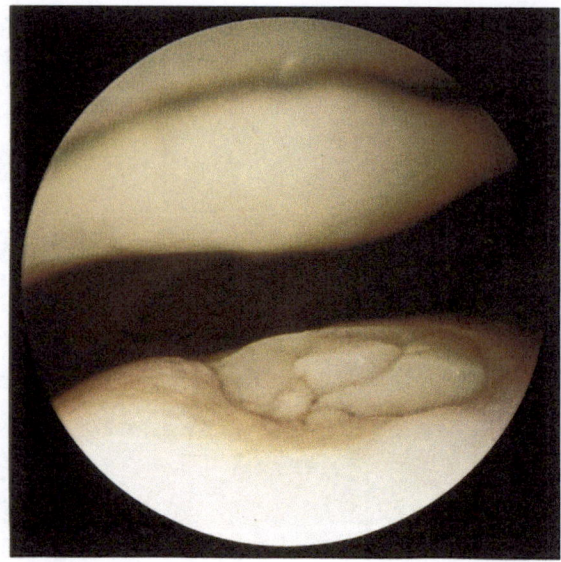 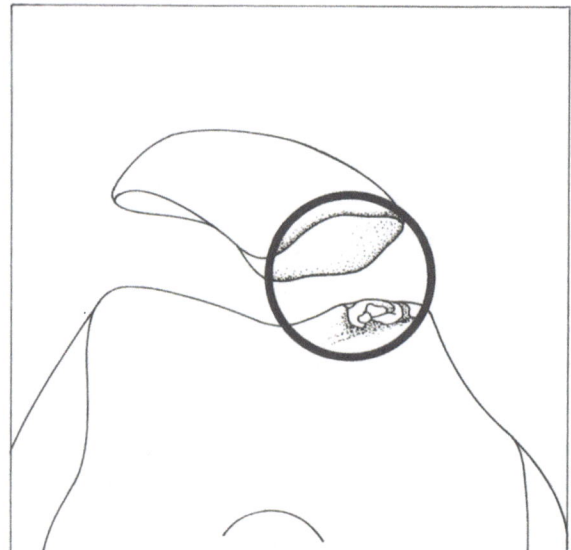

Fig. 80. Recent contusion fracture of the cartilage at the medial femoral condyle (stage I)

A history which has been carefully taken is of great value in interpreting the arthroscopic findings (see Chap. 15).

Changes in the articular cartilage can be assumed with certainty to be degenerative if cartilage lesions are present throughout the joint. The correct arthroscopic interpretation of discoloration of the cartilage requires experience. Healthy cartilage can be induced to take on a wide variety of colors simply by changing the intensity of the illumination. Whenever possible, therefore, one should try to work with a standardized light intensity and avoid excessive illumination of the joint.

14.4.1 Classification of the Cartilage Fracture

Stage I: This is the stage immediately following the accident. The margins of the fracture or gap are characteristically sharp and clearcut. The nature of the injury is apparent from the appearance and site of the defect.

Stage II: After approximately 6–8 weeks the sharp margins of the defect have become rounded off. At this stage it is still possible (but sometimes very difficult) to differentiate between the different types of injury such as contusion, shear, or combined trauma. If the

cant step between the two. Healing of the cartilage gap is sufficiently deep its floor may be reddened; this is a sign of incipient healing of the gap by the connective tissue reaction.

Stage III: At this stage of repair, which is reached approximately 6 months after occurrence of the injury, it is no longer possible to distinguish between the different modes of trauma. However, assessment of the injury in another respect is both easily possible and important. If solid repair and healing of the cartilage gap has occurred, the surface of the cartilage is no longer smooth and glistening but is level with the healthy cartilage at its junction with the latter and there is no signifi-

Fig. 81. Old cartilage damage at the medial femo- ▷ ral condyle with rounded-off edges (stage IIIa)

Fig. 82. Cartilage lesions at the patellar ridge and at the middle of the trochlea

Fig. 83. Long-standing deep cartilage defect in the trochlea with undermined edges (stage IIIb)

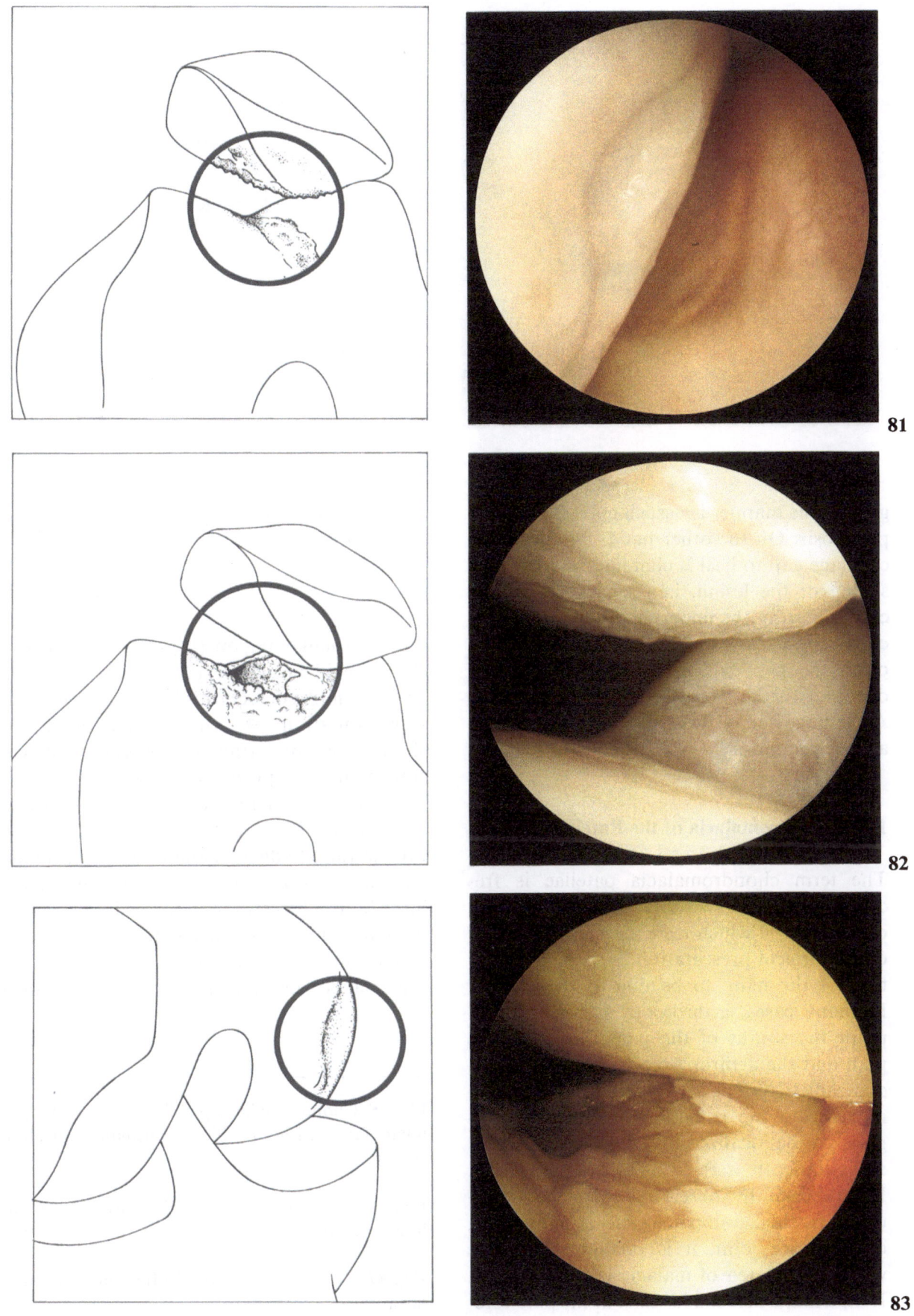

81

82

83

77

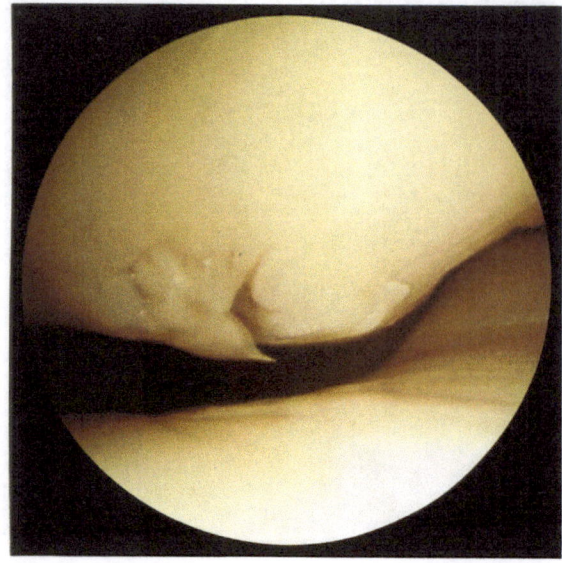

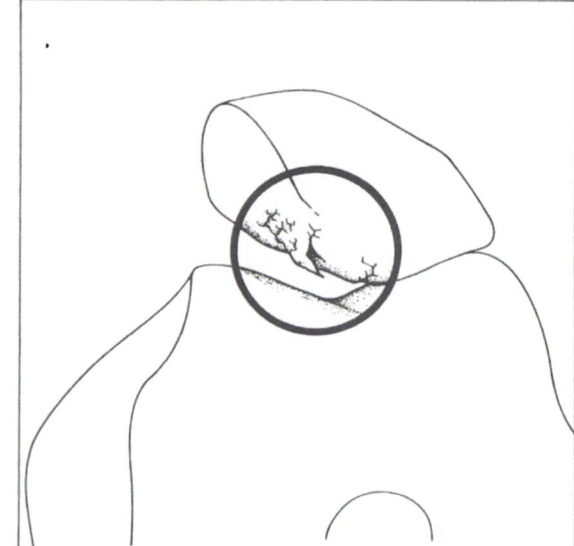

gap in this manner is associated with a good prognosis. On the other hand, failure of the cartilage gap to heal is characterized by worsening of the lesion, i.e., separation of the cartilage from the underlying bone. Arthroscopy reveals raised cartilaginous margins around the gap, which are unequivocal evidence of further separation of the cartilage. A cartilage gap of this type is associated with a poor prognosis.

14.5 Chondromalacia of the Patella

The term chondromalacia patellae is frequently applied to describe "pain at the front of the knee," which we assume on the basis of the clinical presentation, i.e., the localization of the pain, to be due to the patella. In many cases, arthroscopy is able to pinpoint the source of the pain; however, the pain and the arthroscopic findings are often contradictory. The cartilage defect, chondromalacia, in the patellofemoral articular region can be localized by arthroscopy and its size and depth assessed by means of a probe. In addition, by observing the contact between trochlea and patella during movement of the knee joint, it is possible to decide whether the area of malacia is under strain. If a cartilage defect does exist in the patellofe-

Fig. 84. Chondromalacia patellae of moderate severity at the medial patellar facet

moral articular region (Figs. 84–87) and the clinical evidence suggests that the symptoms arise from this defect, this raises the everawkward question of whether an operation should be undertaken. Leaving patellar transplantation procedures out of consideration for the moment, many surgeons may feel more inclined to "nibble" away and smooth off the raised edges of the diseased cartilage with an appropriate instrument, such as a large biopsy forceps or a motor-driven water-irrigated shaver. Even so, the procedure is often quite a radical one and should not be undertaken lightly. The results of open

Fig. 85. Chondromalacia patellae at the lateral patellar facet without villous formation (healing stage) ▷

Fig. 86. Chondromalacia patellae with marked villous formation

Fig. 87. "Cartilage scarring" after surgical patellar abrasion

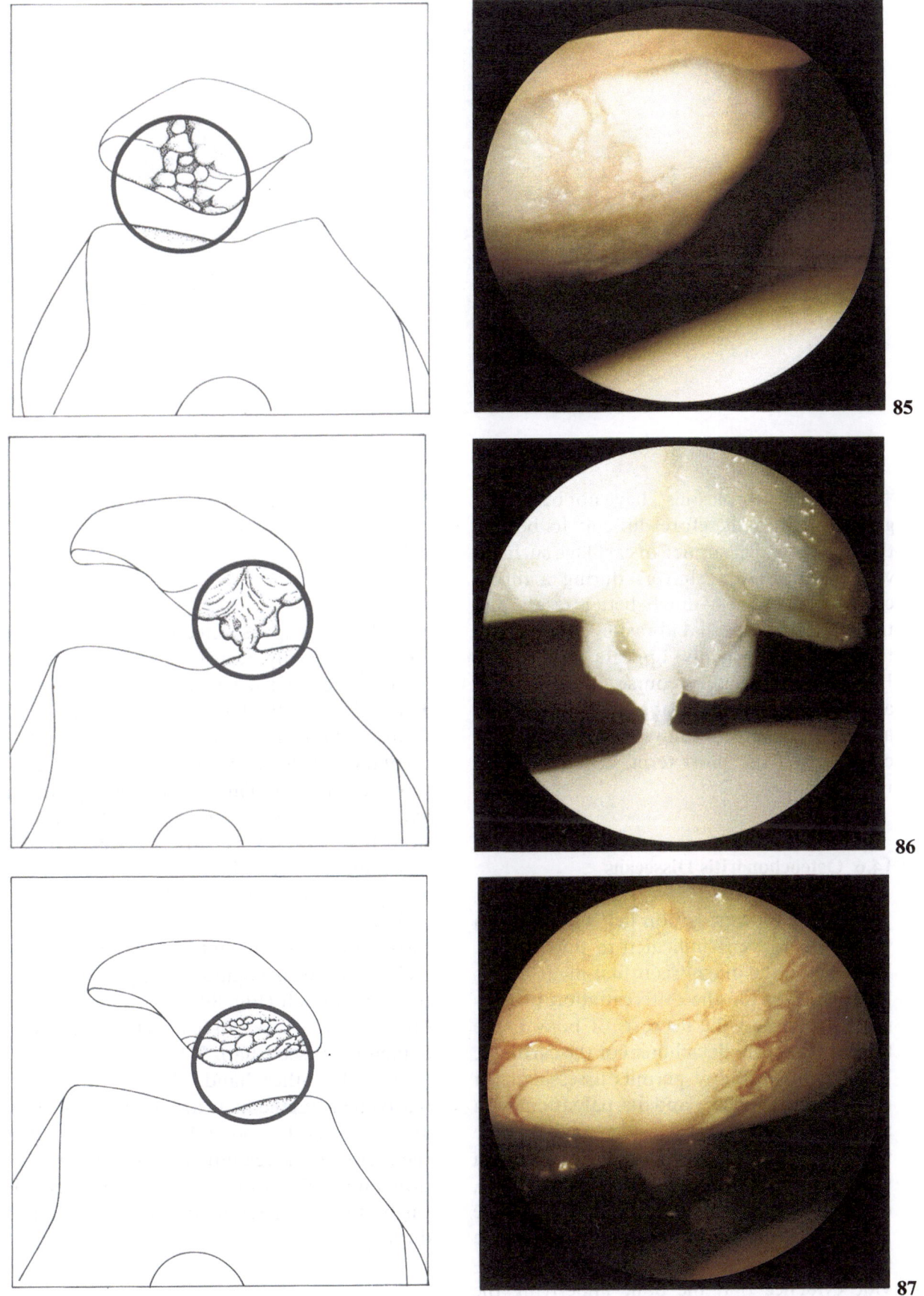

85

86

87

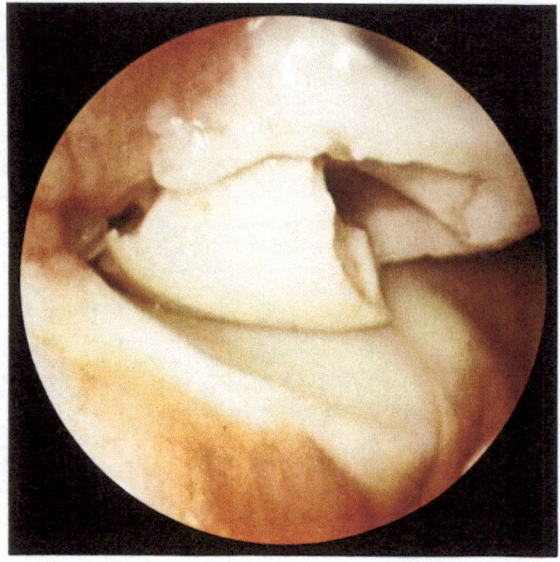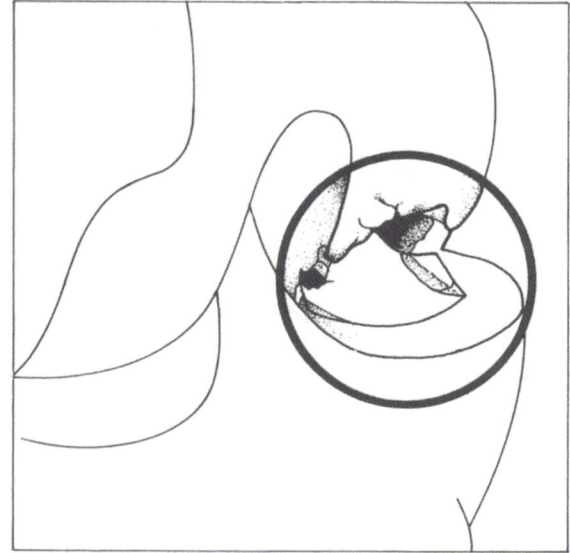

"abrasion arthroplasties" have not been very good and it is therefore difficult to believe that the radical clearance of cartilage surfaces with motor-driven shavers during arthroscopy would give a much better result. On the other hand, partial abrasion of loose cartilage edges certainly appears reasonable. However, the further course of the disease after this procedure is not predictable as such abrasion, though it may well alleviate the condition in the short term, does not eliminate its causes.

14.6 Osteochondritis Dissecans

Arthroscopic investigation helps to establish whether surgery is indicated in this disease. Frequently, the diagnosis is first made radiologically, because the differentiation process in the bone and the necrosis of bony tissue take place before detachment of the cartilage. Because arthroscopy permits assessment of the articular surface and its palpation with a probe, it makes it possible to determine whether the cartilage layer still has some firm substratum. Very often, in its initial stages, osteochondritis dissecans is not detectable from within the joint itself. A strong probe – the blunt trocar often suffices – may provide evidence that the bone underlying the articular cartilage is defective. If the bone is already markedly necrotic, early fissuring of the cartilage and marked ballooning can be detected. Once the loose body has separated from its bony bed, the sharp edges of the cartilaginous defect project against the background (Fig. 88). This process of separation tends to begin in the zone of weight transmission. If separation has already occurred, the observer can assess the exact size of the focus arthroscopically and decide between reattachment or removal of the loose body. Arthroscopic reattachment of a completely detached osteocartilaginous fragment is extremely difficult (Fig. 89), and is indicated in only half the cases of osteochondritis with detachment (see Chap. 21).

On the other hand, the monitoring of reattached fragments is an important task of arthroscopy. It is possible to assess whether the cartilage has readapted to its former position and arthroscopic removal of metal is easily done after reimplantation of adequate duration.

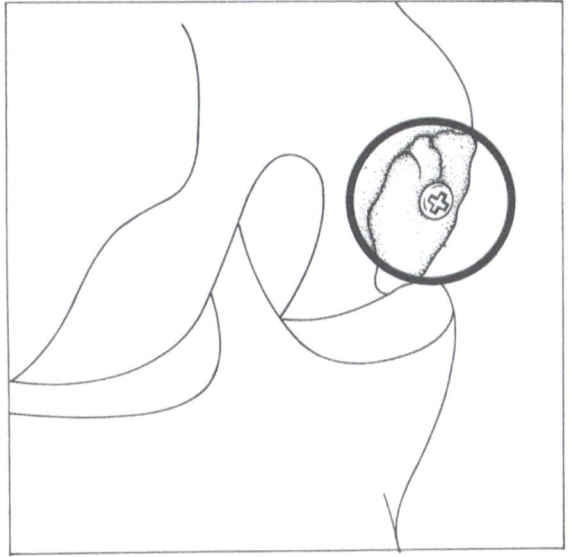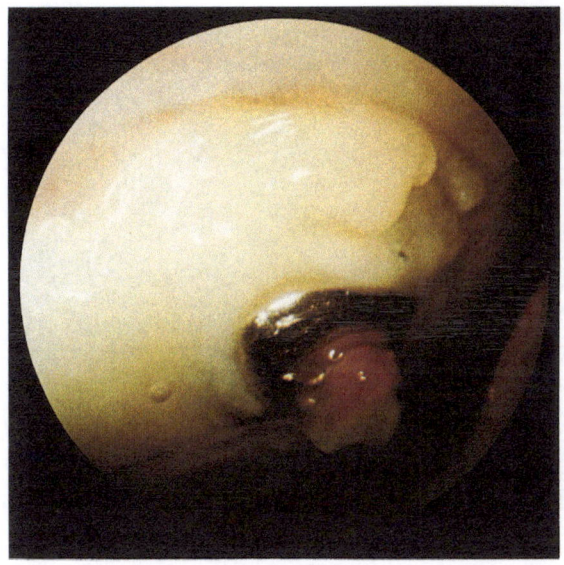

Fig. 89. Reattachment of fragment in osteochondritis dissecans using a small-fragment screw

14.7 Arthroscopic Appearance of Lesions of the Anterior Cruciate Ligament

There are two important uses of arthroscopy in suspected lesions of the anterior cruciate ligament. It is indispensable in recent injuries of the ligament, and it can also provide exact information as to the state of the remnants of the ligament in cases of long-standing instability of the knee joint. In the recently injured knee joint with hemarthrosis and an indefinite clinical picture (especially when the history is vague to the point that there is only the patient's familiar account of subluxation to go by) arthroscopy is capable of providing precise information as to the condition of the anterior cruciate ligament. General anesthesia is advisable for recently injured knees. The surgeon will very often begin with a preliminary examination under anesthesia before taking a decision. Local anesthesia for recently injured knees is sometimes possible, but rather painful for the patient.

The knee joint is thoroughly cleared of blood by intensive fluid irrigation, when it is often easy to locate the anterior cruciate ligament. With gas distension at low pressure (possibly combined with a blood pressure cuff under general anesthesia), the continuity of the ligament can be excellently assessed from the lateral approach. When, as is frequently the case, the ligament is ruptured in its upper third close to its attachment to the lateral condyle, its fibers can be seen lying on the tibial plateau in "cauliflower" fashion; another comparison is with a withered bunch of flowers. The view of the inner aspect of the lateral condyle often reveals blood extravasation and residual stubs of the ligament. Such findings are unequivocal. It is more difficult to assess a partially torn anterior cruciate ligament (Figs. 90–92) which, though inadequate, remains in place. It is essential to compare an internally torn anterior cruciate ligament that still preserves its continuity with the picture of a healthy, firm, cordlike ligament. In such cases palpation with a hook often reveals the existence of partial ruptures at different sites and clinical testing under arthroscopic monitoring often shows up the inadequacy of the ligament. Hemorrhages are common. Obviously, when such findings are present, the menisci must also be carefully inspected. Easy opening-up of the medial side of the joint is indicative of a rupture of the tibial collateral ligament (Fig. 93), in which case hemorrhages are of-

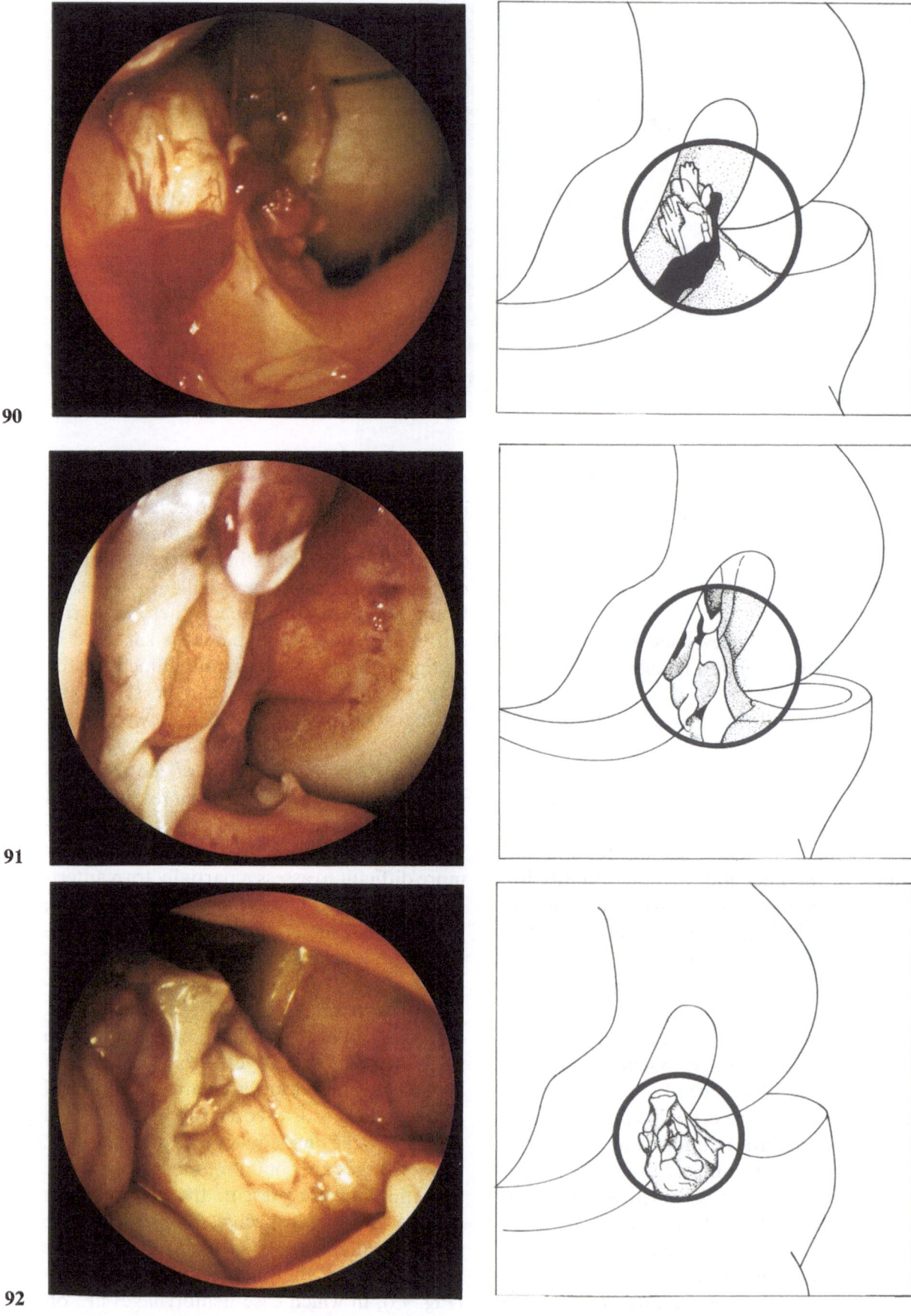

90

91

92

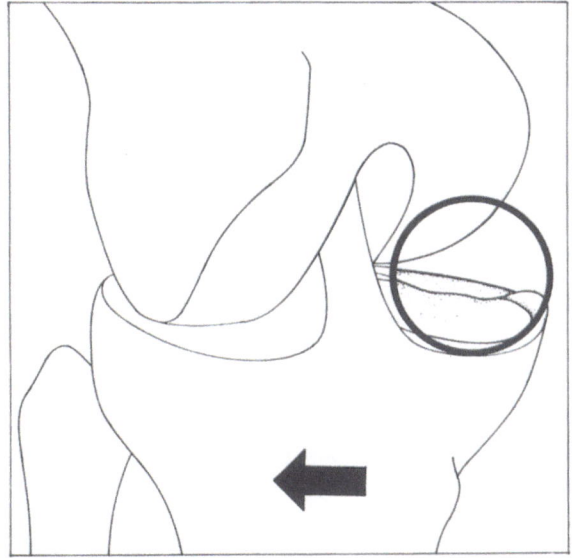

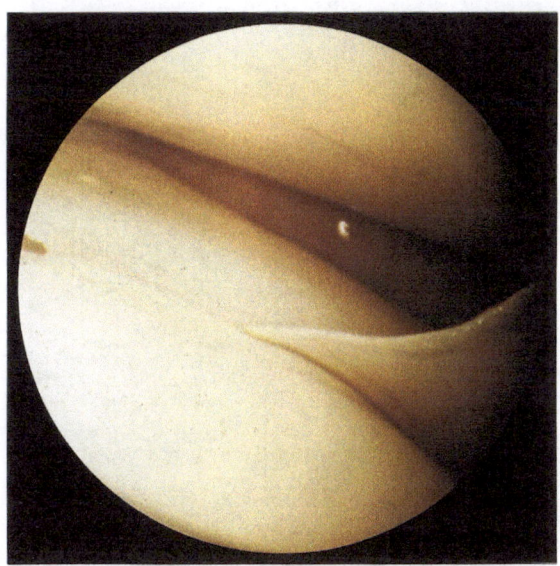

ten found at the synovial attachment of the medial meniscus. Reconstructive measures on the ligamentous apparatus and the torn parts of the meniscus are then indicated.

Chronic inadequacy of the anterior cruciate ligament is somewhat easier to assess. If clinical examination establishes anterior instability, in whatever combination with other lesions, the arthroscopist can obtain a view of the remains of the previously damaged ligament. Often the only findings are small stubs at the attachments, though complete absorption of the ruptured ligament is possible. However, in many cases a stringy, obviously inadequate anterior cruciate ligament is present. Visual comparison with a healthy ligament is enough in itself to suggest inade-

Fig. 93. Complete exposure of medial meniscus allowed by insufficiency of tibial collateral ligament

quacy. Testing under arthroscopic viewing is possible. If the optical system is sufficiently retracted, the effect on the ligament of the anterior drawer sign elicited by the assistant is easy to assess. The observer must always inspect the inner aspect of the lateral condyle with the extensive site of attachment for the cruciate ligament. If a clear view into the posterior recess is possible here, this suggests an old proximal avulsion of the anterior cruciate ligament. Here again, the insertion of a hook aids the assessment of the tension and attachment of the ligament.

14.8 Arthroscopic Appearance of Lesions of the Posterior Cruciate Ligament

Although the diagnosis of anterior cruciate ligament rupture in recent injuries may be difficult, it is often easier to establish rupture of the posterior cruciate ligament clinically. Here again, taking a careful history is of prime importance. When the accident involved a violent impact against the head of the tibia, usually with the knee flexed, this

◁ **Fig. 90.** Recent partial avulsion of anterior cruciate ligament

Fig. 91. Old tear of anterior cruciate ligament. The loose twisted structures of the torn ligament are visible

Fig. 92. Old avulsion of anterior cruciate ligament with complete stump formation

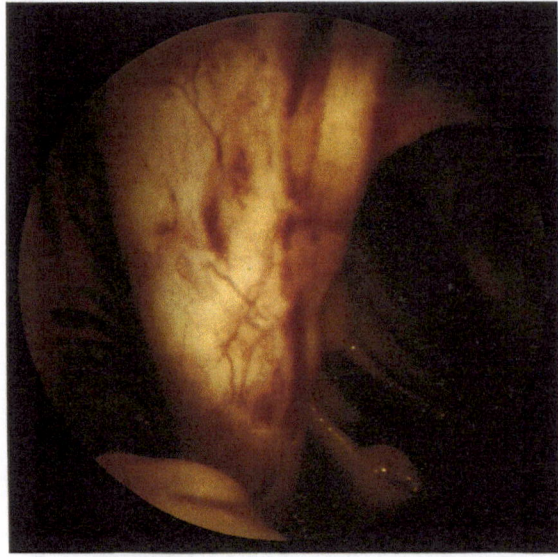

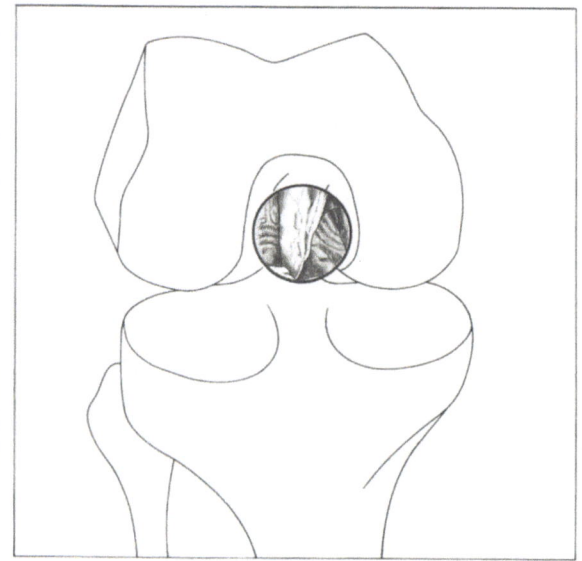

Fig. 94. Rupture of posterior cruciate ligament

should automatically suggest to the clinician the possibility of a posterior cruciate lesion. Traffic accidents are involved in over half the cases. The diagnosis of a posterior cruciate ligament rupture is often overlooked as a femoral fracture or dorsal dislocation of the hip diverts the observer's attention from the only slightly swollen knee joint. Signs of contusion and old scars at the front of the tibial head therefore deserve attention. Although the diagnosis of a posterior cruciate ligament rupture can nearly always be made clinically, arthroscopic investigation is important with both the freshly damaged ligament and chronic posterior instability. Very often there has been an avulsion of the ligament at the posterior aspect of the tibia and arthroscopy is able to clarify whether the ligament is still strong enough for reconstruction and reattachment or whether a plastic procedure should be undertaken.

As a rule, the view of the posterior cruciate ligament from the anterolateral aspect is unsatisfactory; inspection is limited to the attachment to the inner side of the medial condyle, and as this site is very often covered by a fat pad it is not possible to view the posterior cruciate ligament at all. Therefore, it is necessary to illuminate the posterior recess from in front and to advance the optical system dorsally, lateral to and beneath the

anterior cruciate ligament. The change to a 70° optical system is now helpful, as the region of the attachment of the posterior cruciate ligament can be fairly easily inspected in backward view. With fresh injuries extensive irrigation is necessary. As usual – and it is particularly the case here – a medially inserted hook is necessary to test for ligamentous instability.

The situation is made easier when the anterior cruciate ligament is already absent because of earlier damage. This allows a clear view of the posterior ligament (Fig. 94); the entire course of the ligament can then be inspected and the rupture site easily identified.

On the whole, however, in injuries of the posterior cruciate ligament, arthroscopy is more of an aid to planning an operation. The history and the clinical picture remain the decisive factors in diagnosis and treatment.

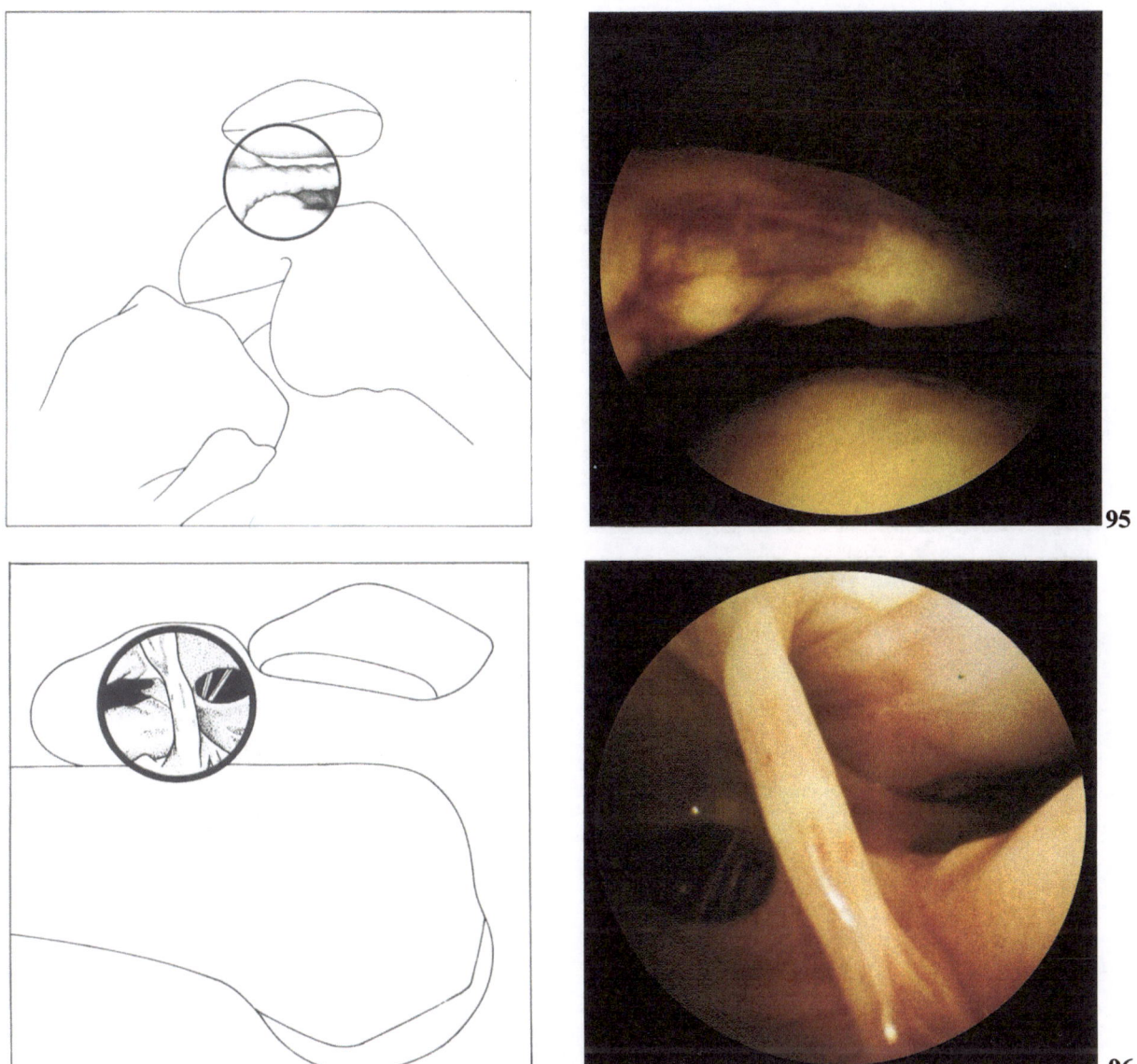

Fig. 95. Thickened medial plica

Fig. 96. Connective tissue bands in the suprapatellar recess restrict free movement of the knee joint

14.9 Lesions of the Plicae – Previously Operated Knee Joints

Various connective tissue bands or plicae occur physiologically in the knee joint and are explicable in terms of the developmental history of the joint. The best-known of these is the infrapatellar synovial plica (alar fold), the connective tissue band running from the tip of the infrapatellar fat pad to the roof of the intercondylar region (see p. 58). Disease of the medial part of the plica is the more important, as inflammatory irritants or even a simple synovitis can give rise to scar-

ring and thickening of the plica here. The plica, though intrinsically delicate (see also p. 165) can become thickened and scarred, giving rise to the so-called "plica syndrome." It is extremely difficult to form an opinion on a plica so altered; whether such thickened connective tissue bands should be regarded

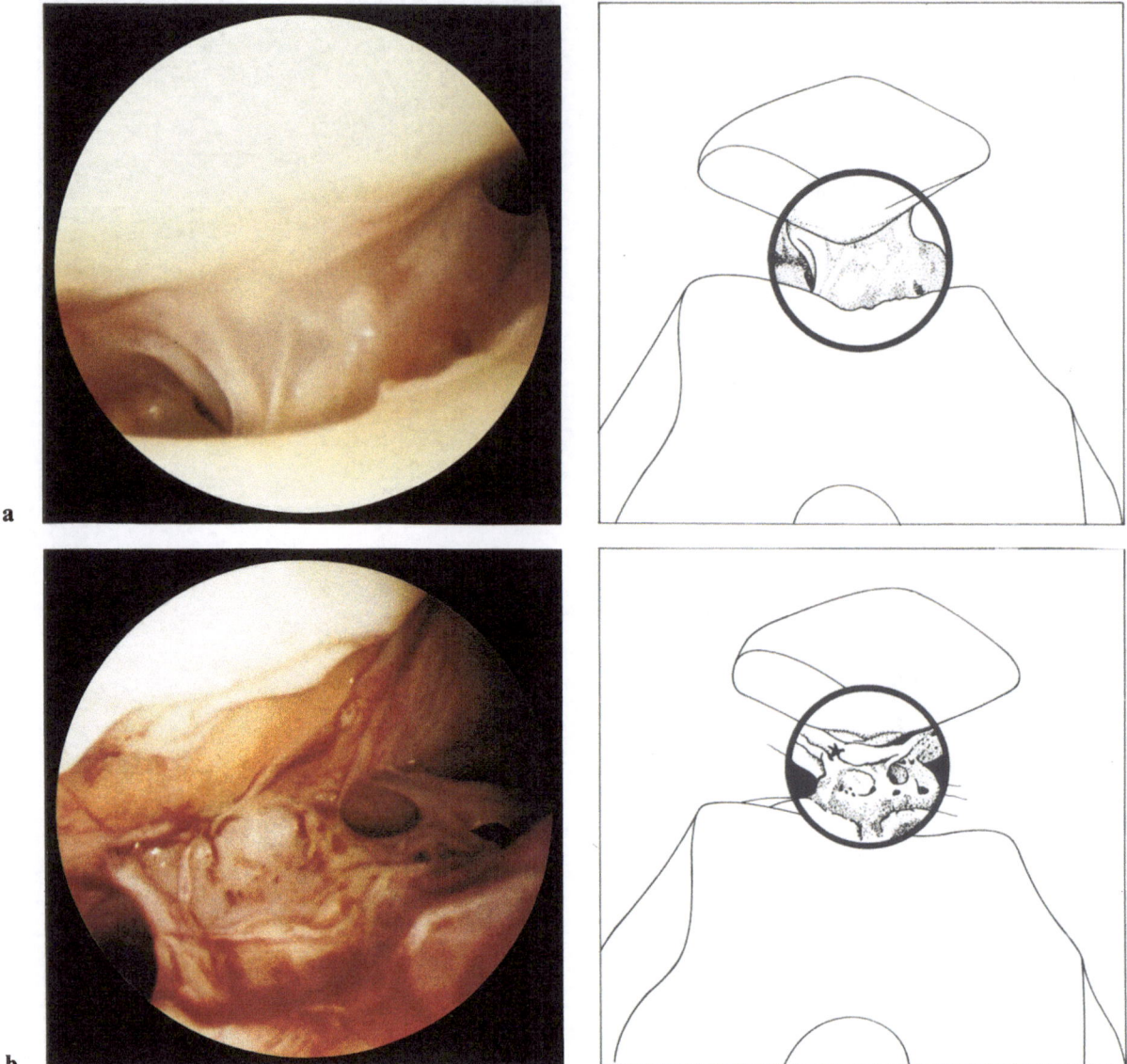

a

b

as sufficient grounds for operation must be related to the clinical picture (Fig. 95).

Knee joints that have previously been operated on frequently display connective tissue bands (Figs. 96–98) in both the lateral and the suprapatellar recesses. These produce a certain stiffness or even actual restriction of movement. The knee joint is markedly more difficult to investigate and the joint cavity cannot be distended with precision. All this impairs the visual conditions and it is therefore often necessary to adoption of various approaches to inspect the entire joint cavity in such a previously operated and

Fig. 97a, b. Parapatellar and suprapatellar connective tissue bands before and after forcible flexion under general anesthesia

scarred knee. It is possible to divide the adhesions by diathermy, sharp dissection, or even by forcible mobilization under anesthesia.

86

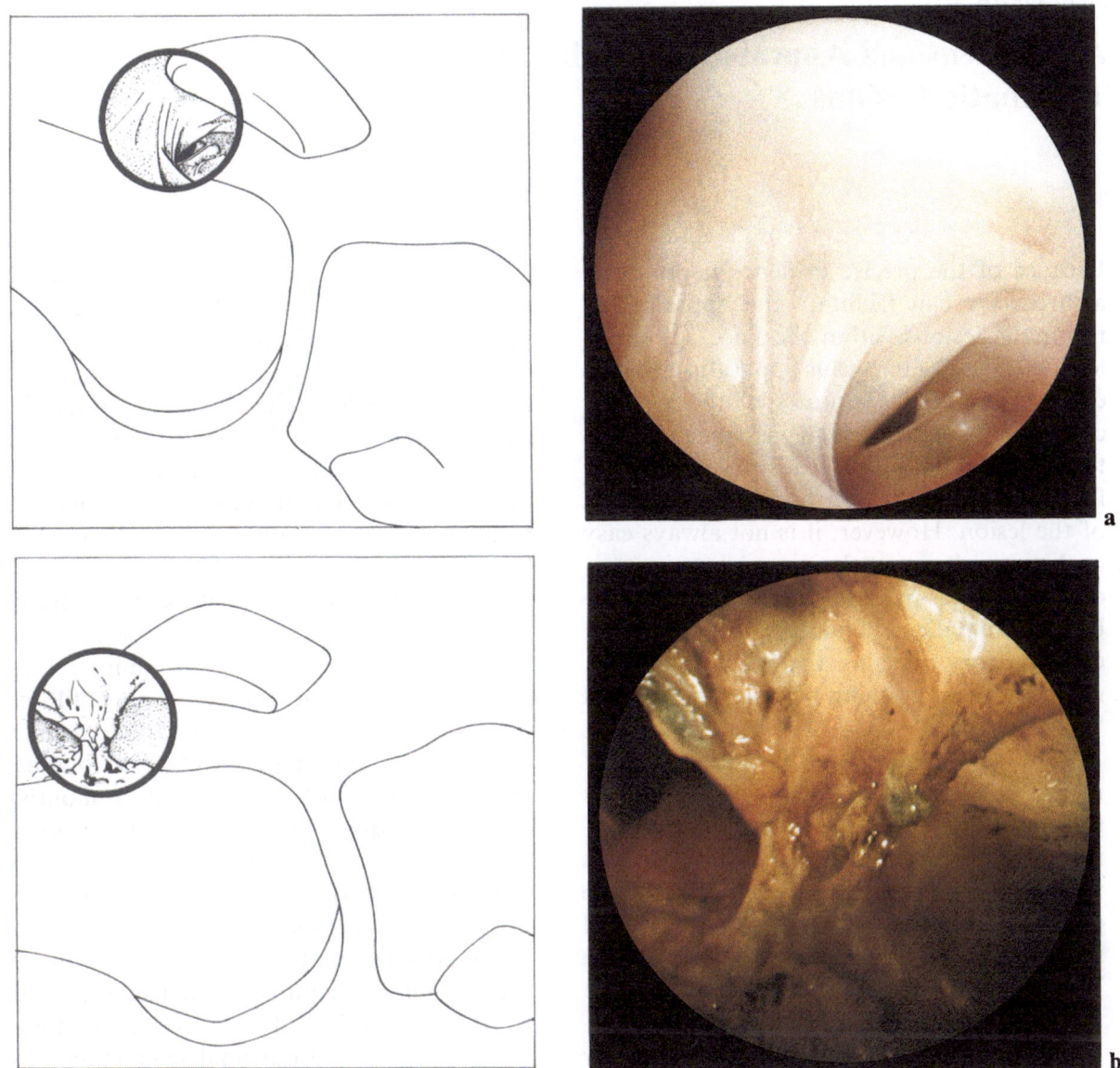

Fig. 98 a, b. Diathermy division of connective tissue bands in the suprapatellar recess; there is no bleeding, though transection is not yet complete

CHAPTER 15
Assessment and Appraisal of Problematic Internal Traumatic Lesions

Because of the precise evidence it provides, arthroscopy can facilitate the appraisal of traumatic lesions within the knee. Of these, lesions of the ligamentous apparatus are pre-eminent, especially ruptures of the anterior cruciate ligament. Here the assessment is often straightforward as the history gives a sufficient indication of the mechanism of origin of the lesion. However, it is not always easy to distinguish a recently injured anterior cruciate ligament from an already inadequate but retraumatized ligament. Therefore, an exact history remains the most important means of distinguishing between "new" and "old" lesions.

The same applies to the assessment of meniscus lesions. With an intact ligamentous system and an isolated meniscus lesion, judging whether there is a lesion or not depends very much on the history and the age of the patient. Truly isolated lesions of the medial meniscus must be regarded as rather rare. With preexisting problems of instability, a meniscus tear that develops later must be regarded as the consequence of the instability and so assessed. Here again, arthroscopy helps to determine the exact findings.

The assessment of posttraumatic damage to the articular cartilage is notably more difficult. Here again, the previous history is extremely important. The nature of the injury must be precisely reconstructed and assessed. The patient often reports a pain-free interval of several months, but if the injury dates back for more than 6 months a connection between it and articular cartilage damage can no longer be drawn. A pain-free interval of some 3 months is typical. During this period the damaged tissue fragments are discharged even in bradytrophic cartilage tissue, leading to painful irritation of the knee joint.

As a rule, X-ray films show no evidence whatever of arthrosis when examined for signs of traumatic articular cartilage damage. Obviously, other types of lesions, such as those of osteochondritis dissecans, should be ruled out. In addition, certain anomalies of the knee joint such as a marked patella alta or a dysplastic patellofemoral joint make a traumatic origin of the cartilage lesion less likely.

A closely circumscribed cartilage defect found during arthroscopy is more likely to be of traumatic origin. Depending on the date of the accident, the defect may still exhibit sharp edges, though the fracture margins of these traumatic cartilage lesions become rounded off after about 2 months. After 6 months or more it is no longer possible to determine with certainty whether a cartilage lesion is of traumatic or degenerative origin (see Sect. 14.4).

Besides traumatic injury to the cartilage, the differential diagnosis of incipient generalized osteoarthrosis of the knee joint should include patellar chondromalacia and femoral chondromalacia. Impressions in the cartilage, which are particularly obvious to the arthroscopist, present special problems in this respect. Impressions in the medial condyle can be physiologic. A certain amount of experience is needed for anatomic identification of these frequently deeply indented areas of car-

Fig. 99 a–c. Deep impression on medial femoral condyle caused by apex of patella, exposed by maximal extension of the knee joint. The arthroscopic figure in (**b**) is turned through 180° from the normal orientation; please view it upside down

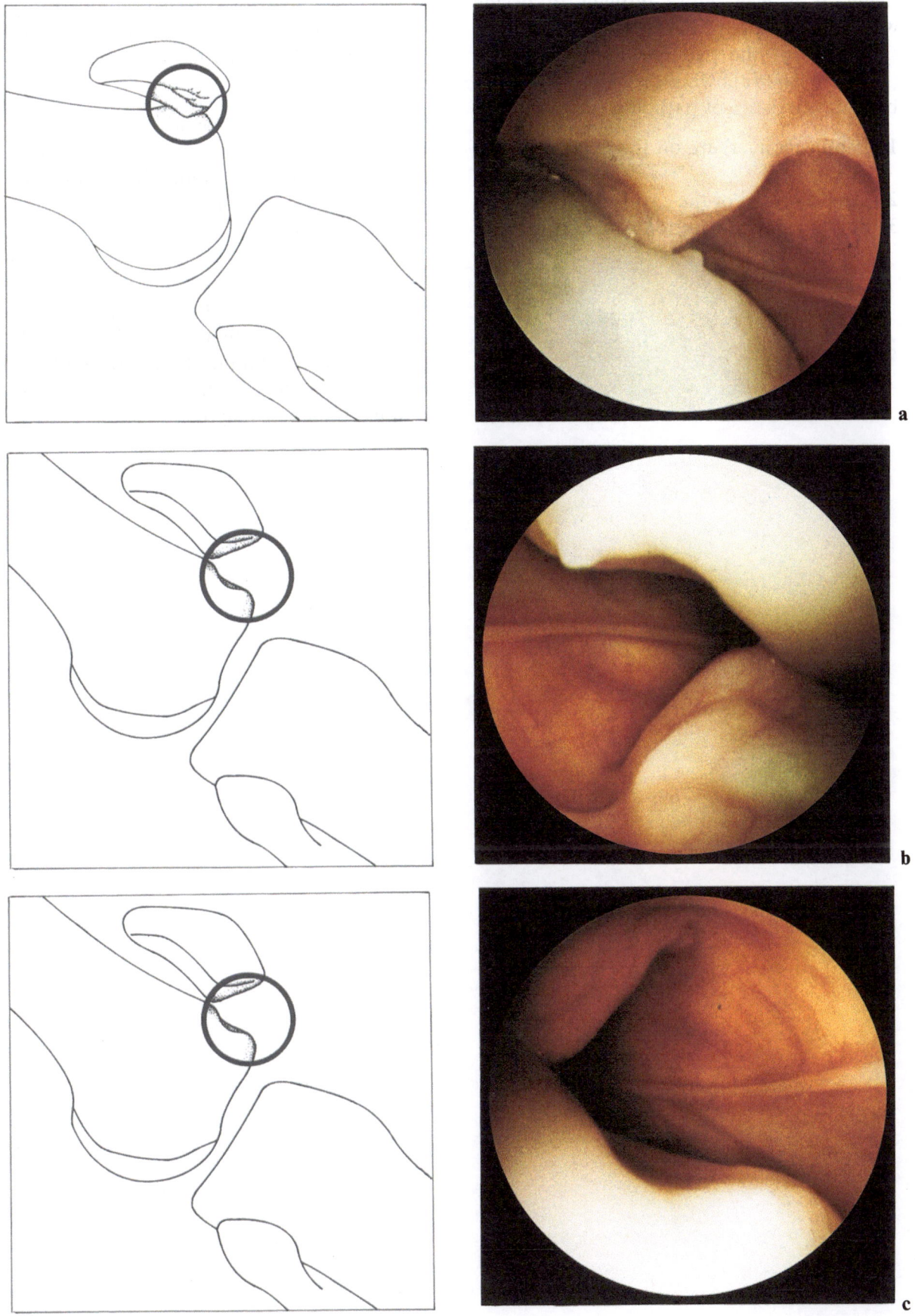

tilage. It is even more difficult to decide whether an impressed area of cartilage is responsible for the patient's knee symptoms (Fig. 99). The following are visible or tangible characteristics of pathologic change:

1. Pannus converging on the depressed area of cartilage
2. Discoloration of the cartilage
3. Softening or dissolution of the cartilage

In the assessment of cartilage lesions in the knee joint for the purpose of financial compensation, arthroscopy has two great advantages over arthrotomy:

1. One is less likely to have qualms about performing arthroscopy, which is a relatively small and harmless procedure, for the investigation of a suspected posttraumatic cartilage lesion.
2. The arthroscopic findings can be very easily documented. A photograph of a sharp-edged chunk of cartilage which has broken away from a femoral condyle provides far more information than any number of written sentences, however well formulated the latter may be.

Arthroscopic Operations

CHAPTER 16
Conditions for Operative Arthroscopy

Increasing experience with diagnostic manipulation of the arthroscope stimulates orthopedists and surgeons not to confine themselves to mere inspection of the joint cavity with the instrument, but also to operate arthroscopically on the lesions so displayed, without recourse to conventional arthrotomy.

Inspired by the Japanese, the forerunners of this operative technique were the Americans. In the middle of the 1970s, some European surgeons embarked on operative arthroscopic procedures. By the end of the 1970s and the beginning of the 1980s meniscectomy with the aid of the arthroscope had become a routine procedure in Anglo-American, Scandinavian, and German-speaking countries.

Arthroscopic diagnosis and especially the possibility of operating with the aid of the arthroscope have revolutionized knee joint surgery in recent years. The outstanding factor here is that it involves a relatively minor procedure which nevertheless provides significantly more diagnostic information on the overall condition of the knee joint than does a unilateral arthrotomy. The therapeutic results of sound arthroscopic operative techniques are similar to those of open knee joint surgery.

Apart from exact diagnosis of internal derangements of the knee by means of the arthroscope, the decisive advance lies in the possibility of treating these lesions by a relatively minor operative procedure. However, as with other endoscopic techniques, arthroscopic surgery presents the surgeon with specific difficulties when compared with open procedures.

The technique of arthroscopic operation is one that is difficult to pass on; the surgeon must himself develop his techniques for the various procedures, gather his own experience, and perfect his own style. The main difficulty with endoscopic operating lies in the narrowness of the space in which relatively bulky instruments must be manipulated right next to sensitive articular cartilage. Another considerable technical problem is getting used to "one-handed" operating, for as a rule the other hand must hold the arthroscope.

The following exposition should be regarded as a "cookbook" to help the beginner, and as an extra aid to the more advanced students in dealing with problems as they arise. A reliable mastery of diagnostic arthroscopic technique and a corresponding routine for the assessment of the findings within the knee joint are absolute prerequisites for the first attempts at arthroscopic operative procedures. To make the technically difficult operation easier for the surgeon, or even just to make it possible, the external conditions and the technical procedure must be optimized. Maximal relaxation of the patient by correct choice of anesthesia, appropriate positioning and fixation of the leg in a support, the application of a tourniquet to prevent bleeding obscuring vision, distension of the joint cavity by means of a fluid medium, and correct siting of the incision are all decisive factors contributing significantly to the success of an arthroscopic operation. All these apparently incidental technical factors are fundamental to the most important condition for endoscopic operations, i.e., good vision.

It should be made as easy as possible for the beginner to ensure adequate vision, and so the operating conditions will be further discussed here. The ideas mentioned result

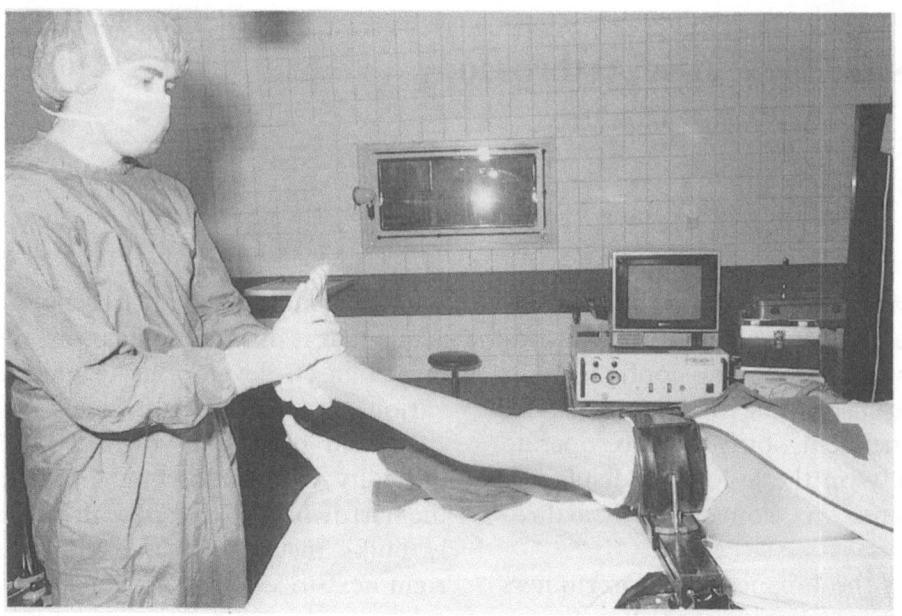

from years of experience involving more than 2500 arthroscopic operations. The routinely used procedure should, however, be continually and critically reappraised. Technical developments will certainly lead in the future to further improvement and perhaps simplification of arthroscopic operative procedures.

16.1 Anesthesia

The possible anesthetic techniques have already been discussed in Chap. 9. General anesthesia has notable advantages for the arthroscopic surgeon, especially a beginner. Muscle relaxation and freedom from pain are maximal and the individual joint compartments, especially at the back of the knee, are easy to open up. One essential for an arthroscopic operation is now possible; a tourniquet can be applied painlessly to the thigh. The upper thigh can be firmly fixed to an adjustable support. The duration of the operative procedure is not limited from the outset, as it is with a local anesthetic.

The negative psychologic effects, both on the patient and on a still inexperienced surgeon, of an operation undergone while the patient is fully conscious should not be underestimated.

Fig. 100. Hyperextension of the knee for inspection of the superior recess and the patellofemoral joint

16.2 Positioning

Correct positioning and fixation of the leg is of prime importance in an arthroscopic operation. Certain structures in the knee joint cavity are visible and accessible to the operative instrument only when the knee is in a particular angle of flexion or held under forcible varus or valgus pressure.

The use of a special (nonsterile) leg support, which can be applied over the pneumatic tourniquet while leaving sufficient room for thorough skin sterilization and toweling, guarantees optimal fixation of the thigh. By manipulating the lower leg alone to exert varus or valgus pressure, and by maintaining flexion or extension and lateral or medial rotation, the assistant can render the separate compartments of the knee joint visible to the arthroscope and accessible to the operative instruments. The suprapatellar recess, the patellofemoral joint, and the lateral and medial recesses are best inspected with the joint in maximum extension (Fig. 100).

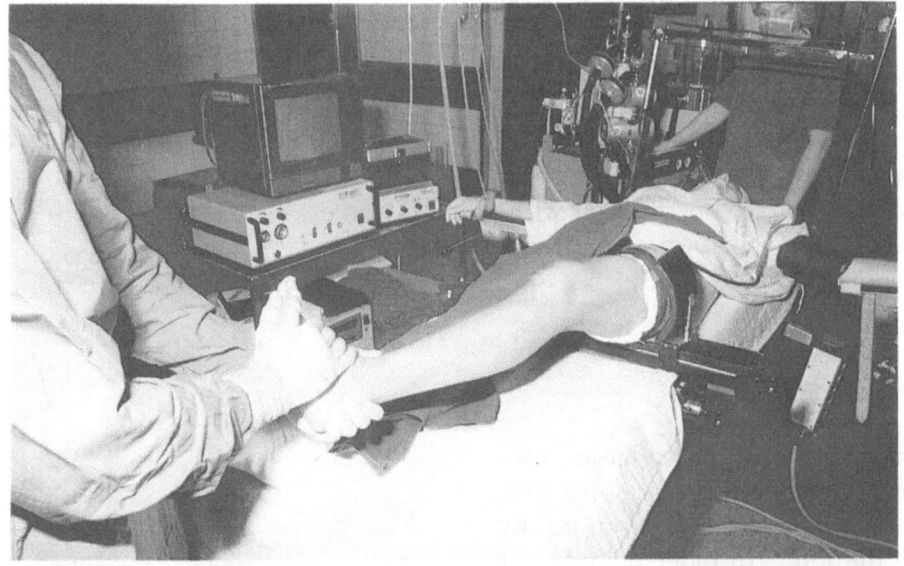

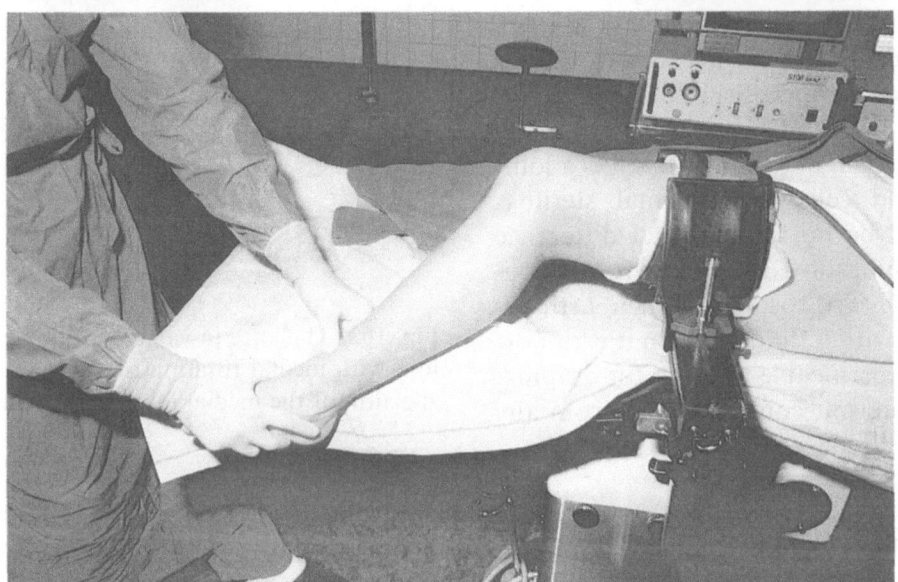

The lateral compartment is best visible in the varus position, with medial rotation and 10°–30° flexion of the joint (Fig. 101). The intercondylar fossa with the cruciate ligaments is best displayed at between 20° and 60° of flexion and with no rotation and no varus or valgus pressure (Fig. 102).

The medial joint compartment is most easily inspected with the knee under valgus strain and in 10°–30° of flexion with the lower leg laterally rotated (Fig. 103). The posteromedial and posterolateral compartments are best visualized in only slight flexion (5°–10°) and with corresponding valgus or

Fig. 101. The knee in varus position and 20° flexion, with the lower leg medially rotated, for inspection of the lateral joint compartment

Fig. 102. Knee in about 50° flexion for inspection of the intercondylar fossa with the cruciate ligaments

varus strain. These statements are for general guidance. Obviously, in individual cases, such as if there is variation in the shape of the condyles, the posterior horn of the medial or lateral meniscus may be better displayed in other flexion positions. While arthroscopic operations can certainly be performed without a leg support, firm fixation of the thigh is nevertheless of considerable help.

16.3 Tourniquet, Drapes

Application of a thigh tourniquet has considerable advantages, especially for operative procedures, as vision is not obscured by bleeding into the joint. In older patients, or when marked varicosities are present, a tourniquet should be avoided because of the increased risk of thrombosis. Although the incisions are small and the morbidity of the procedure very slight, it is nevertheless a joint operation and cells for maximal sterility. There should be no fundamental difference between draping of a knee joint for arthrotomy and for arthroscopy. When arthroscopy is done with a fluid medium it is important to use impermeable material for draping, in order to prevent contamination from any exudation of fluid.

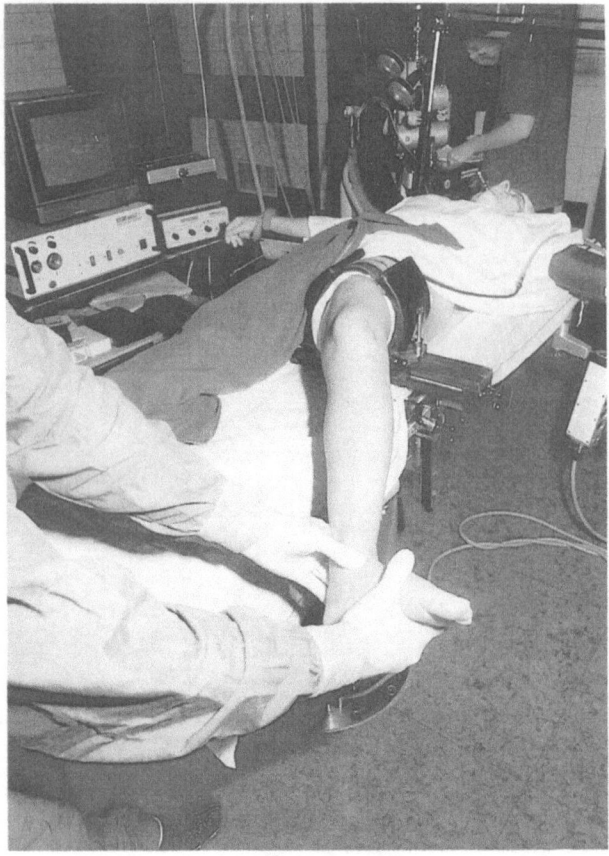

Fig. 103. The knee in valgus position and 20° flexion, with medial rotation of the lower leg, for inspection of the medial joint compartment

16.4 Gas Filling, Fluid Irrigation

Discussion of the type of medium to be used for distension of the joint cavity – whether gas or fluid – is as old as arthroscopy itself. In purely diagnostic arthroscopy both methods have their advantages and disadvantages and the arguments over which medium is to be used are presumably endless. Each surgeon must decide which method best suits his inclinations and convictions.

However, it cannot be disputed that fluid distension of the knee has quite marked advantages over gas insufflation in operative arthroscopy, for the following reasons:

1. The uncomplicated nature of fluid irrigation is proven. For the beginner, arthroscopy is already difficult enough; he should not be further burdened with the more trouble some details of gas insufflation. An infusion bottle with Ringer or saline solution suspended from a transfusion stand about 50–80 cm above the knee joint exerts sufficient hydrostatic pressure to thoroughly fill and distend the knee joint.

2. Basically, at least two incisions are required in arthroscopic operations; a fall in pressure during distension of the joint with gas may always occur as the system is not a closed one.

3. Continuous irrigation of the knee is indispensable in cases of hemarthrosis or when there is a turbid serous effusion if struc-

tures are to be clearly recognized at all. The continuous introduction of fluid via the arthroscope and its drainage via the distantly attached special drainage cannula ensure that the visual field remains unimpaired during the operation, despite any bleeding or the presence of detached fragments of menisci or articular cartilage.

4. The risks with fluid irrigation are slight and there is no danger of emphysema. The articular cartilage cannot dry out in the course of a long operation.

5. By means of irrigation and suction at intervals, concealed loose bodies or separated portions of menisci can be brought into the arthroscopic visual field. Only fluid distension of the knee permits unhampered working, and allows change of instruments or change of arthroscopy site from a lateral to a medial incision to be done without problems.

16.5 Incisions

The standard incisions for operative arthroscopic procedures are anterolateral and anteromedial. Each is some 8 mm long and placed vertically close to the patellar ligament and about 1 cm above the anterior margin of the tibial head (Figs. 104, 105).

Almost all arthroscopic operations can be performed via these two incisions. The frequently advocated "central approach" through the patellar ligament is not recommended, providing no better view than the anterolateral approach and causing damage to the ligament. Moreover, transligamentous insertion of an arthroscope or other instrument greatly hinders the surgeon's freedom of maneuver.

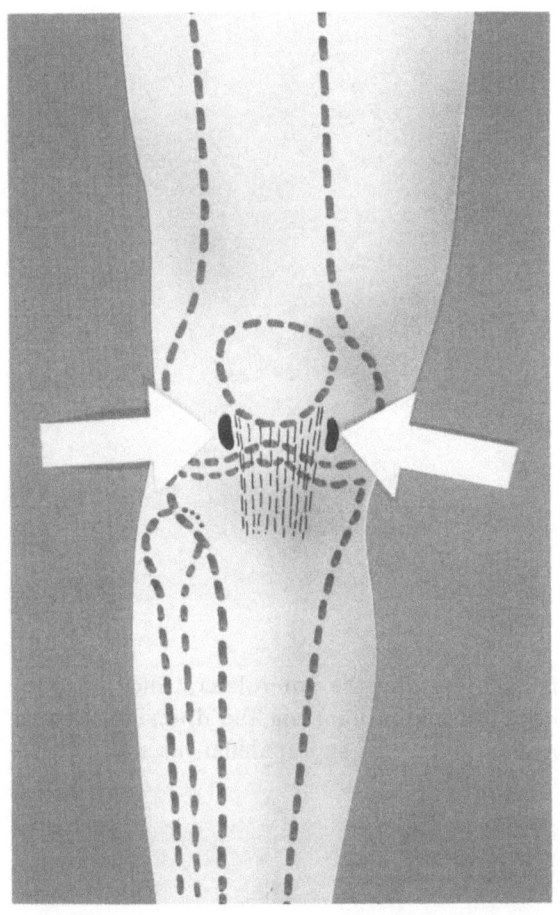

Fig. 104. Sites of the standard anterolateral and anteromedial incisions about 1 cm above the anterior margin of the tibial head at the edge of the patellar ligament

In many knee joints where the ligaments are very tight, it may be necessary to add to the standard incisions mentioned above a posteromedial incision behind the tibial collateral ligament in order to reach the posterior horn of the medial meniscus or a loose body in the posteromedial recess. This incision is made behind the tibial collateral ligament and somewhat above the joint space with the knee flexed to 90°, and the outer tube with the sharp trocar is then inserted with the joint maximally distended (Fig. 106). It is very important to proceed with caution and to flex the knee to at least a right angle, so as to avoid damaging the popliteal vessels or nerves. In rare cases it

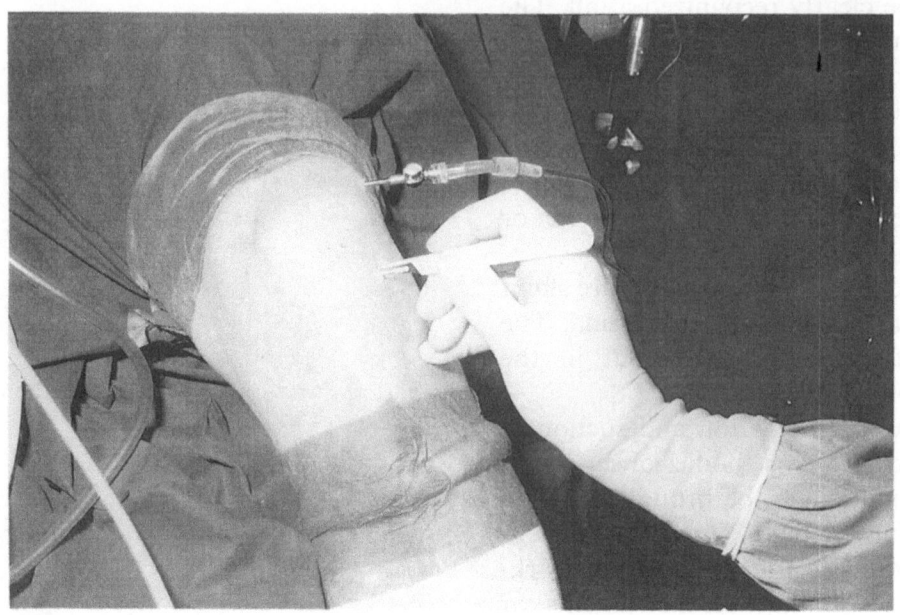

Fig. 105. Making the anterolateral incision after distension of the joint via the drainage cannula introduced into the suprapatellar recess

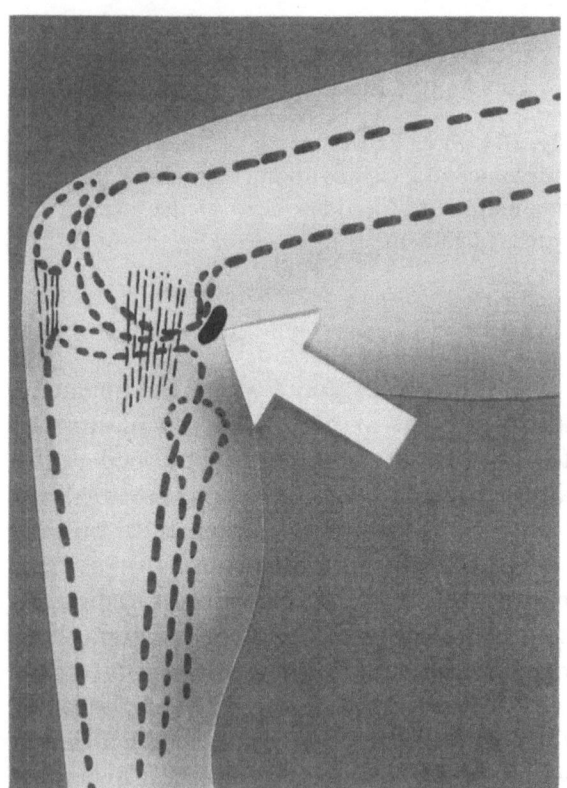

Fig. 106. Site of posteromedial incision behind the collateral ligament at the posterior margin of the femoral condyle

may even be necessary to consider a posterolateral approach, such as when a large loose body in the posterolateral recess cannot be displaced forward into the anterior joint compartment.

More often, however, it is found necessary to extend the puncture for the drainage cannula at the upper outer margin of the patella into an actual incision. If there is extensive damage to the articular cartilage at the back of the patella, or if it is necessary to resect a hypertrophic medial synovial plica or to remove a very large loose body in the lateral part of the superior recess, a superolateral approach facilitates the proceedings (Fig. 107).

As a rule (in 95% of cases in our series), all arthroscopic operations including subtotal meniscectomy can be performed via the two standard anterolateral and anteromedial incisions.

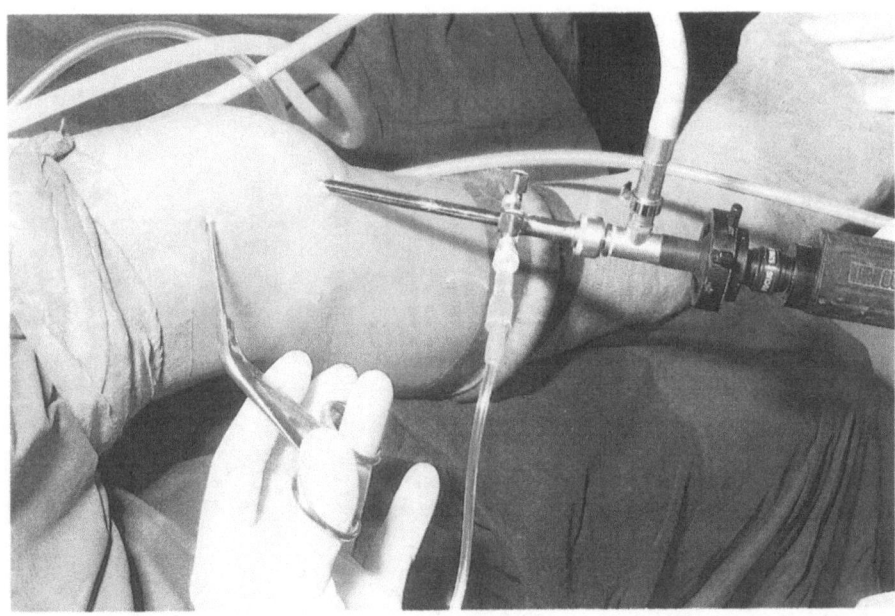

Fig. 107. Arthroscope in the anterolateral incision and operation instrument in the superolateral incision

16.6 Operative Equipment

The routine investigative procedure using a probe hook, the operative instruments, the video system, and the special requirements for sterility has already been throughly discussed in the diagnostic part of this book. Therefore, special attention will be paid here only to the equipment used by the authors, which will be repeatedly mentioned in the detailed description of techniques for the different meniscus lesions.

Faced with the profusion of instruments supplied by different firms, it is essential for the novice to decide on what is reasonable, what is required for a basic outfit, and what would be unnecessarily burdensome. The opinions even of experienced arthroscopists differ greatly on these problems. Whereas some prefer motor-driven instruments such as shavers, planers, edgers, and cutters, and others work almost exclusively with knives, the beginner, in our view, should as much as possible confine himself to instruments which minimize the risk of joint damage.

These include all those instruments with blunt rounded heads whose insertion into the knee joint causes no damage to the articular cartilage. The most important instruments therefore, for all resections and smoothing procedures are the cutting basket forceps. These should be available in various grades of strength, shaft curve, and angle on every operating table. Scissors are also indispensable. Not only are the various hooked scissors very helpful, but ordinary narrow fine dissecting scissors may be used more often and with better results within the joint, as experience increases.

Appropriate grasping and gripping forceps for the removal of loose bodies or large portions of menisci are obvious components of the equipment; forceps with pointed teeth certainly cannot prevent the slipping of smooth meniscus fragments or loose bodies during extraction through the narrow incisions but they can make such extraction more difficult. A sharp narrow gouge for smoothing articular cartilage lesions is another sensible piece of equipment. It is very difficult to lay down firm rules regarding instruments, but it can be stated in general that every surgeon should use those instruments which most closely approach the ideal of enabling "one-piece resection" and with which the

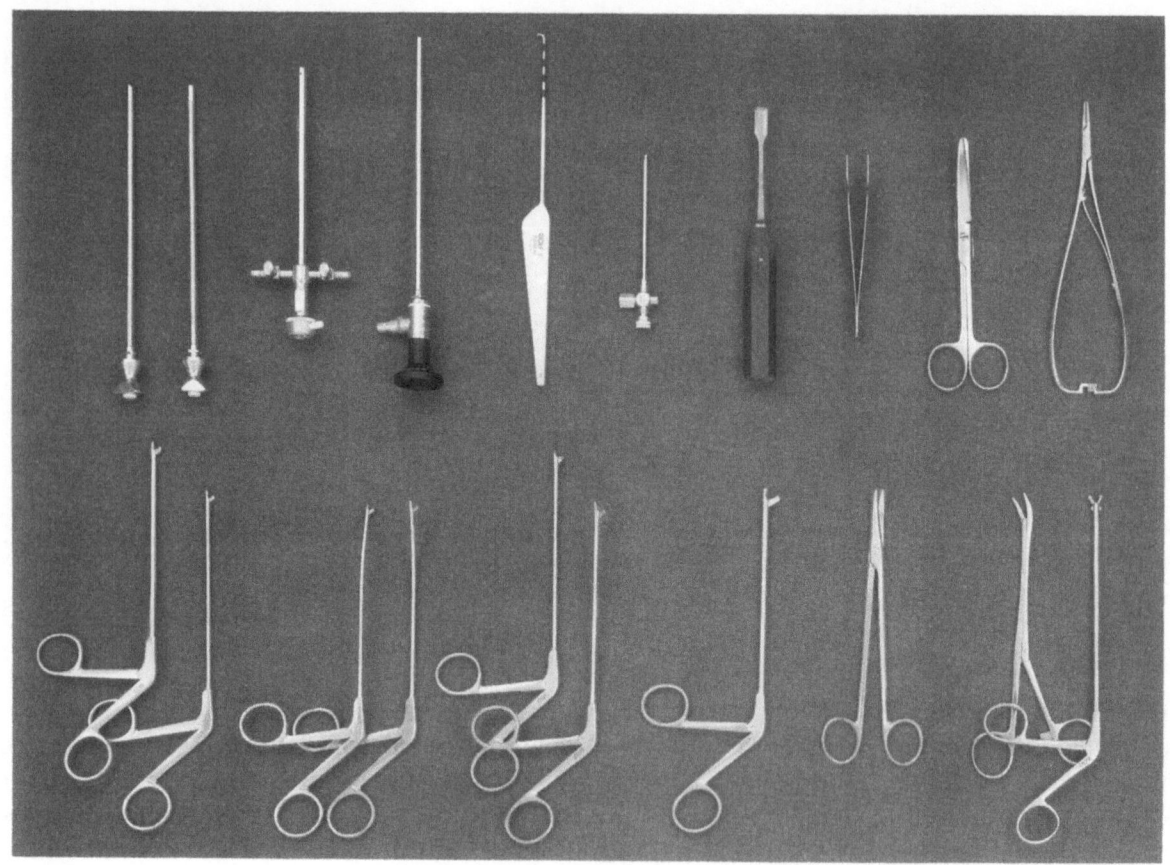

Fig. 108. The set of instruments used by the authors for operative arthroscopy (details in text)

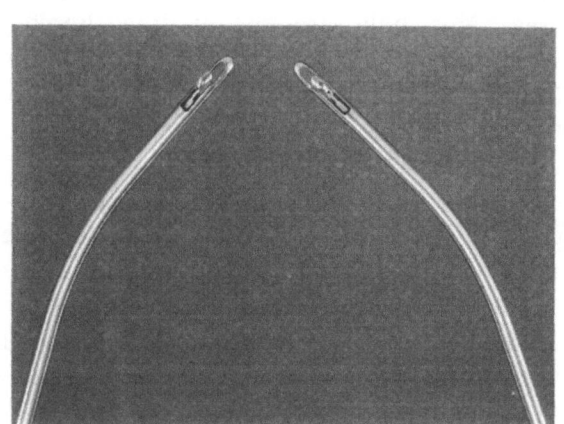

Fig. 109. 3.4-mm basket forceps, curved right and left

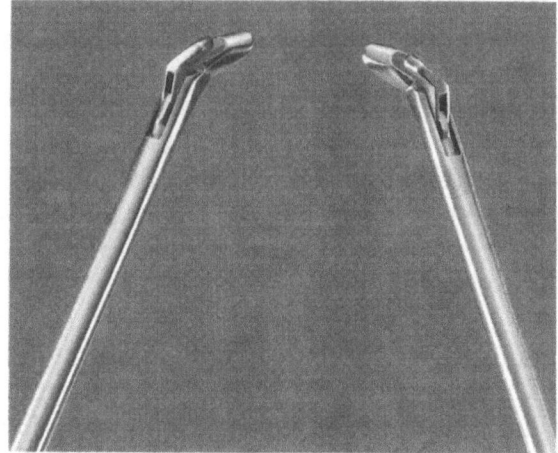

Fig. 110. 3.4-mm basket forceps angled to right and left

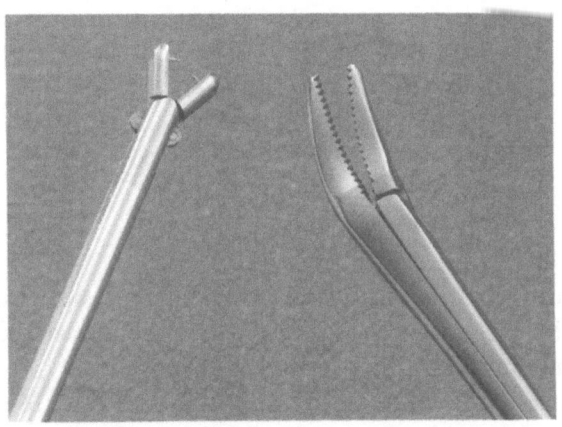

Fig. 111. Slender, slightly curved meniscus-grasping forceps and large toothed forceps with double-spoon bite

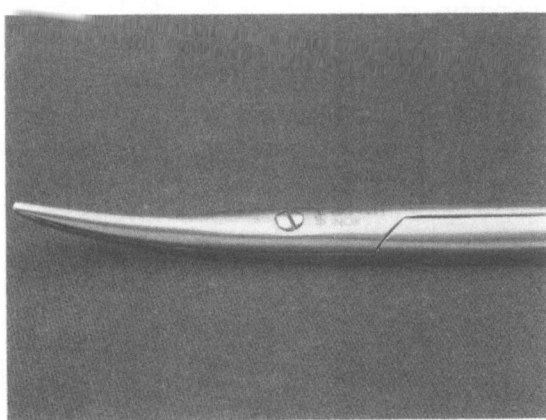

Fig. 112. Dissecting scissors

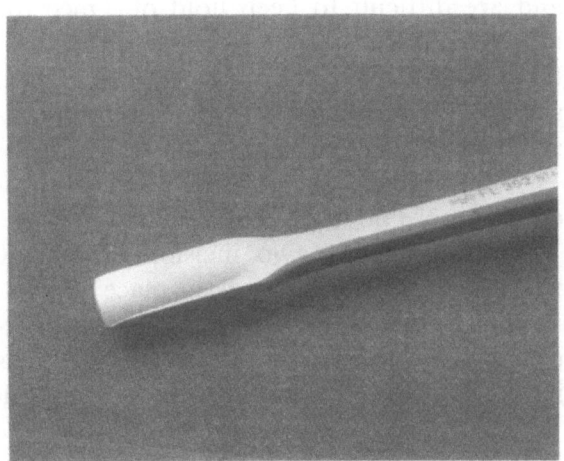

Fig. 113. Gouge for cartilage smoothing

least possible damage is inflicted on the knee joint.

Besides the basic diagnostic equipment (outer arthroscope tube, pointed trocar, blunt trocar, 5-mm arthroscope with 10° angle of view, special drainage cannula, and probe hook), the following instruments should be available on the instrument table (Fig. 108):

basket forceps:

4.5 mm, straight
3.4 mm, straight
3.4 mm, right-hand curve
3.4 mm, left-hand curve   (Fig. 109)
3.4 mm, angled right
3.4 mm, angled left   (Fig. 110))

hooked scissors:

4.5 mm, straight
3.4 mm, straight

grasping forceps:

4.5 mm, double spoon bite
slender, easily separated grasping forceps (Fig. 111)
normal, small, easily manipulated dissecting scissors (Fig. 112)
8-mm-wide sharp gouge (Fig. 113)

CHAPTER 17

Removal of Loose Bodies

The removal of loose bodies from the joint is the "simplest" arthroscopic operation. If a loose body is imprisoned in the lateral recess and has been well visualized with the arthroscope, it appears easy to grasp it with suitable forceps and remove it from the joint, the operation being concluded in the shortest possible time (Figs. 114–118). However, these smooth rounded bodies often roll into a corner where they are difficult to see and to grasp. Even when, after several attempts, they have been grasped, they often slip out of the forceps or are difficult to extract through the small incision because of their size.

With arthroscopy, just as with arthrotomy, the problem is not so much to lay hold of the loose body as to locate it. The knee joint contains preferred sites or "catchment basins" in which the loose bodies usually lie. These preferred sites for radiopaque loose bodies as confirmed at diagnostic arthroscopy are as follows:

1. The suprapatellar recess and its medial and especially lateral expansions alongside the condyles
2. The dorsomedial recess
3. The dorsolateral recess above and below the meniscus
4. The intercondylar fossa.

Removal of loose bodies from the suprapatellar recess and its medial and lateral expansions as well as from the intercondylar fossa usually presents no problems. It is sometimes difficult, however, to displace them into the anterior joint compartment from the posterior medial and lateral recesses by manipulations such as external pressure, movement, irrigation, or suction. Occasionally, the arthroscope has to be introduced behind the tibial or fibular collateral ligaments; this is more often the case on the medial side as the posterolateral recess is smaller than its medial counterpart. It is also more easily inspected from in front and loose bodies within can then be more easily displaced forward.

The extraction of a loose body requires no more than good grasping forceps, which must have a ratchet handle as most loose bodies have very smooth rounded surfaces and are difficult to keep hold of. Once the loose body has been seized, its withdrawal through the small incision is the next critical stage as the resistance of the surrounding tissue tends to make it slip out of the forceps.

The arthroscopic procedure in the presence of loose bodies is as follows.

To begin with, two incisions are made while a thigh tourniquet is in place so that, as soon as the loose body is sighted, the forceps can be moved to the exact spot. This is done under continuous irrigation with Ringer solution or saline. As soon as the loose body enters the field of vision, irrigation and drainage are discontinued so that it does not float away. A grasping forceps is inserted through the second incision and the loose body seized by gradual closure of the blades of the forceps. A useful dodge is to attempt to drive the loose body into a "corner" so that it is to some extent fixed and cannot elude the forceps or escape when gripped.

Fig. 114. Large loose body in lateral joint recess ▷

Fig. 115. Exposure of a loose body with the probe hook

Fig. 116. Approximation of the large grasping forceps to the loose body

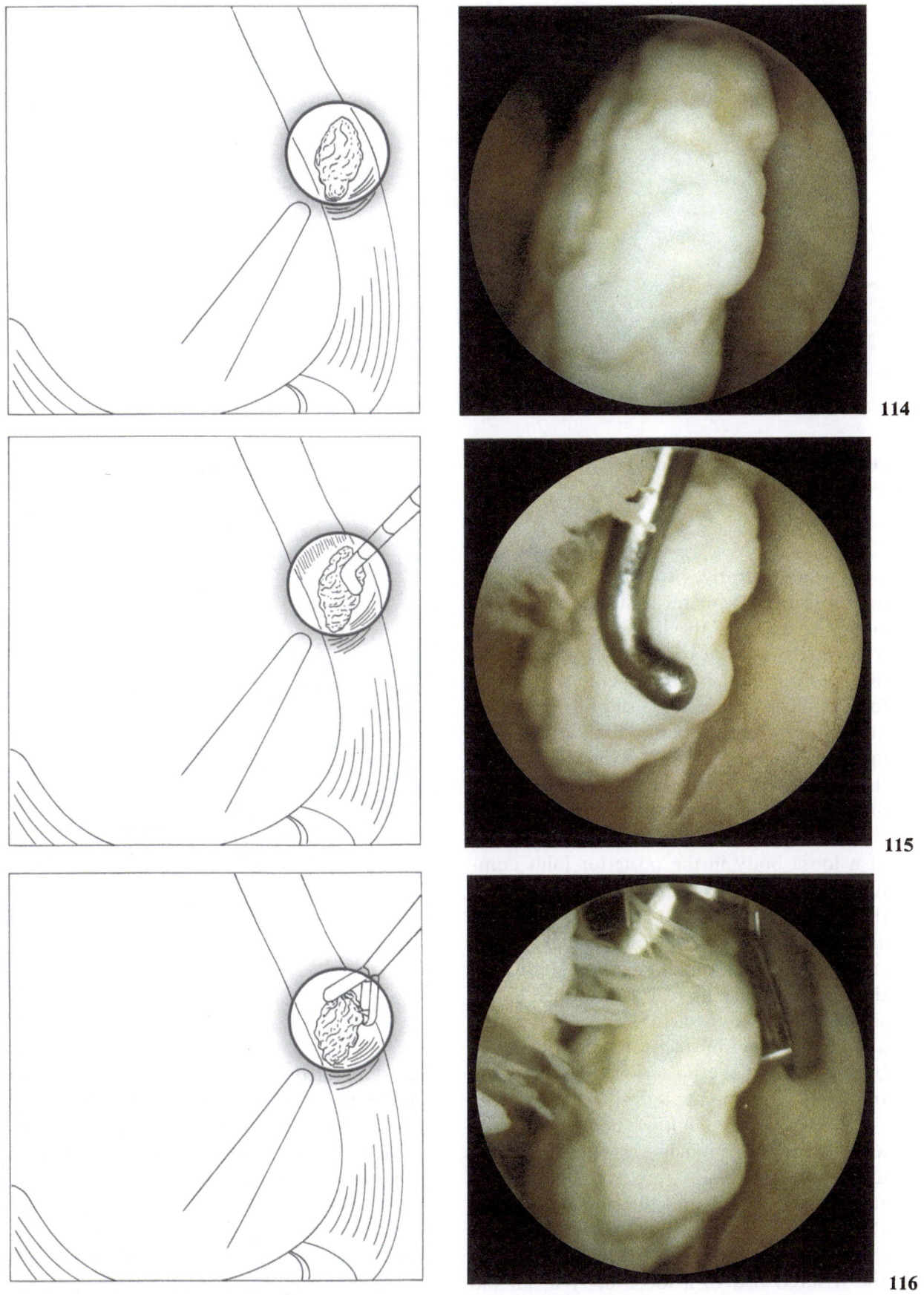

114

115

116

103

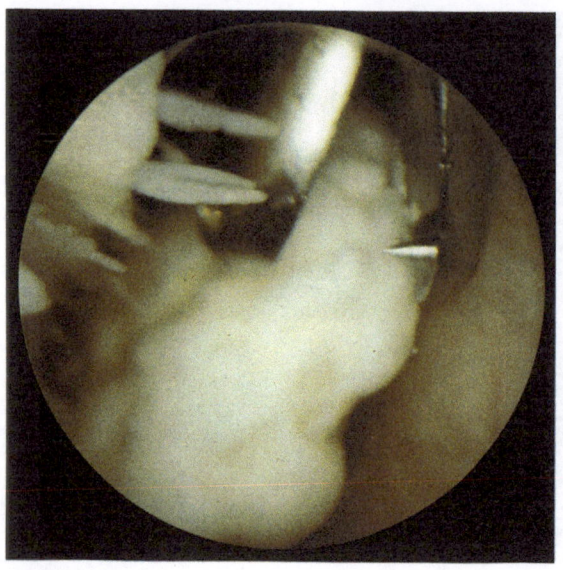
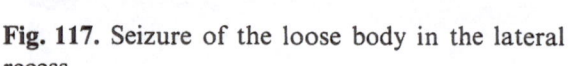
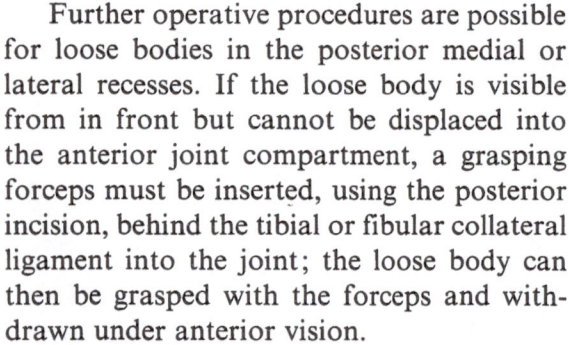

Fig. 117. Seizure of the loose body in the lateral recess

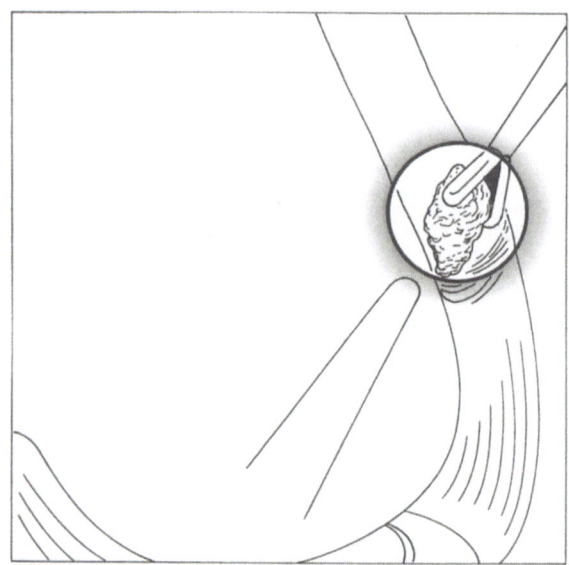

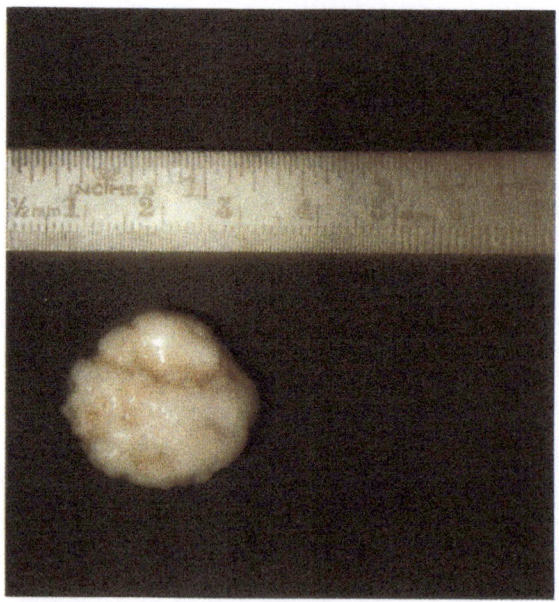

Further operative procedures are possible for loose bodies in the posterior medial or lateral recesses. If the loose body is visible from in front but cannot be displaced into the anterior joint compartment, a grasping forceps must be inserted, using the posterior incision, behind the tibial or fibular collateral ligament into the joint; the loose body can then be grasped with the forceps and withdrawn under anterior vision.

If there has been radiologic confirmation of a loose body in the posterior joint compartment which has not been visualized arthroscopically via the standard incisions, the arthroscope must be introduced behind the collateral ligament in an endeavor to display the body. A grasping forceps can then be inserted parallel to the arthroscope or through a second posterior incision and the loose body seized in the posterior recess and extracted from the joint.

After removal of a loose body, diagnostic arthroscopy is routinely performed and the entire joint surface carefully palpated with the probe hook to find the site of origin of the loose body. This is not always successful, despite every effort. However, if, for instance, the fissured bed of a loose body in an old osteochondritis dissecans is found, this should be tidied up arthroscopically or by open arthrotomy to prevent further development of loose bodies. Foreign bodies such as glass splinters and metal fragments that have penetrated the joint, as may occasionally happen after open joint injuries, are removed in the manner described above. An instrument may even break within the knee during an arthroscopic operation. The broken portions of the instrument are removed from the joint with a grasping forceps under arthroscopic visual monitoring. Recently, small magnets have been developed which can be introduced into the joint to remove small metal fragments very elegantly.

Despite every care, the loose body may become free and get lost as it is withdrawn through the various layers of the incision. If the joint is thoroughly but unsuccessfully searched and the loose body cannot be retrieved, it must be assumed that it has "gone missing" in the subfascial or subcutaneous layers. By cautious palpation near the incision, and also by diaphanoscopy with the light at the tip of the arthroscope, the position of the loose body in the tissue layers may be pinpointed and it can then be removed.

Small loose bodies up to a diameter of 4 mm need not be extracted as they can be flushed out under pressure through the stem of the arthroscope.

CHAPTER 18
Arthroscopic Meniscus Operations

The commonest and most important arthroscopic operation is resection or partial resection of a meniscus. In this procedure, all avulsed, torn, or frayed portions of the meniscus are resected, leaving the leargest possible healthy and functionally effective residual portion of meniscus.

Total meniscectomy has now been completely abandoned because of the subsequent premature development of arthrosis, and partial meniscectomy is now customary. Routine subtotal meniscectomy without regard to the extent of the meniscus lesion is also a thing of the past for most surgeons. The general tendency is to be sparing as regards resection, whether the meniscus is resected by arthrotomy or miniarthrotomy, or by means of the arthroscope under local or general anesthesia. The attitude to be adopted should always be to resect as little as possible and as much as necessary.

It is fascinating for both patient and surgeon to see how quickly symptoms can disappear and a normal gait return after arthroscopic meniscectomy. With the aid of the arthroscope, an experienced endoscopist can achieve the same therapeutic results as with an arthrotomy. The great advantages of an arthroscopic operation are the much reduced trauma to the joint and the more thorough and precise examination of the entire knee joint.

However, the arthroscopist, especially the beginner, should set himself a time limit and should be prepared, if technical difficulties arise during the procedure, to discontinue the planned arthroscopic operation and open the knee joint. Under no circumstances should the surgeon attempt to "force through" the arthroscopic operation as the joint may only sustain additional damage thereby. An arthroscopic operation that takes longer than an hour is inferior to an open arthrotomy. Thanks to arthroscopic diagnosis and the possibility of arthroscopic treatment – with a much shorter operative procedure in comparison with conventional open arthrotomy – indications for meniscectomy are now much more circumspect and differentiated. Previously, many subtotal meniscectomies were performed "just because the joint was already open," even though resection was not actually necessary on objective grounds.

In contrast, it is very much easier for the modern surgeon to take the decision to withdraw the endoscope from the small incision without having performed any sort of resection, and he is also better placed to gain the understanding of his patients. The surgeon should also consider during the procedure whether a frayed or degenerative lesion that has been found is really the cause of the patient's symptoms, whether meniscus resection is necessary, and whether such a procedure will actually relieve the patient's symptoms.

Arthroscopic procedures have also greatly transformed methods of treating the very common lesions of the posterior horn. By means of the arthroscope it is possible to perform a partial resection of the posterior horn in a region that is very difficult to inspect from the usual large arthrotomy incision.

Basically, any type of meniscus lesion can be operated on arthroscopically, the only limiting factors being the skill, flexibility, and experience of the surgeon. As in arthrotomy, the task consists of resecting and extracting the part of the meniscus to be removed, as far as possible in one piece. At least two incisions, one for the arthroscope and one for the instrument, are needed for this. This so-called two-point technique is preferred by many surgeons, including the authors, and will be described in detail below. Many surgeons, inspired by the Swedish school of arthroscopy, add the central transligamentous approach of Gillquist to the anterolateral and anteromedial incisions. This allows two instruments in the joint besides the arthroscope. The indisputable advantage of this method lies in the many situations when a portion of meniscus that was previously grasped in the forceps can be resected under traction. A disadvantage of this procedure is the need for a "third hand," since an assistant must hold either the arthroscope or the forceps and this is not always a simple matter. The presence of two instruments within the knee impairs the visual field and further constricts what is already a confined space.

This emphasizes the main problems for the arthroscopic surgeon: potentially poor vision and the confined space in which he has to work. These problems apply as much to the "two-point" as to the "three-point" technique. How these difficulties may be overcome, and what technical procedure should be used to deal with the various types of meniscus lesion by the two-point method, will now be discussed in detail.

CHAPTER 19

Technique of Arthroscopic Medial Meniscus Operations

The operative technique described below for the different types of meniscus lesions is that of the authors, and makes no claim to be the only possible technique. There are certainly other ways to resect a meniscus and remove it from the joint. However, the beginner in particular needs a "cookbook" type of introduction, and even the more advanced surgeon can overcome many a problem by using a systematic approach.

Before going into the technical details, here is a simple practical hint for the beginner. When operating on the medial meniscus the arthroscope is nearly always in the lateral incision and the operative instrument in the medial incision. Therefore, a right-handed operator should select mainly right knees for his first arthroscopic operations as he can operate on these in the usual way with his right hand. The previously described position of the surgeon lateral to the leg to be operated on makes it considerably more difficult for a right-handed operator to resect a left medial meniscus.

19.1 Medial Bucket-Handle Tear

A bucket-handle tear of the medial meniscus is one of the most common meniscus lesions. This type of lesion is easily dealt with by arthroscopic operation as large portions of the meniscus are already avulsed and only a small incision is required to detach the entire meniscus. However, the surgeon may encounter considerable difficulty in properly exposing the attachments of the bucket-handle portion to the main body of the meniscus in both the posterior and anterior horn regions.

Resection of an avulsed bucket-handle portion of a medial meniscus takes place systematically in six stages:

Stage 1: Exposure and Repositioning

An absolute prerequisite for any operative procedure is the exact exposure of the extent of the lesion and a precise arthroscopic diagnosis. The arthroscope is inserted from the lateral side and the medial joint compartment is inspected over the anterior cruciate ligament; the probe hook is positioned via the anteromedial incision. If only the meniscus is visible – and not, as is usual, the joint space with the condyle, tibial head, and free margin of the meniscus – this suggests that there is a displaced bucket-handle tear, and this suspicion is confirmed if the displaced portion can be replaced with the probe hook and the meniscus after such repositioning appears "normal." The reverse state of affairs may obtain, the apparently normal meniscus suddenly becoming displaced into the intercondylar fossa when tested with the probe hook (Fig. 119).

When the bucket-handle portion of the medial meniscus has already been displaced for a long period, repositioning – usually a simple matter – may occasionally encounter difficulties. Here, help may be obtained from the blunt trocar of the arthroscope and the meniscus may be restored to its original position with the more powerful instrument.

Repositioning is indispensable for precise diagnosis and exposure of the tear. Only after repositioning can the exact extent of the tear be determined with the aid of the probe hook, the persisting connections of the torn part of the meniscus with the main body be properly inspected, and its planned resection

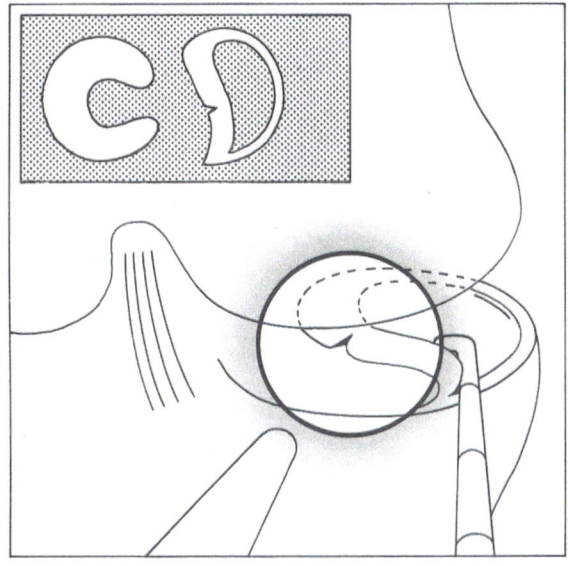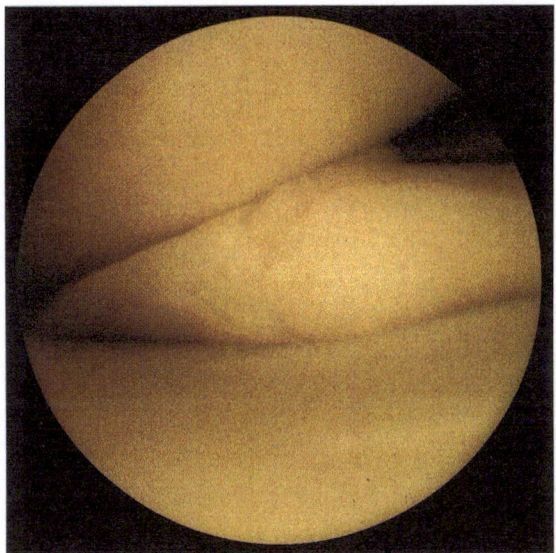

Fig. 119. Displaced bucket-handle tear of medial meniscus

be determined. The resection, too, must be performed in the restored state as it is then very much easier to visualize the position of the joint and there is no temptation to cut blindly.

Stage 2: Section of the Posterior Horn

Nearly all authors supplying detailed information on arthroscopic procedure recommend that in dealing with a medial bucket-handle tear the anterior horn should first be divided, the meniscus displaced and held under traction, and the basal connection at the posterior horn then divided. In the authors' opinion, this procedure has considerable disadvantages. After transection of the anterior horn, it occasionally happens that the large meniscal flap, whose only basal attachment is now at the posterior horn, slips into the posteromedial recess and is often no longer accessible to the arthroscope from the two anterior incisions. Further, transection of the posterior horn in the displaced state under forceps traction is notably more difficult than in the replaced condition, as the

view of the site of attachment and the precise sectioning are greatly hampered.

With the bucket-handle tear of the meniscus reduced, it is usually best to detach it first at the posterior horn. The bridging zone in the posterior horn region is easily demonstrable with the probe hook. The arthroscope, with its tip close to the anterior cruciate ligament and the lateral side of the medial condyle, is introduced from the lateral approach and kept in this position. This region is best displayed if the lower leg is held in strong valgus strain and lateral rotation, with the knee in 5°–10° at most of flexion.

The probe hook is then replaced by a strong, curved 3.4-mm basket forceps (curved to the right for the right knee, to the left for the left knee), and the connection of the bucket-handle portion to the body of the meniscus in the posterior horn region is severed with the fewest possible cuts and without leaving a large stump (Figs. 120, 121). When the bucket-handle portion is reduced, it is under so much tension in this position that further tension by traction is unnecessary, and sectioning can be done without difficulty.

Note that only the bridging zone is transected, and that further cuts in the remaining body of the meniscus in the posterior horn region are not to be made blindly after the

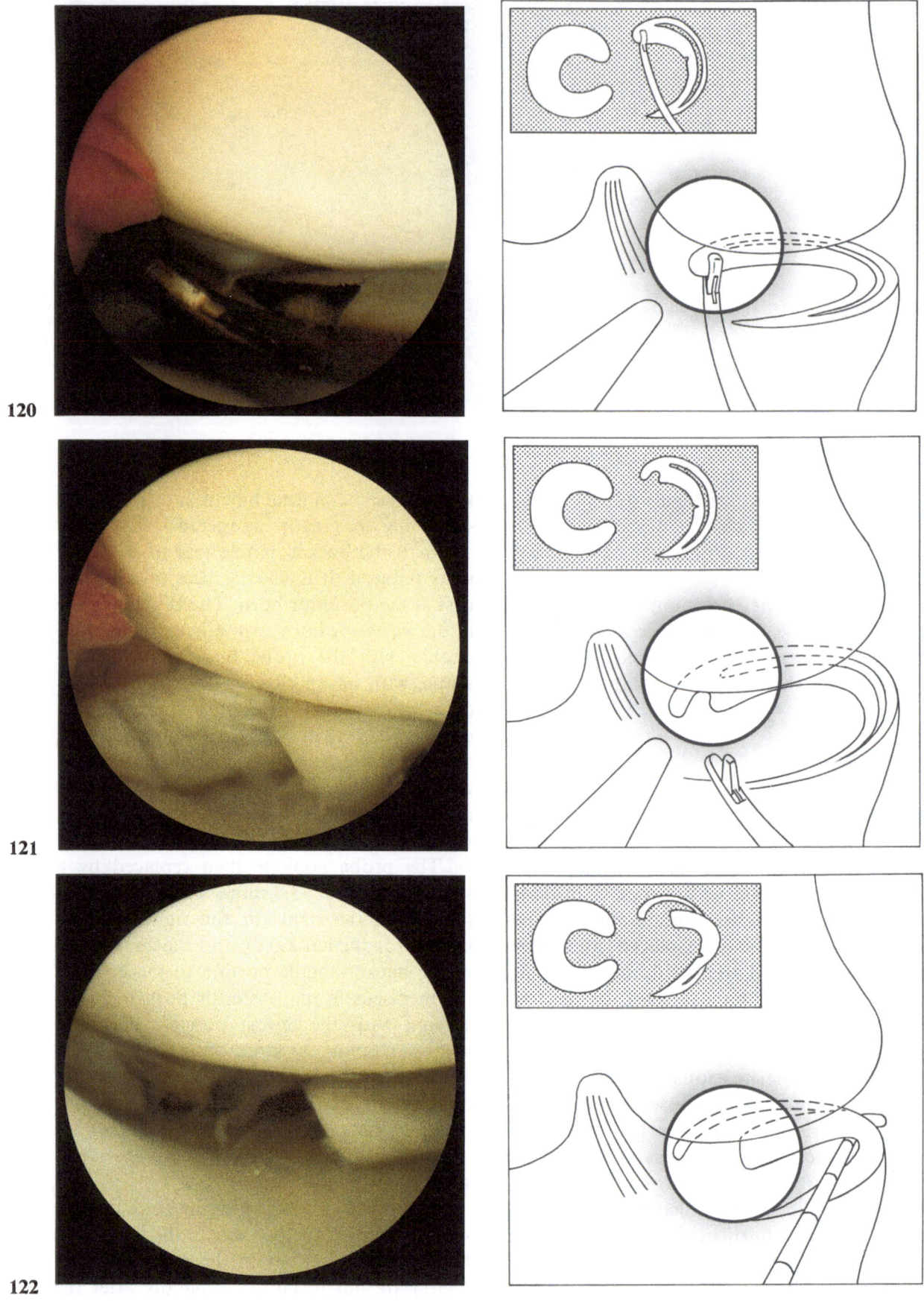

connection of the bucket-handle portion has been severed. As soon as the bridge at the posterior horn has been transected, the bucket-handle portion of the medial meniscus can be displaced inward (Fig. 122).

Stage 3: Displacement into the Medial Recess

When the connection to the body of the meniscus at the posterior horn has been transected, the basket forceps is replaced by the probe hook and the bucket-handle portion, now transformed into a meniscus flap, is displaced into the medial recess. Next, keeping the site of section in the visual field, the probe hook is passed under the bucket-handle portion and an attempt is made to displace it inward. At this point it will be at once apparent whether all the fibers have been transected at the site of section at the posterior horn. The bucket-handle portion of the meniscus can be drawn medially without effort if this is the case, giving free exposure of the site of the tear and the remaining meniscus body (Figs. 123, 124).

The bucket-handle portion, still attached to the body of the meniscus at the anterior horn, is then displaced up into the medial recess. There are two reasons for doing this. First, in this position of the meniscus the connection to the base at the anterior horn is very much better displayed than with the meniscal portion lying in the joint; further, in addition to this better exposure, the up-

ward displacement of the meniscal portion produces increased tension on the part to be resected, so facilitating its section. Second, should the portion of meniscus float away once divided completely from the body of the meniscus, thus not remaining in its original position, it comes to lie in the much more accessible superior recess and not in the posteromedial recess. Therefore, the bucket-handle portion should be displaced medially and as far forward as possible with the probe hook. Then the connection with the body of the meniscus in the anterior horn region is brought into the arthroscopic visual field and the planned resection is demonstrated with the probe hook (Fig. 125).

Stage 4: Section of the Anterior Horn

Now large hooked scissors or dissecting scissors are introduced from the medial approach and brought, still closed, into the visual field of the arthroscope and approximated to the remaining meniscus bridge. When dividing the bucket-handle portion at the anterior horn, care must be taken to stay as close as possible to the body of the meniscus and not to proceed so carelessly as to leave behind a meniscus stump perhaps as long as 1.5 cm. It is therefore better to cut from in front, from the free edge of the meniscus to the tear, and not from the tear forwards. This method makes it easier to avoid leaving too large a stump. If the anterior horn has been well displayed and the initially closed scissors have been brought into the visual field, the meniscus bridge is seized between the now opened scissor blades and then pressed with the open blades in the direction of the joint capsule; the resection is begun and then completed in a few cuts (Fig. 126).

During the section care should be taken to stay in the initial incision line, placed exactly in the line of the tear. After complete transection the portion of meniscus to be resected is free in the joint. If the surgeon is afraid of complete separation of the meniscus, he can leave an absolutely minimal

---

◁ **Fig. 120.** Beginning of resection of bucket-handle portion at the posterior horn with the curved basket forceps

Fig. 121. Partial transection of the posterior horn bridge at the base of the medial meniscus with a bucket-handle tear

Fig. 122. Medial displacement of the bucket-handle portion after transection of the posterior horn bridge

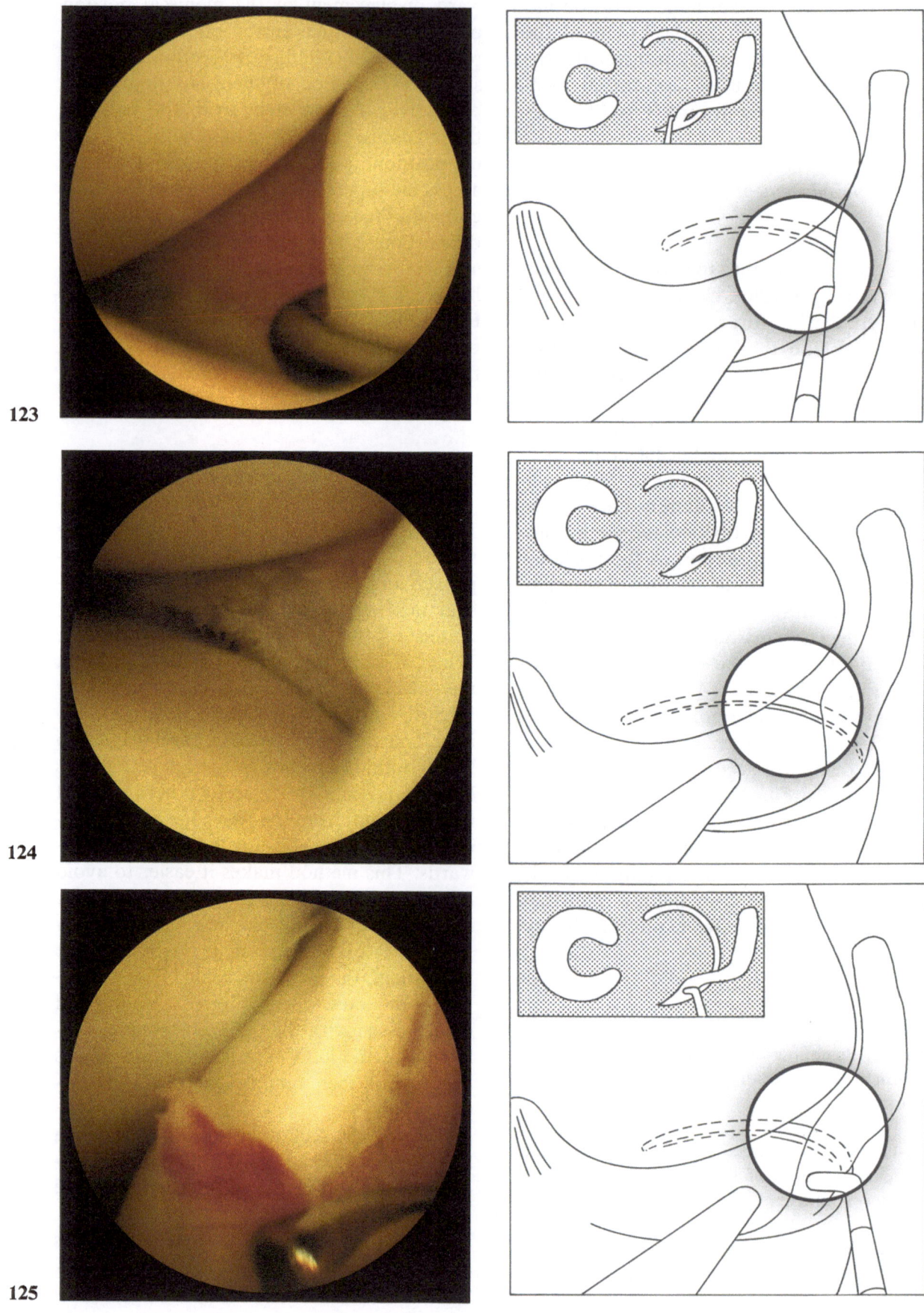

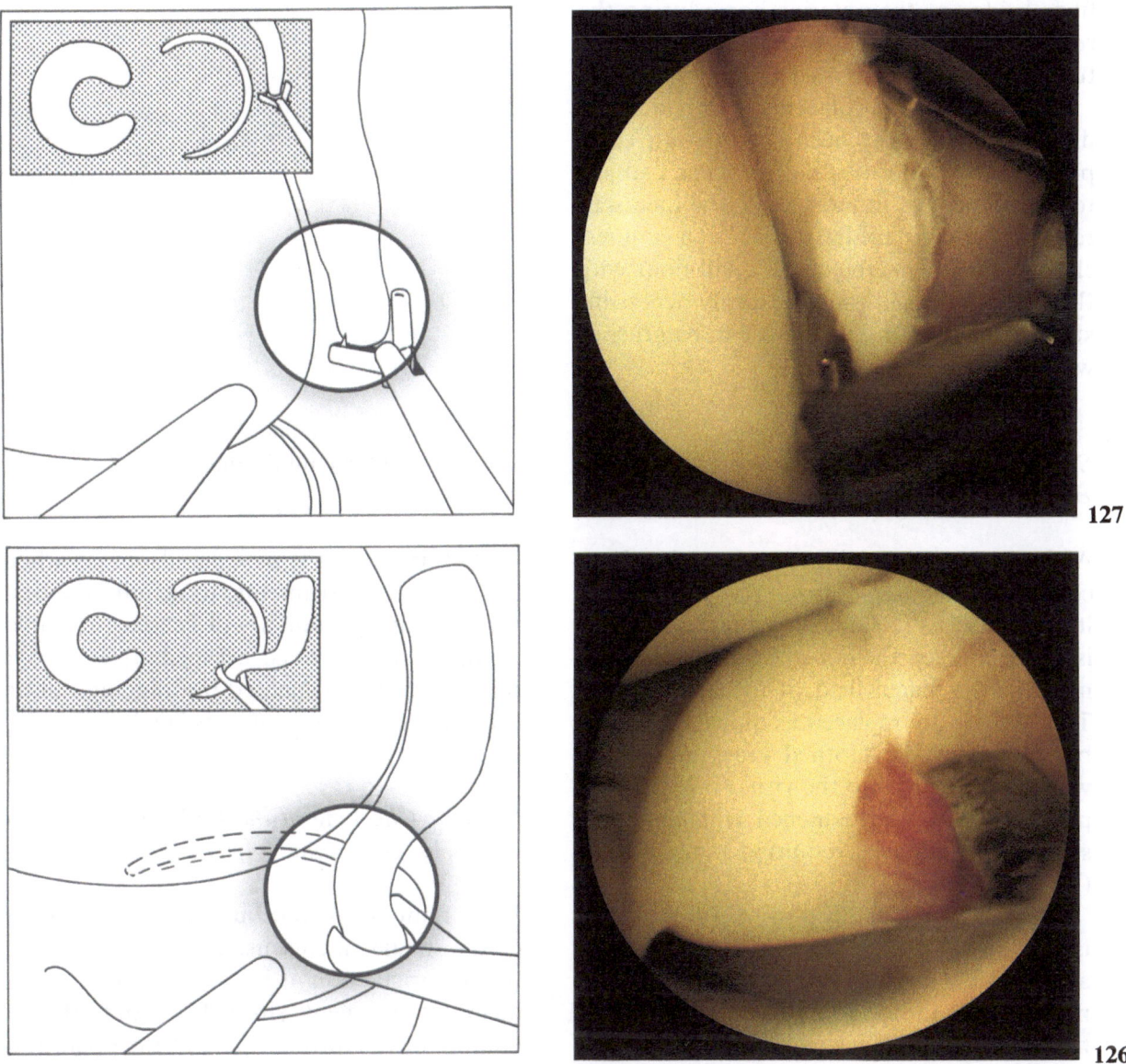

127

126

Fig. 123. Upward reflection of the bucket-handle portion with the probe hook into the medial joint recess

Fig. 124. View of the meniscus tear at the base after upward reflection of the bucket-handle portion

Fig. 125. Outlining the incision at the anterior horn bridge of the medial meniscus with the probe hook

Fig. 126. Transection of the anterior horn bridge of the bucket-handle portion with the large hooked scissors

Fig. 127. Seizure of the detached bucket-handle portion with the large toothed forceps alongside the medial femoral condyle

fiber bridge at the anterior horn during the resection which he can then tear off with a tug after grasping the medial meniscus.

When precise displacement into the medial joint recess has been carried out, complete transection raises no problems (subject to experience) as in most cases the meniscus remains in the medial recess. Of course, should this not be the case, it will float with the irrigation fluid into the easily accessible suprapatellar recess, where it can be grasped without difficulty.

Stage 5: Seizure and Extraction of the Bucket-Handle Portion

After the torn part of the meniscus has been completely separated from the main body, it is essential to remain calm while an attempt is made to keep the detached meniscus fragment in the visual field of the arthroscope. The scissors are replaced as quickly as possible by a suitable toothed grasping forceps which is brought into the visual field and approximated to the detached fragment very speedily, a maneuver requiring some practice (Fig. 127).

The bucket-handle portion of the meniscus, usually 4–5 cm long (Fig. 128) and relatively thick, must be grasped at one end and not in the middle to facilitate its extraction through the small incision. It is really very important not to grasp it anywhere in the middle but deliberately at its narrow end if one is not to lose hold of it again during the extraction. Once it has been grasped precisely at its narrow end, the surgeon now concentrates exclusively on the extraction and ceases to peer through the arthroscope at this point. The toothed forceps can be taken in both hands and with gentle rotary movements and regulated traction the meniscus is extracted entire from the joint through the small incision.

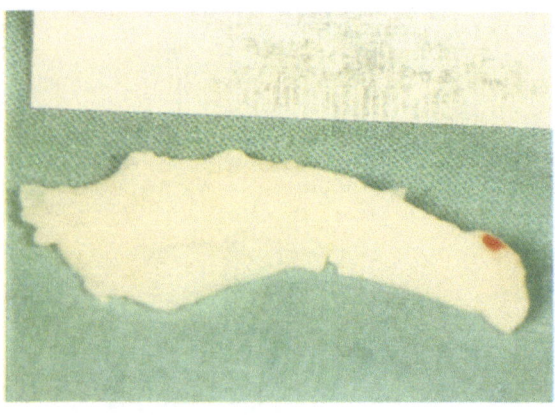

Fig. 128. The medial meniscus with bucket-handle tear shown in the joint in Figs. 119–122

In this context it pays handsomely, when buying one's instruments, to acquire the best possible forceps which will keep a firm hold on the meniscus once grasped. It is always very satisfying to succeed in dragging out an entire meniscus through this small incision.

Stage 6: Checking of the Body of the Meniscus, Smoothing, Afterresection

After removal of the bucket-handle portion of the medial meniscus, there should be no undue satisfaction at having removed a large meniscus fragment, since this is only the beginning of the difficult part of the operation. Next, the probe hook must be reintroduced through the medial incision and the remaining body of the meniscus must be carefully inspected and palpated, including the site of the tear which was previously well covered by the large bucket-handle portion and not open to careful inspection.

The following possibilites exist. There may have been a smooth avulsion which calls for no further smoothing of the body of the meniscus. There may be extensive fringing and fraying calling for careful rounding off. In addition there may be flaplike radial or horizontal tears in the body of the meniscus, and one or two further tears of the bucket-handle type which require resection may be encountered. In most cases one finds a rather

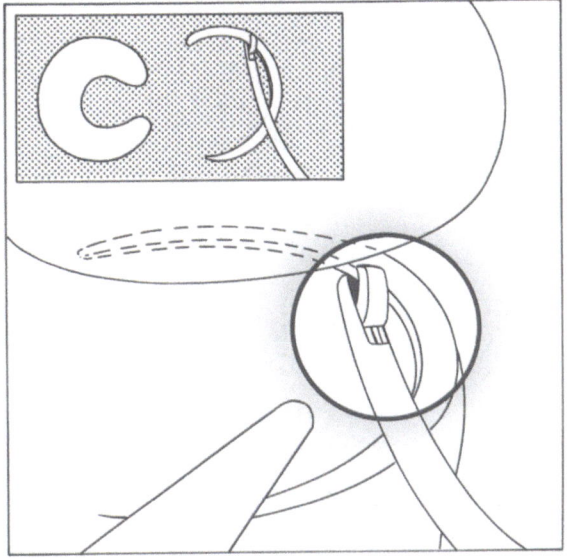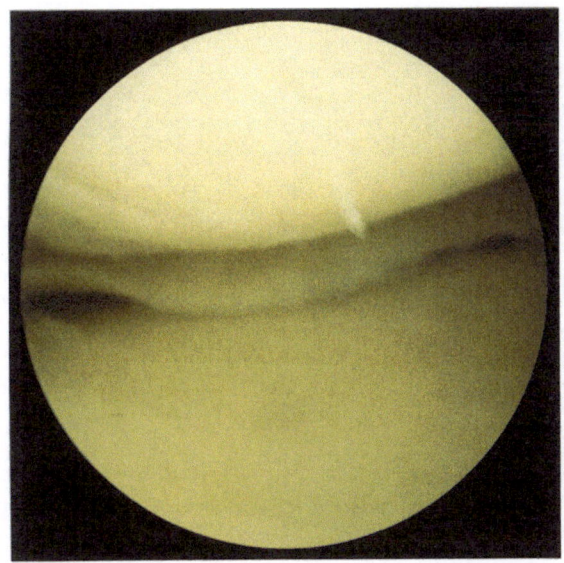

Fig. 129. Smoothing the residual base of the medial meniscus with the basket forceps

frayed meniscus body which is subsequently smoothed round with a cutting basket forceps (Fig. 129). If flaplike, transverse, or bucket-handle tears are present, these are resected as explained in the relevant chapters. Further, one should once again ensure that no large stubs have been left behind in either the posterior or anterior horn region where sectioning has taken place. If this has happened, despite every precaution, these stubs have to be afterresected, which is usually not easy as they are unstable and elude the cutting instrument. In the posterior horn region, one can manage very well with a curved and angled 3.4-mm basket forceps or, in straightforward cases, i.e., a joint that can be opened up widely, with a straight 4.5-mm basket forceps. The anterior horn is usually best managed with the dissecting scissors, or possibly with the 4.5-mm basket forceps.

After the bucket-handle portion has been extracted and the body of the meniscus checked with the probe hook, it is usual to smooth around the base of the meniscus with a cutting basket forceps so as to leave a well smoothed edge. However, the magnifying effect of the arthroscope should be borne in mind; at some point the smoothing process must stop, and the clinical relevance of a few small slender fibers is questionable.

The operative procedure for bucket-handle lesions as detailed above in the six stages should be regarded as a basis for the arthroscopic surgeon to work from. This technique has been of proven value to the authors, but this should not prevent individual surgeons from exercising their skill in varying the details or even the entire procedure.

It is not possible to use the procedure as described for an irreducible bucket-handle tear. In such a case the resection is begun at the anterior horn, the bucket-handle portion is reduced after transection of the anterior horn, and then the bridge at the posterior horn is divided. The authors have encountered an irreducible medial bucket-handle tear in much less than 1% of cases. Occasionally, however, it is very tiresome and complicated to reduce a chronically displaced bucket-handle portion.

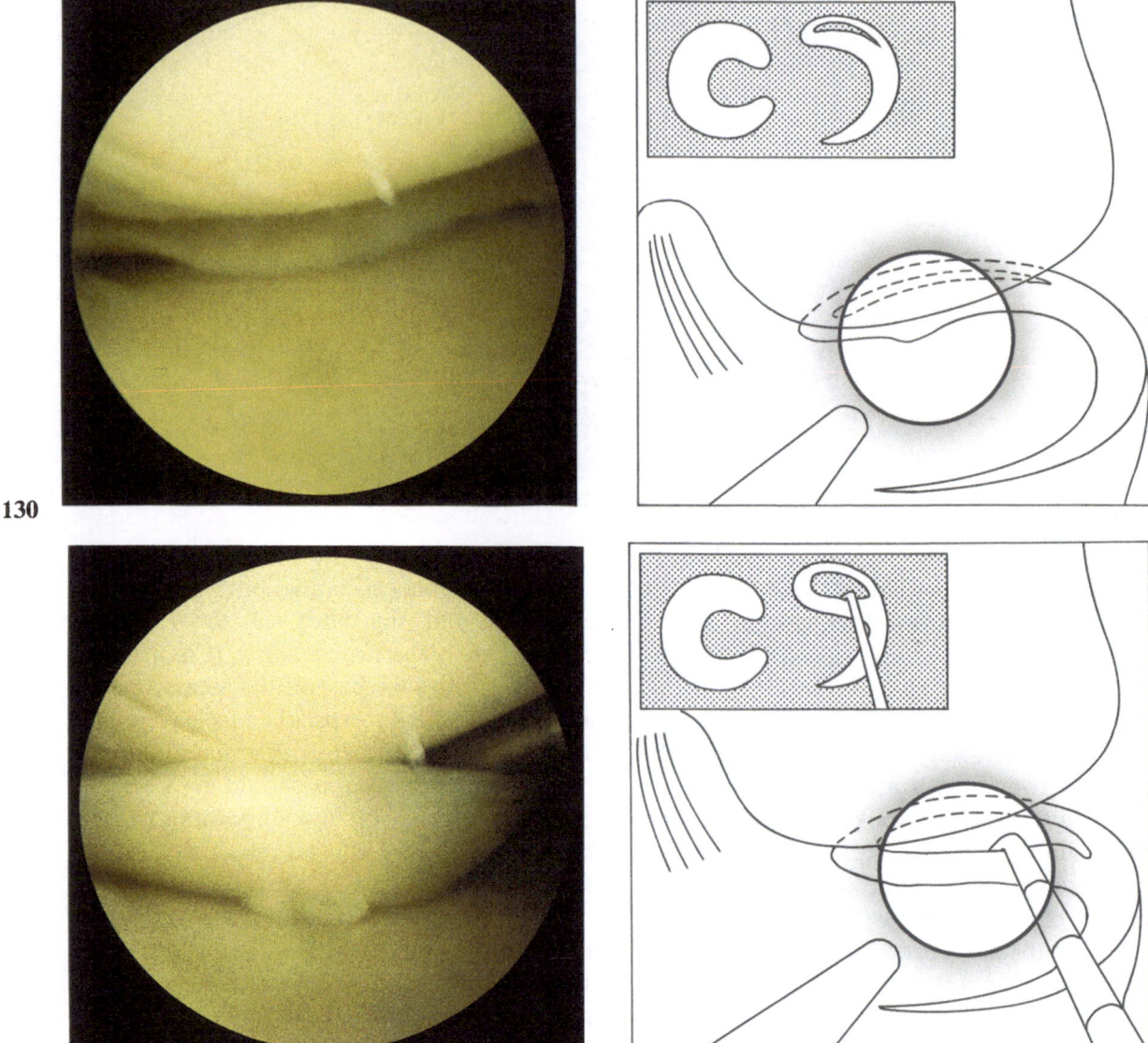

19.2 Longitudinal Tear of Posterior Horn

The most common meniscus injuries of all are posterior horn lesions of the medial meniscus, which can occur in every possible form. A relatively common injury of this severely stressed region is the longitudinal tear, which is particularly difficult to diagnose and whose excision is occasionally complicated.

There is no doubt that arthroscopic misdiagnosis, as a result of inspection without use of the probe hook, is most common with this type of lesion. What is seen is an altogether unremarkable meniscus with a smooth free margin; no abnormality is visible at its

Fig. 130. Posterior horn of medial meniscus with circular basal tear not diagnosable by inspection

Fig. 131. The same tear as in Fig. 130, now displayed with the probe hook

base, insofar as this is not hidden by the medial condyle. Only insertion of the probe hook will show the instability of the posterior horn, display the tear, and confirm the diagnosis (Figs. 130 and 131). The operative procedure may be described in stages analogous to those for a bucket-handle tear.

116

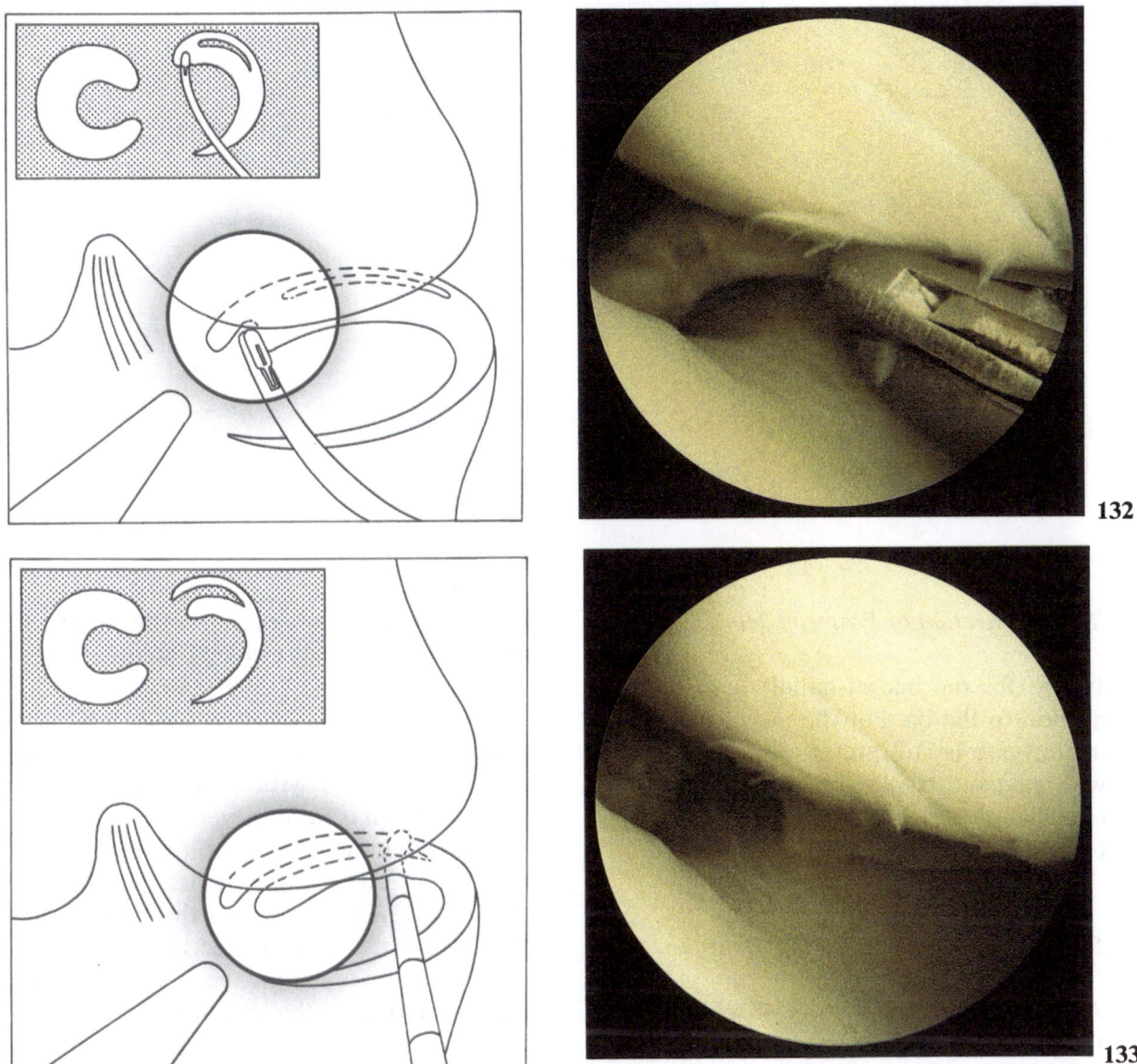

132

133

Stage 1: Exposure

As already mentioned, insertion of the probe hook is extremely important with this type of tear. Without exact palpation, diagnosis and operative arthroscopic procedure are not possible. As with the bucket-handle tear, the extent of the damage must be precisely demonstrated. It is important to establish the anterior limit of the tear towards the intermediate part of the meniscus or anterior horn to ensure too much of the meniscus is not resected.

Fig. 132. Beginning of resection at the posterior horn with the curved basket forceps

Fig. 133. Medial displacement of the posterior horn after detachment

117

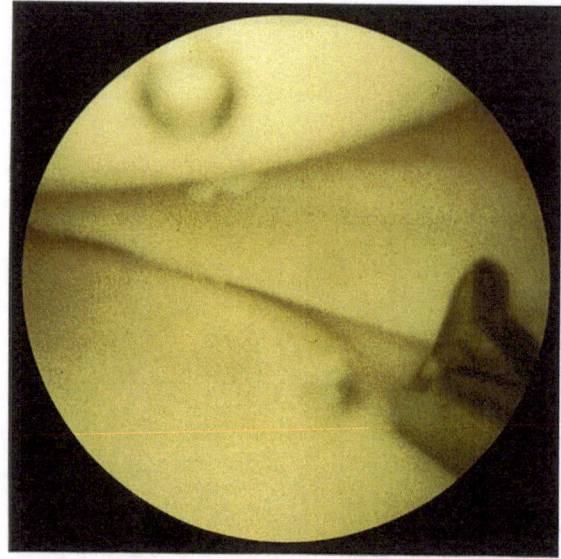

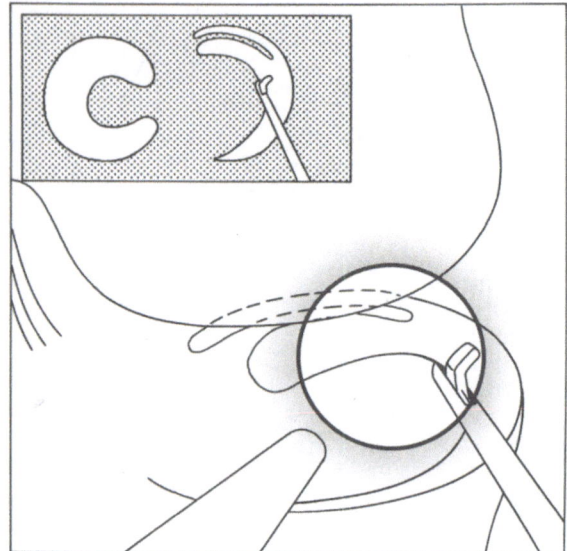

Stage 2: Section of Posterior Horn

Just as for the bucket-handle tear, the connection to the base of the meniscus – which in this case is still preserved – is transected with a curved basket forceps from the intercondylar fossa (see Chapter 19.1, stage 2) (Figs. 132, 133).

Stage 3: Arrangement of the Meniscus

After posterior transection, displacement of the torn portion of meniscus from the intercondylar fossa into the medial recess depends on the extent of the tear in the intermediate zone. If merely the posterior horn of the meniscus is affected, i.e., the posterior third of the meniscus, stable displacement into the medial recess is not possible or sensible. By the time section is begun in the intermediate zone, the posterior horn will have resumed its original position. If the posterior half of the meniscus is affected, upward displacement into the medial recess is often possible; and if the posterior two-thirds is affected, displacement as with a complete bucket-handle tear is possible.

Unfortunately, isolated posterior horn lesions, together with complete bucket-handle tears, are by far the most common meniscus

Fig. 134. Beginning of resection at the intermediate zone with the angled basket forceps

injuries. Therefore, in this case, a further operative procedure with replacement of the posterior horn is necessary.

An advantage of resection in the reduced state is that no turning or twisting at the free edge of the meniscus occurs through upward displacement, so a very precise minimal incision can be made from the free edge to the tear at the base in the intermediate zone.

Stage 4: Separation in the Intermediate Zone

As with the bucket-handle tear (see Sect. 19.1, stage 2), if the connection to the base of the meniscus is detached from the inter-

---

Fig. 135. Abrupt stepped transition between pre- ▷ served and resected portions of the meniscus

Fig. 136. Continuation of the incision at the intermediate zone with the dissecting scissors after notching

Fig. 137. Cutting away the posterior horn to the site of the tear with the dissecting scissors

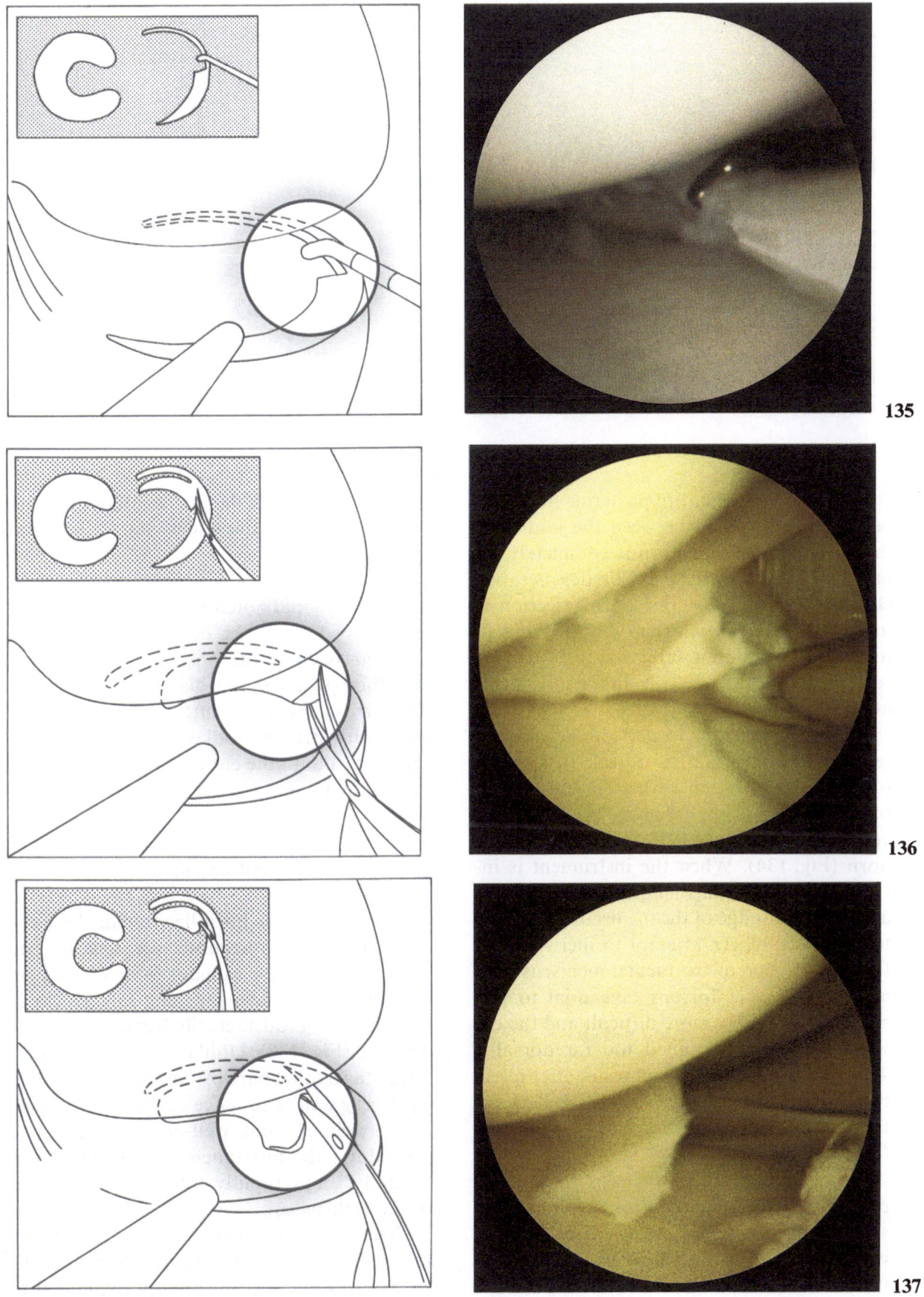

135

136

137

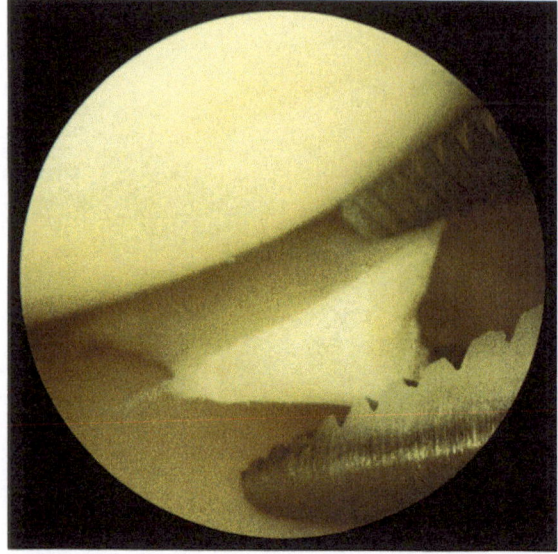

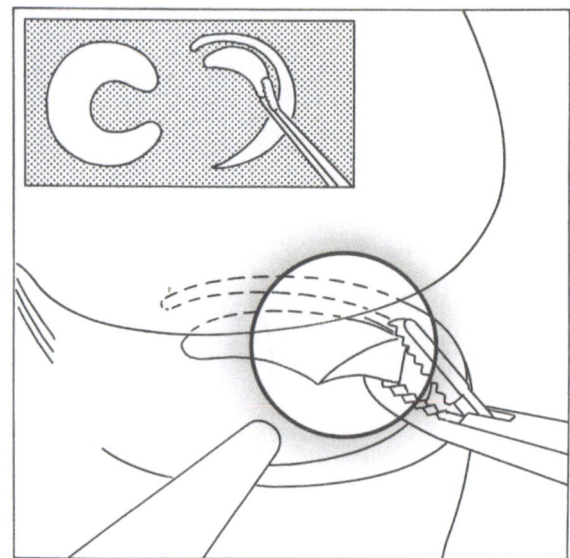

Fig. 138. Seizure with the grasping forceps of the posterior horn lying free in the joint

condylar fossa, the entire posterior horn can be turned like a flap between the joint surfaces. If the posterior horn is completely intact (no color, consistency, or degenerative changes), partial posterior horn resection is indicated. Then the posterior horn lying in its original position is subjected to a tapering resection from the free edge in the intermediate zone.

The object here is to perform an incision tapering from ventral to dorsal. It is useful to begin the resection with a sharply angled basket forceps at the free edge about 1–2 cm ventral to the end of the tear at the posterior horn (Fig. 134). When the instrument is introduced from the medial incision in this situation, the free edge of the meniscus is encountered vertically. An attempt to incise the intermediate zone of the medial meniscus with a straight basket forceps tangential to this site is considerably more difficult and the cut will usually be continued too far dorsally. This leads to the unpleasant result after resection of an abrupt stepped transition between the resected and retained portion of meniscus (Fig. 135).

After incising the free edge in the intermediate zone with the basket forceps, small dissecting scissors with a slightly bent tip (this is not a special arthroscopic instrument) are used to make a very neat and complete cut from the original notch to the site of the tear (Figs. 136, 137). If the beginning of the tear is so far back in the posterior horn region that the space for the dissecting scissors is too narrow, the last connecting fibers are divided with straight hooked scissors or a basket forceps until the entire posterior horn lies free in the joint.

Stage 5: Seizure and Extraction

Once the posterior horn lies free in the joint after completed resection, the scissors (or basket forceps) are exchanged as quickly as possible for a slender grasping forceps capable of opening satisfactorily between the joint surfaces (Fig. 138). Unlike many other operative stages, this part of the procedure lends itself very well to practice on the model knee. For a reliable and well-directed operative procedure, the instrument has to be moved "blindly" and rapidly into the visual field of the arthroscope.

The free portion of meniscus is held by the arthroscope in the visual field and the closed grasping forceps are approximated to it as quickly as possible. It should become routine not to have to search for the instrument with the arthroscope but to keep the operative field or free portion of meniscus in the visual field and to guide the instrument there without effort. Searching for the instrument in the joint with the arthroscope is not a good idea as this causes too much disturbance and the view is easily lost.

The danger at this stage of the operation is that the posterior horn may float away into the back of the medial recess, which is very difficult to reach. After complete transection the grip must be applied as described above to lessen the risk of disappearance into the dorsal recess.

If the posterior horn threatens to slip away dorsally so that it can no longer be grasped with the slender forceps, one can attempt either to redisplace the free meniscus fragment into the anterior joint compartment with the probe hook, or to suck it forward with a narrow sucker. It is then seized with the grasping forceps, again taking care to seize it at its free end and not in the middle to ease its extraction through the small incision. The separated meniscus portion is then cautiously withdrawn from the joint through the small incision.

If, however, despite every caution, the meniscus fragment does disappear into the posteromedial recess, an additional incision must be made behind the tibial collateral ligament and the arthroscope and grasping forceps inserted there to remove the fragment.

Stage 6: Checking, Smoothing, Afterresection

After removal of the large posterior horn fragment, the remaining base of the meniscus is again palpated with the probe hook and any residual fibers or large meniscus flaps are cleared away with a transecting basket forceps.

The object of partial meniscectomy is to remove as much meniscus tissue as necessary and preserve as much as possible. Thus, when partial resection of the posterior horn is performed as described above, the posterior horn is usually subtotally removed while the anterior horn is completely preserved. In this type of resection there is a critical point at which torn meniscus portions at the intermediate zone of the meniscus may be left behind. Therefore, after the posterior horn has been removed from the joint and the remaining base has been smoothed, the probe hook must be employed to make a precise check of whether a residual step has been formed or there are unstable portions of meniscus. Meticulous, even resection and smoothing of the base of the meniscus significantly reduce the recurrence rate.

It is therefore necessary in the intermediate zone of the medial meniscus to make a tapering resection of the meniscus extending 1.5–2.0 cm, i.e., to even out the 8- to 10-mm wide anterior horn and the residual 2- to 3-mm wide base of the posterior horn in the transition zone. If partial posterior horn resection is correctly performed, the medial meniscus has an intact normal anterior horn in its anterior third; in the intermediate zone it becomes increasingly narrow and the posterior horn has been subtotally removed.

It is nearly always still necessary, after removal of the posterior horn, to even out the intermediate zone. An attempt should always be made to bring the basket forceps up to the free edge of the meniscus as nearly as possible at right angles, as this gives a better working surface for resection. It is essential to feel that the transition between the posterior and anterior horn regions, which have very different transverse thicknesses, is

121

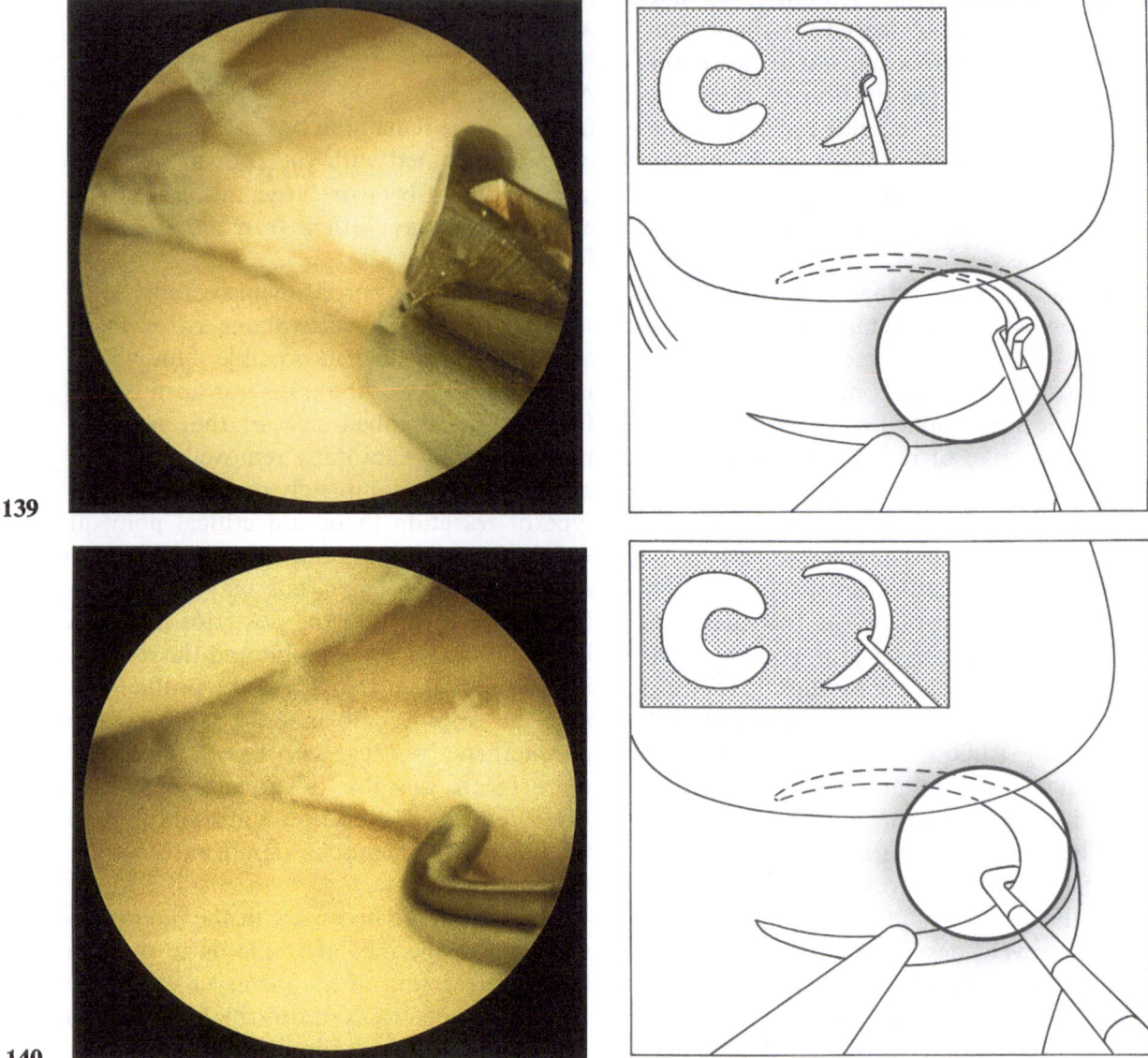

139

140

as smooth as possible and that no step or instability remains; at the same time too much meniscal tissue should not have been removed.

This is most easily achieved using the medial incision as the working passage with a curved or, better still, an angled basket forceps (Fig. 139). If adequate resection from the medial side is not possible because the tangential contact of the forceps with the free margin does not provide enough of a working surface, the arthroscope will have to be introduced from the medial side and the instrument manipulated from the lateral inci-

Fig. 139. Smoothing and evening-out resection at the intermediate zone of the medial meniscus

Fig. 140. Checking the residual portion of the meniscus with the probe hook after partial menisectomy

122

sion. In particular, it is possible from this position to perform a resection to even out the transition from the posterior horn to the middle third of the meniscus, using either straight or angled basket forceps.

The meniscus fragments obtained in this type of forceps resection are removed from the joint from time to time with a sucker. Finally, the resection and the stability of the residual portions of meniscus are once again checked with the probe hook (Fig. 140).

19.3 Flap Tear

Flap tears of the medial meniscus are very common; they may occur in any part of the meniscus, but are far more frequent in the posterior half of the meniscus. An extensive flap tear of the posterior horn region of the medial meniscus which is pedicled at the intermediate zone is simple to operate on arthroscopically and is ideal for a beginner's first steps. The pedicle of the flap must be severed, the flap seized and extracted from the joint, and the body of the meniscus subsequently smoothed.

Stage 1: Exposure

With a flap tear of the medial meniscus, the torn-off part of the meniscus is moved to and fro in the joint with the probe hook. Then a search is made for the exact site of the tear and the pedicle of the flap is precisely exposed before planning further steps (Figs. 141, 142). By far the most common lesions are flaplike tears of the posterior horn, pedicled on the intermediate zone. The operative procedure for this type of tear is described below.

Using the probe-hook, the posterior horn portion of the medial meniscus should be examined particularly carefully; this is best accessible from the intercondylar fossa, even to the most laterally situated posterior horn portion of the meniscus. Very often unstable meniscus fragments or additional flaps of meniscus are found here, as this area of the

posterior horn is seldom torn quite smoothly. These flaps may be deceptively tucked away dorsally or by the posterior cruciate ligament and exposed only by deliberate manipulation with the probe hook.

It also happens occasionally that a large posterior horn flap, pedicled at the intermediate zone, is packed away completely under the body of the meniscus and that, with a chronic rounded-off tear, no strikingly abnormal appearance is initially noted apart from some splaying and a clear change of the transverse thickness in the intermediate zone. The extent of the lesion is exposed only by pulling out the torn flap from beneath the body of the meniscus with the probe hook.

More infrequent situations should be borne in mind during diagnosis and exposure. Thus, a longstanding bucket-handle tear may also be avulsed at its attachment to either the anterior or posterior horn, with a smooth slender regenerated structure at the body of the meniscus as after meniscectomy. If the avulsion is at the posterior horn, the large flap may be tucked away in the posterior recess and not exposable, or only exposed with difficulty, from in front. It may also be difficult to expose a flap pedicled at the anterior horn and tucked up in the medial recess if there is a rather hypertrophied infrapatellar fat pad or large synovial villosity in the joint; in these cases the possibility of such a lesion should be borne in mind.

In particular, a large meniscus flap pedicled at the posterior horn and tucked away in the posterior recess may easily be overlooked. It should be evident during diagnostic survey and testing with the probe hook that the meniscus is abnormal in size and consistency, that one is dealing with a regenerated structure, and that somewhere in the joint an avulsed portion persists. If a completely avulsed meniscus fragment cannot be located anywhere in the joint and if, despite all efforts, the large meniscus flap cannot be exposed from in front, the arthroscope must be introduced behind the medial collateral ligament to inspect the posteromedial recess and expose any meniscus fragment tucked

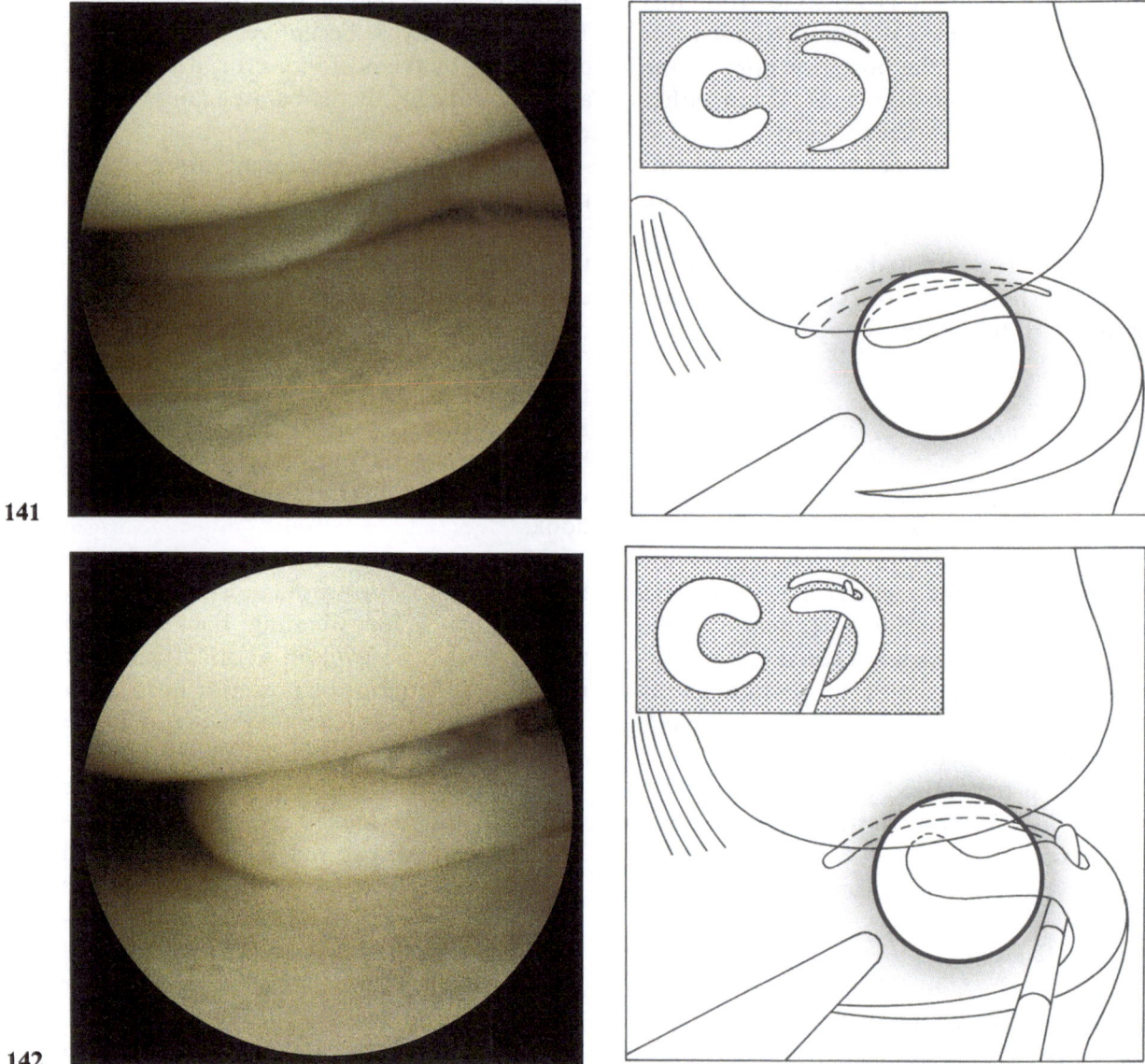

Fig. 141. Flap tear of posterior horn of medial meniscus

Fig. 142. Exposure of the rounded-off posterior horn flap with the probe hook

away there. Even isolated posterior horn flaps – whose attachment to the body of the meniscus is not at the intermediate zone but usually much further lateral in the direction of the intercondylar fossa – may be tucked into the posterior recess and be difficult to expose.

Though these are exceptional cases, it is important to consider them at the critical moment and not to be content with what appears to be a healthy meniscus. However, there is usually a step-formation or small flap at the lateral site of attachment of the medial posterior horn and a large flap of posterior horn pedicled at the intermediate zone.

Stage 2: Posterior Horn Section

With flap tears, using the correct sequence of individual operative stages is not as important as with the lesions previously described. One can begin straight away to remove the large flap pedicled at the intermediate zone and then devote one's attention to the posterior horn portion now accessible from the intercondylar fossa. In many cases this may even be an advantage, such as when the anterior flap is very large and hampers vision and manipulation in this region.

Mostly, however, the step-formation can be progressively nibbled away with a curved basket forceps from the intercondylar fossa, or the connection of the small flap to the body of the meniscus can be transected. If a larger meniscus fragment has been pulled out, this is seized with the grasping forceps and extracted from the joint. Even if one is unsuccessful with the slender toothed forceps in this posterior part of the joint, the meniscus fragment can be brought into the anterior compartment with the probe hook or sucker and then removed from the joint with the grasping forceps.

Stage 3: Repositioning of the Meniscus Flap

A large flap pedicled at the intermediate zone and giving rise to symptoms is very often displaced between the joint surfaces. It is replaced in its proper position with the probe hook. With experience, this is the best method of exposing the exact extent of the tear and the residual pedicle to the body of the meniscus.

Stage 4: Separation at the Intermediate Zone
(See also Sect. 19.2, stage 4)

The pedicle of the flap is cut away from the free edge of the meniscus with angled basket forceps or dissecting scissors, tapering back to the original site of the tear, until the flap is free in the joint (Figs. 143–145). Time is saved if the incision is chosen so that the meniscus tapers from ventral to dorsal and no step is left behind.

Fig. 143. Tapering resection in the intermediate zone with the dissecting scissors

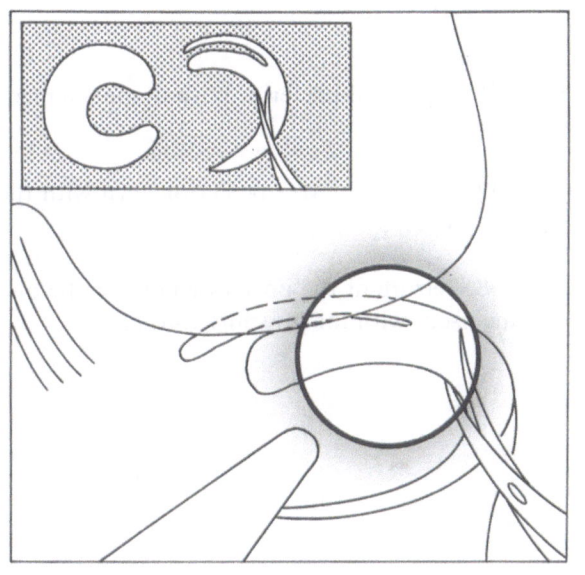
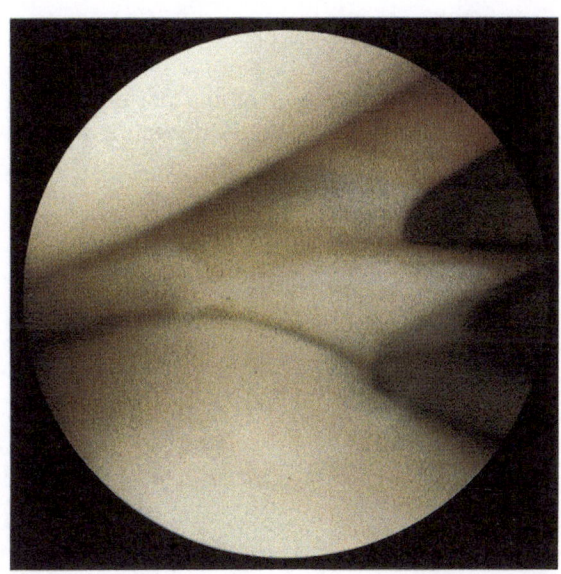

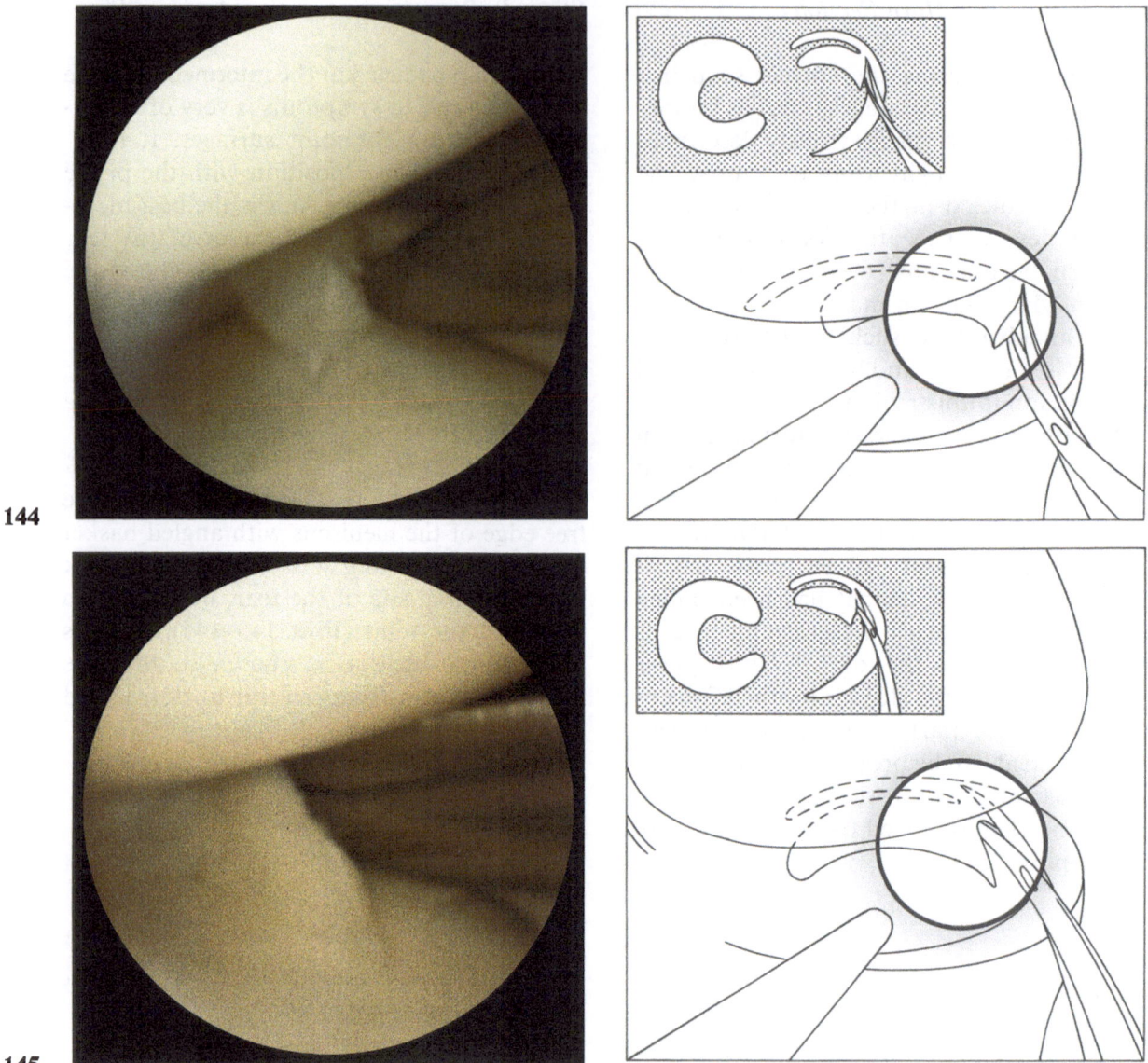

Fig. 144. Partial resection of the posterior horn of the medial meniscus with the dissecting scissors

Fig. 145. Completion of posterior horn resection

Fig. 146. Separated posterior horn of medial men- ▷ iscus free in joint

Fig. 147. Seeking the free posterior horn with the grasping forceps

Fig. 148. Seizure of the posterior horn of the medial meniscus with the grasping forceps

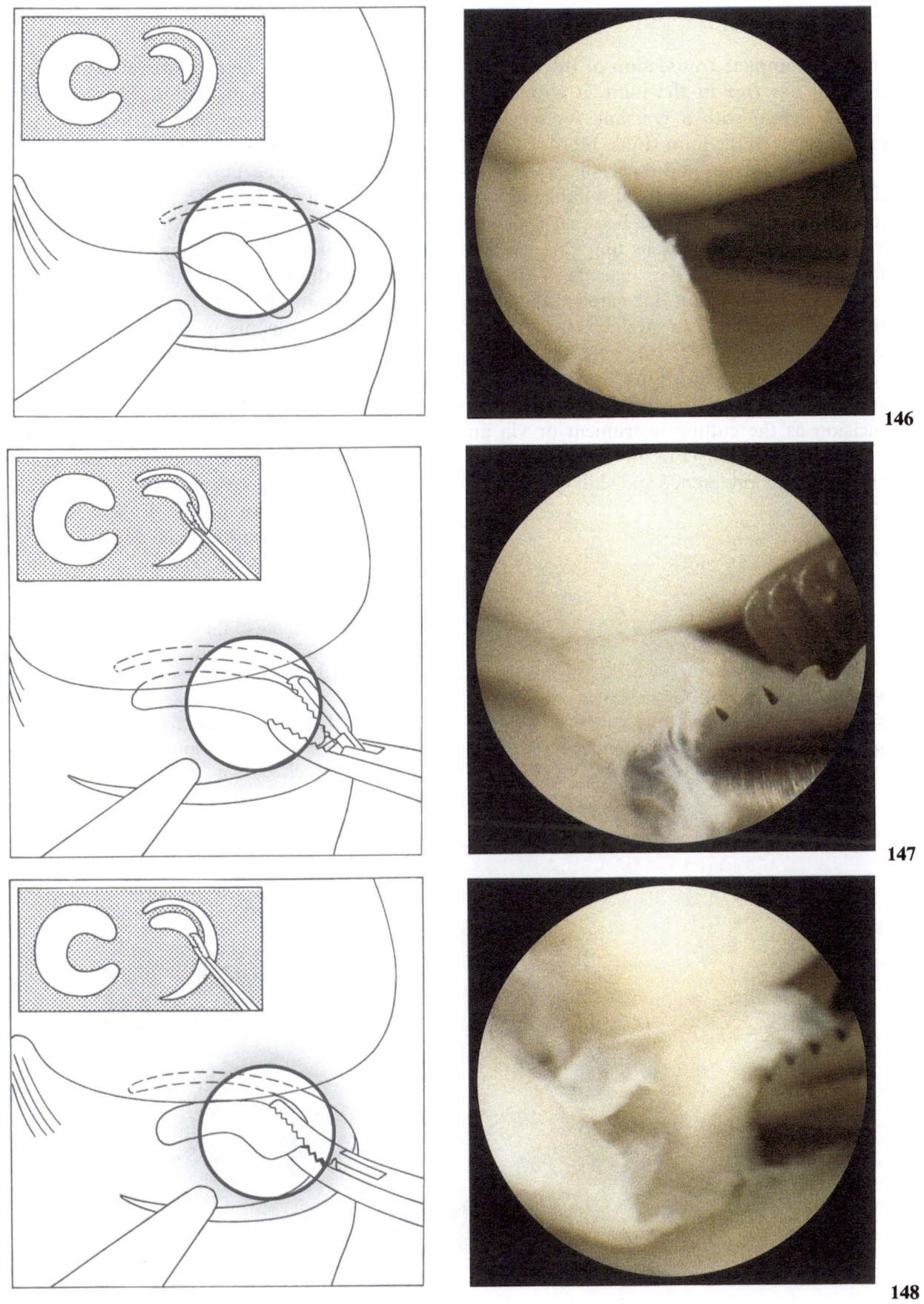

146

147

148

Stage 5: Seizure and Extraction

If, after complete transection of the pedicle, the flap lies free in the joint, it should be directly seized with a grasping forceps and extracted from the joint (Figs. 146–148).

If manipulation and especially triangulation of the instruments is not reliable, a very narrow bridge can be left between the flap and body of the meniscus and this can be torn off once the flap has been firmly grasped, provided that due care is taken not to let the loose body so produced float away. Another possibility is to seize the flap before transecting the pedicle. For this, the grasping forceps can be introduced through the same incision as the cutting instrument or via an additional incision (Fig. 149), according to the surgeon's preference and skill.

Stage 6: Checking, Smoothing, Afterresection

After removal of one or more large meniscus flaps, repeated and meticulous checking with the probe hook is necessary. Other large, unstable portions may persist in the body of the meniscus. The body of the meniscus is smoothed all around with the basket forceps (straight, curved, or angled, as the situation may require) and tapering, afterresection, and smoothing carried out, particularly at the section site (Fig. 150).

With small meniscus flaps where there is merely a small isolated avulsion at the free edge of an otherwise generally stable and intact meniscus, nibbling away of the step-formation ventrally and dorsally is the most important part of the operation. Here again, the object is to remove as much as necessary and as little as possible to leave a smooth stable residual meniscus (Fig. 151).

Fig. 150. Smoothing of the intermediate transition ▷ zone after partial resection of the posterior horn with the basket forceps

Fig. 151. Medial meniscus after partial posterior horn resection with intact anterior horn and narrowed intermediate zone

Fig. 149. Arthroscope in anterolateral incision, slender grasping forceps and cutting instrument in anteromedial incision for simultaneous grasping and section of part of the meniscus

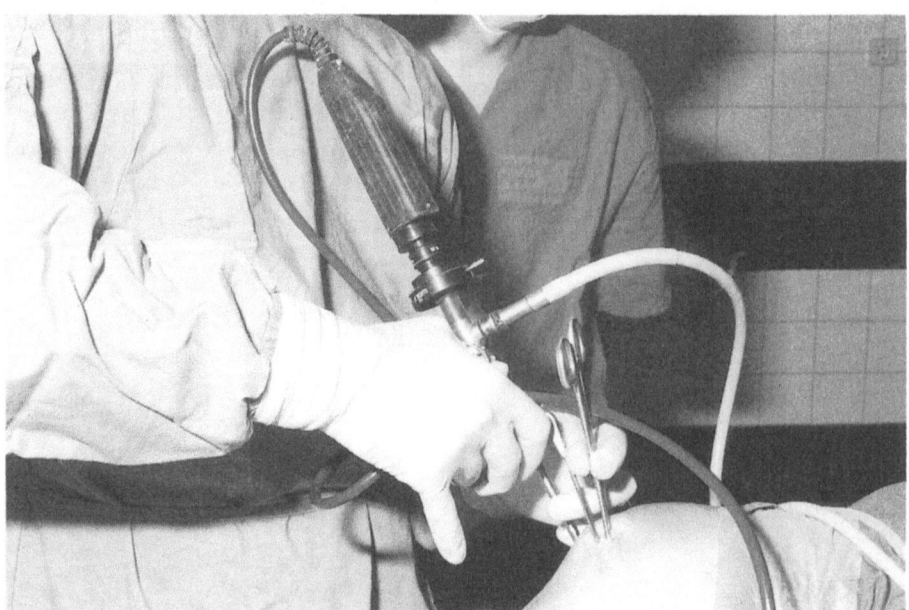

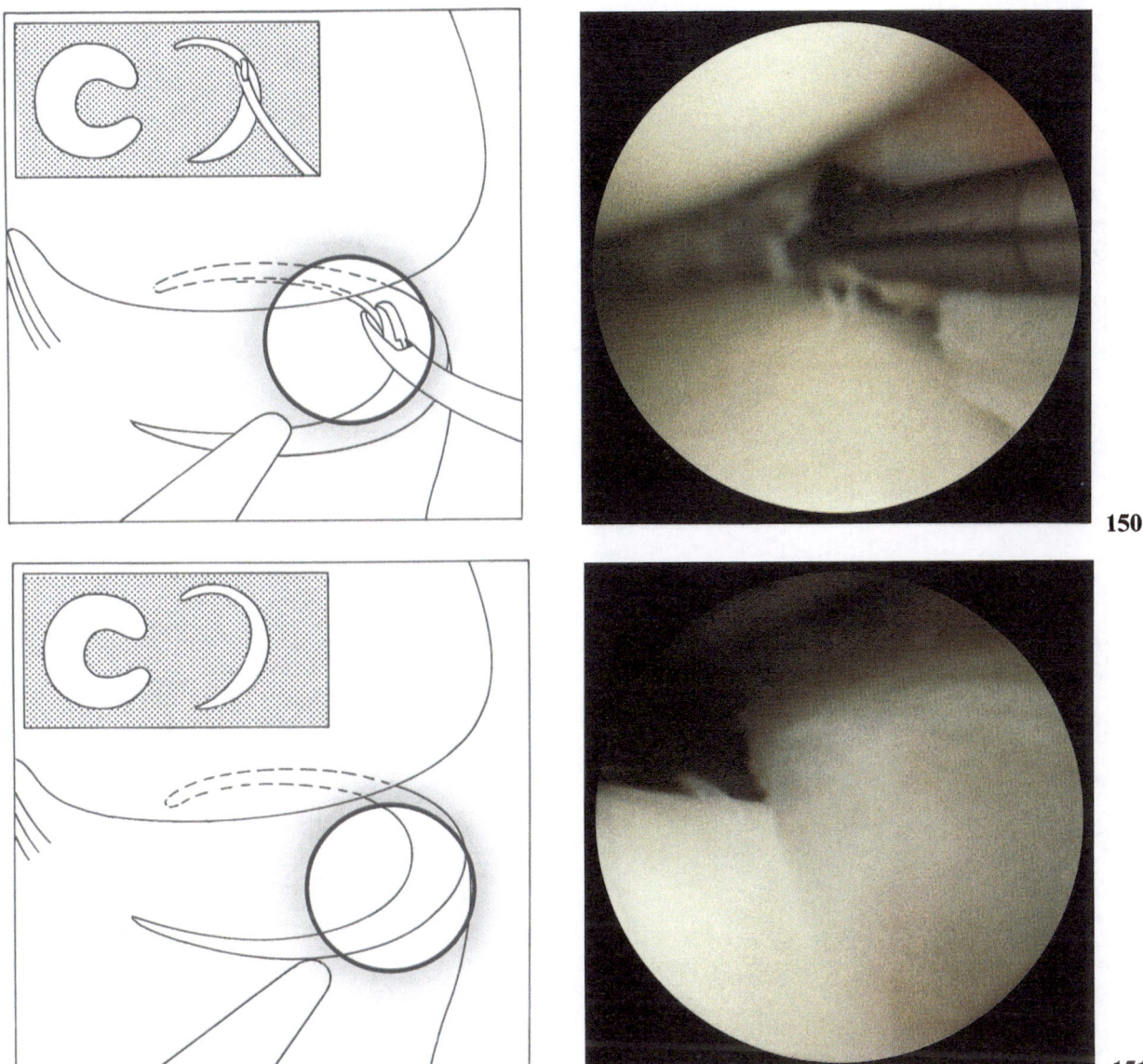

150

151

19.4 Transverse Fissure

With a transverse fissure the body of the meniscus is torn radially. This type of tear is more common in the lateral than in the medial meniscus. The extent of the tears and their clinical importance are very variable; they range from a small, clinically unimportant transverse fissure at the free margin to complete segmentation of the meniscus if the tear involves the base. However, this is only very rarely the case; as a rule, when this type of tear has become clinically relevant, half to two-thirds of the body of the meniscus has been torn inwards from the free margin.

It happens relatively often that a further longitudinal tear extends from the apex of the transverse tear into the meniscus, so producing a flaplike tear. This type of tear formation, including purely transverse fissures and mixed forms combining longitudinal basal tears, is very suitable for partial arthroscopic meniscectomy and this usually makes it possible to preserve large, functionally effective portions of the meniscus. When the circular base is completely preserved, all that is required is resection at the free edge up to the apex of the tear, tapering off ventrally and dorsally.

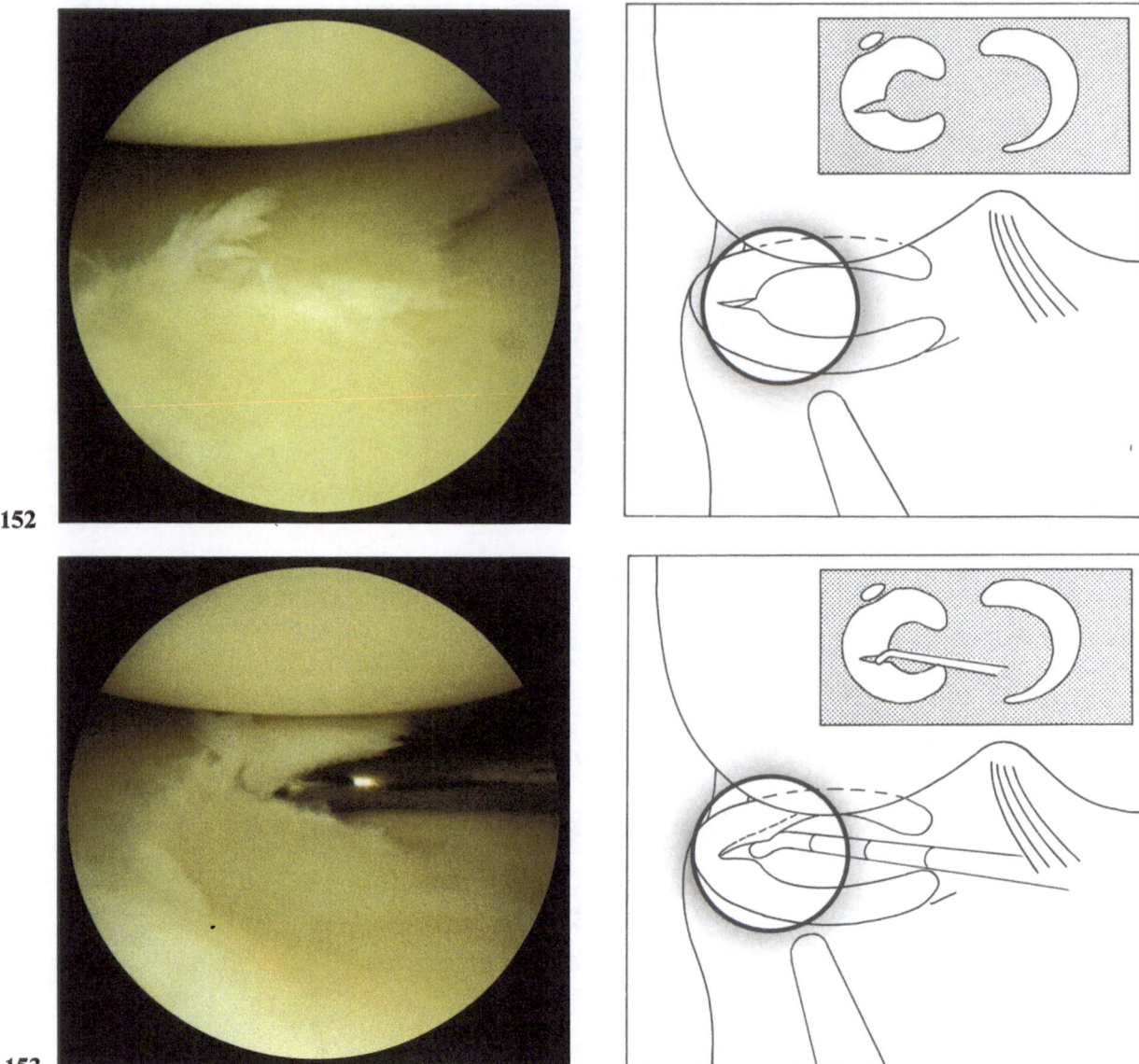

Stage 1: Exposure

Here again, the transverse fissure is not always immediately apparent to the less-experienced arthroscopist (Fig. 152). Therefore it
is important to palpate with the probe hook
to discover how far the tear extends into the
body or base of the meniscus (Fig. 153). It
is likewise essential to probe further ventral
and dorsal to the transverse fissure, and
especially at its apex, to check the meniscus
for additional tears and degenerative changes. Once the exact extent of the lesion is
clear, the individual operation stages can be
planned and carried out.

Fig. 152. Transverse tear of intermediate zone of
meniscus

Fig. 153. Exposure of transverse tear with probe
hook

Stages 2–4: Posterior Horn Section,
Repositioning, Anterior Horn Section

When the investigation is concluded, the meniscus is restored to its original position with the probe hook before incisions are made using the basket forceps most appropriate to the site of the transverse fissure. The sequence of procedure chosen depends on which gives the most favorable visual possibilities. The object is to perform a tapering resection from the free edge of the meniscus to the apex of the transverse fissure, and naturally both ventrally and dorsally, or medially and laterally, from the fissure.

Most commonly, the posterior horn or posterior half of the medial meniscus is affected by this type of tear. The more dorsal the tear, the more difficult is the arthroscopic operative procedure. If the transverse fissure involves two-thirds of the body of the medial meniscus from its free edge and is situated in the intermediate zone, the arthroscope is initially introduced from the lateral side. Then a tapering resection is performed with a sharp angled basket forceps from the ventral aspect of the free edge of the anterior horn 1.0–1.5 cm in front of the tear to its apex (Fig. 154). This large triangular meniscus fragment is seized with the grasping forceps and removed from the joint. A tapering

resection of the meniscus is now done in a ventral direction and evened out, still leaving a rough step dorsal to the site of the transverse fissure (Fig. 155).

In principle, the evening-out in this region can be achieved in either of two ways. A tapering cut can be made either from the apex of the fissure to the free edge or from the edge to the apex of the fissure (Fig. 156). If the cut is made outwards from the apex of the fissure, there is a danger of resecting too much healthy meniscus. It is therefore advisable to cut from the free edge to the apex of the fissure under good vision with an appropriately angled basket forceps, possibly after changing the arthroscope to the medial incision (Fig. 157). Here again, the resulting portion of meniscus that is seized with the grasping forceps and removed from the joint is rather triangular in shape.

The procedure is similar, but technically rather more difficult, when the tear is situated further back, right at the posterior horn, and the apex of the fissure is concealed by the condyle. In order not to sacrifice too much of the meniscus, precise investigation

Fig. 154. Beginning of resection ventral to the transverse tear with the angled basket forceps

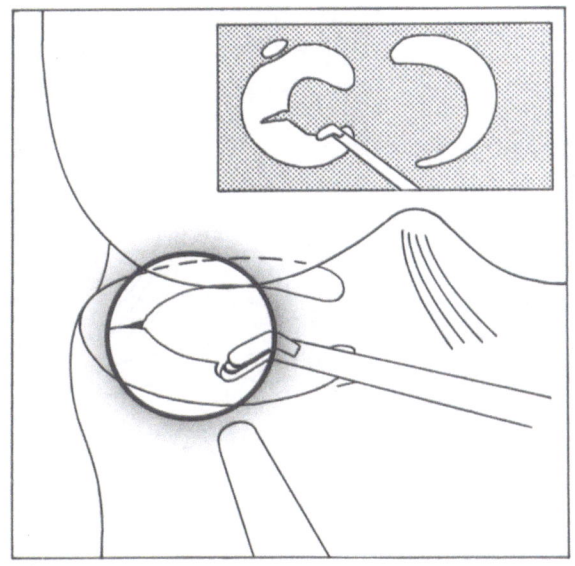

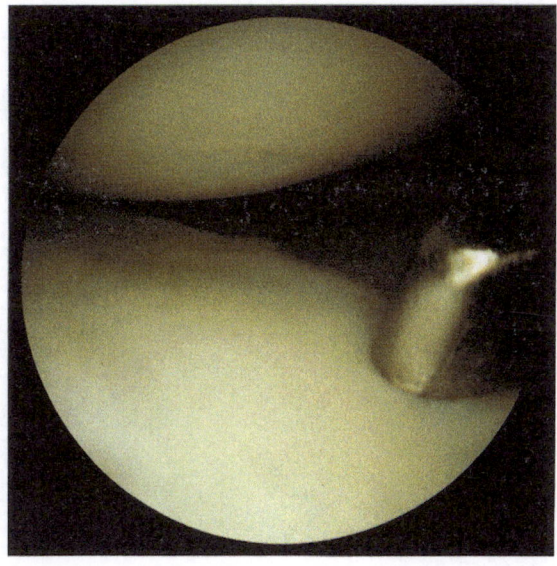

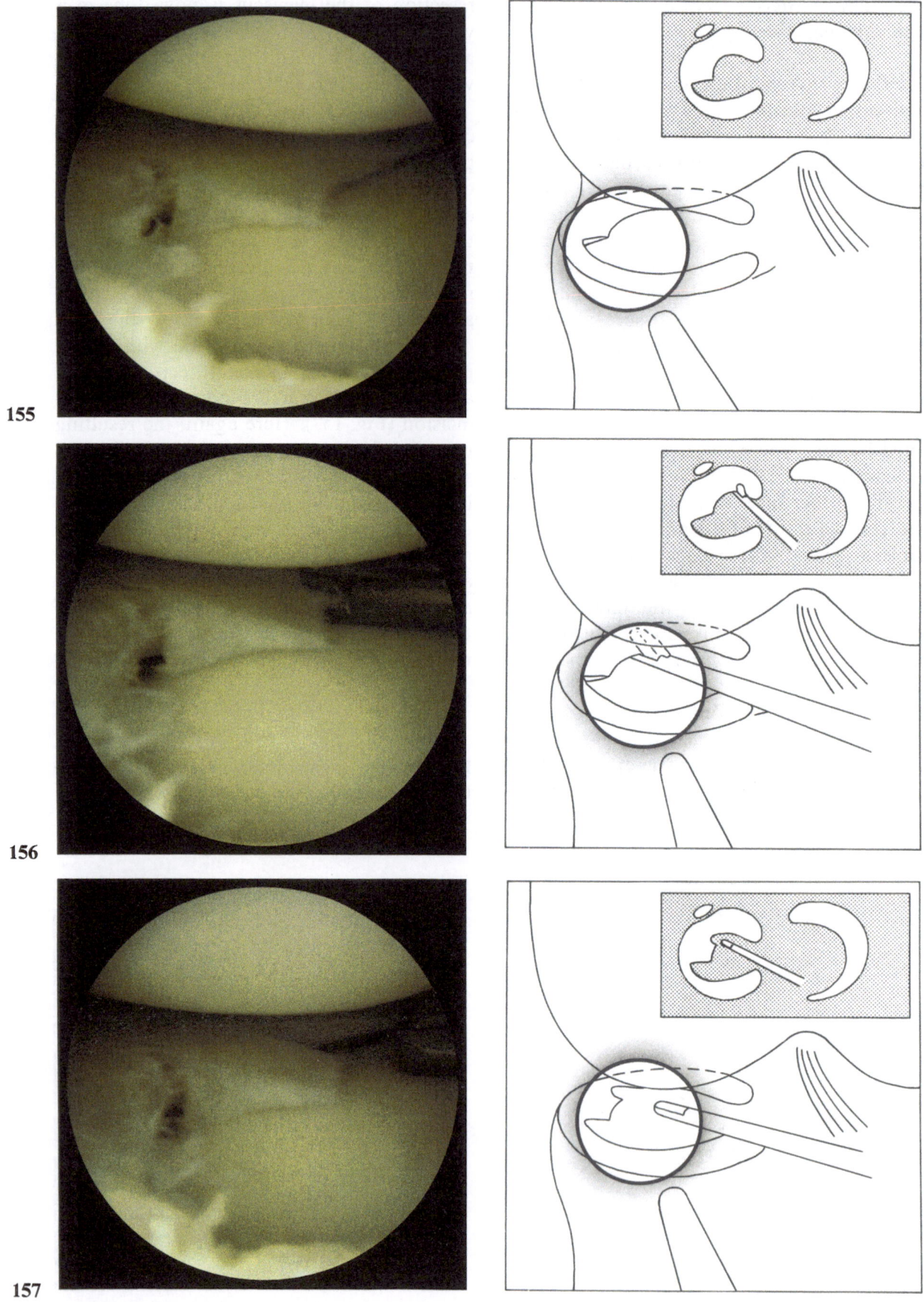

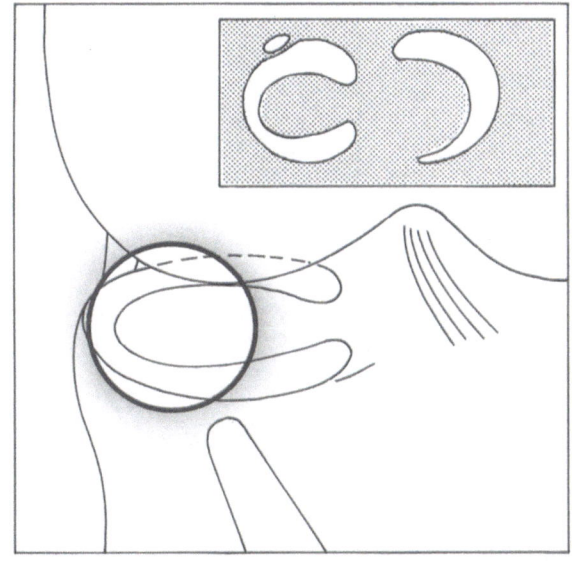

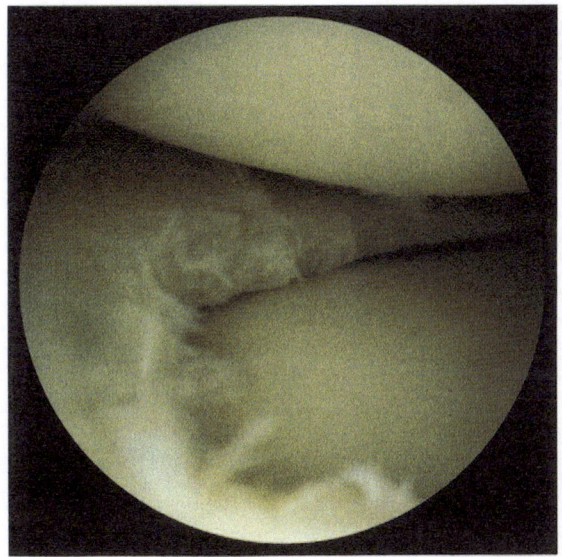

and exposure with the probe hook together with the surgeon's intuition during the incision are essential.

With a transverse fissure in the posterior horn region, a tapering resection is performed 1.0–1.5 cm medial and lateral to the tear, from the free edge of the meniscus to the apex of the fissure. For this a 3.4-mm basket forceps is inserted: it may be curved, angled, or straight, the instrument selected being that with which the cut can be made rapidly, precisely, and at a favorable angle to the meniscus.

Stage 5: Seizure and Extraction

When these resulting large meniscus fragments are either free in the joint or still attached by a slender bridge, they are sezied with the grasping forceps and extracted from the joint. Smaller fragments are removed from the joint with a sucker.

◁ **Fig. 155.** Completed tapering resection ventral to the transverse tear

Fig. 156. Beginning of resection dorsal to the transverse tear

Fig. 157. Tapering resection from dorsal to the transverse tear

Fig. 158. Partial meniscectomy completed for transverse tear, with base of meniscus intact

Stage 6: Checking, Smoothing, Afterresection

After cutting out the transverse fissure with its surrounding, starting from the free edge, the probe hook is used again to check the base of the meniscus, its free edge, and especially the meniscus tissue at the site of section and at the apex of the fissure. Any persistent fraying or residual corner- or step-formations at the incision site are smoothed off with the appropriate cutting basket forceps. No unstable or degeneratively altered portions of the meniscus should remain behind after the partial resection and as much of the meniscus as possible should be preserved (Fig. 158).

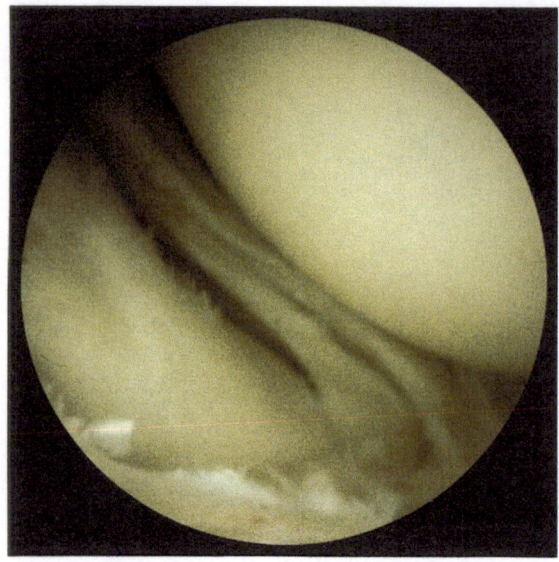 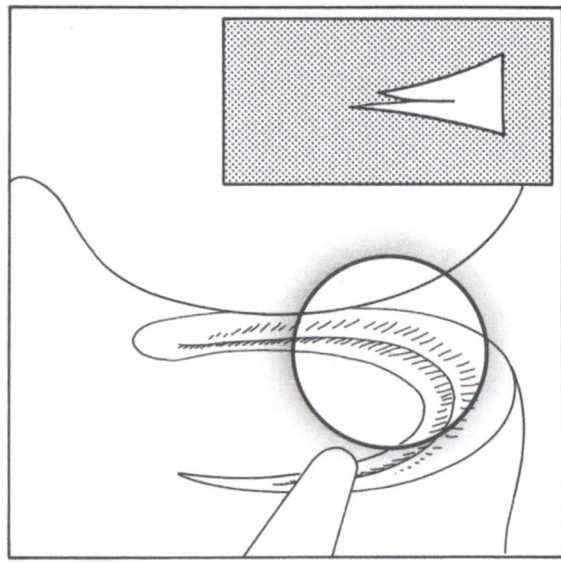

19.5 Tangential, Horizontal, and Incomplete Fissures

A "cookbook" introduction to the operative procedure for every type of tear of the medial meniscus is impossible because of the great number of different types. Therefore, only the main types of tear and their operative management will be described in detail.

With tangential, horizontal, and incomplete tears the operative procedure depends to a very great extent on the site of the lesion, the extent of the tear, and its clinical relevance. Not every small meniscus tear causes clinical symptoms and needs to be operated on.

A tangential tear may occur at any part of the meniscus and is a form of combined transverse, horizontal, and flap tear. Unstable and degenerative parts of the meniscus are resected, though there are certainly borderline cases in which it is difficult to decide whether to remove or to leave a part of the meniscus.

Horizontal fissures of the medial meniscus such as labiate tears at the base or horizontal avulsions of the upper surface of the meniscus are a relatively common type of tear (Figs. 159–163). In many cases the larger stable portion of the horizontally split meniscus can be preserved, though there must be

Fig. 159. Labiate horizontal tear of base of meniscus

a good chance that this residual meniscus will not be avulsed by the first strain.

Incomplete vertical fissures at the lower or upper surface of the meniscus are found very frequently and should not always be taken as automatically indicating that the entire meniscus should be removed. Here again, the extent of the tear and its clinical importance are decisive.

The technique for the operative arthroscopic procedure combines individual stages used for the types of tear described above, and for the fraying and degenerative changes as well as the subtotal meniscectomy described below.

Fig. 160. Posterior horn resection with horizon- ▷ tally torn meniscus

Fig. 161. Resection of anterior horn of horizontally split meniscus with the basket forceps

Fig. 162. Progressive resection of horizontal tear

134

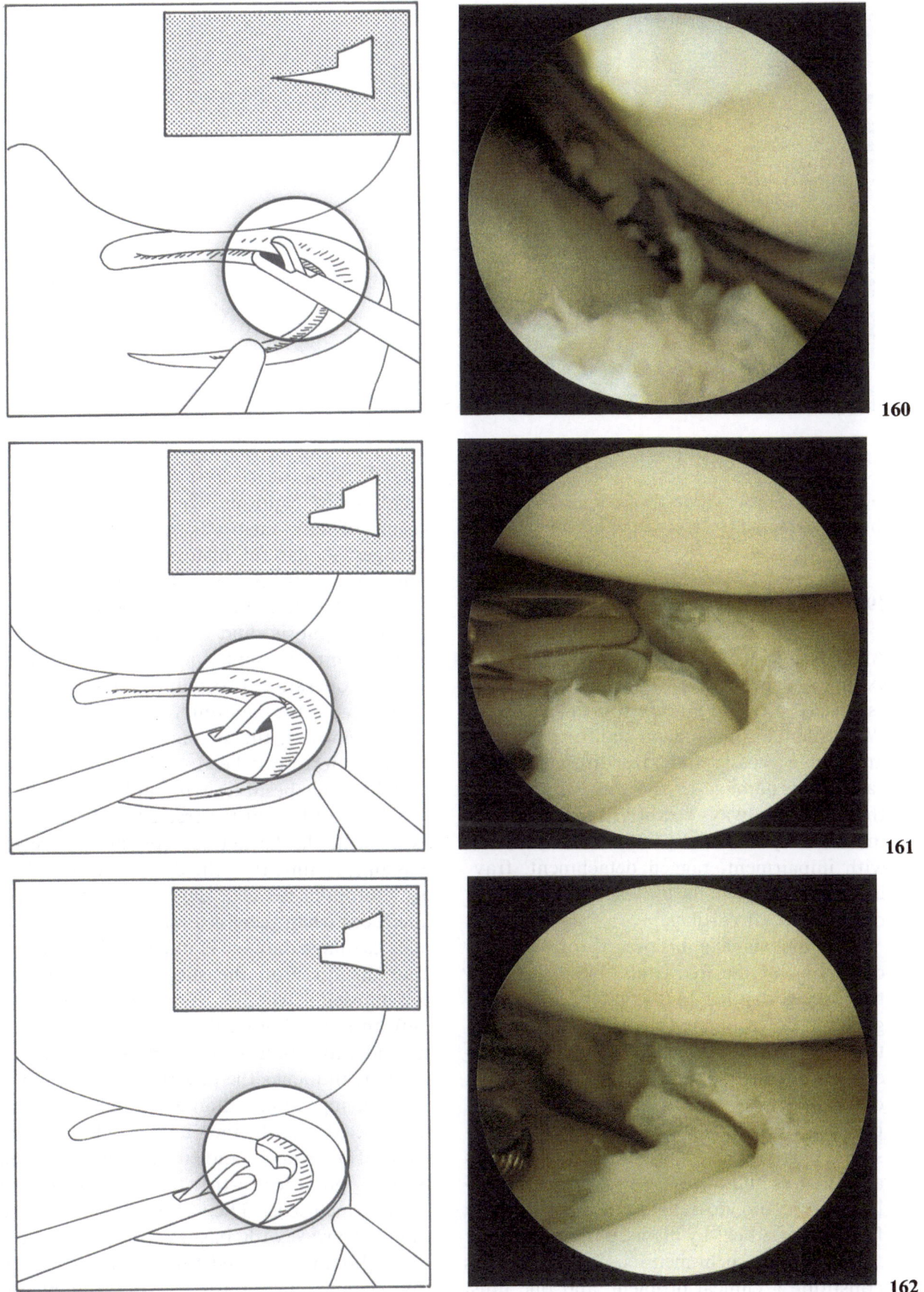

160

161

162

135

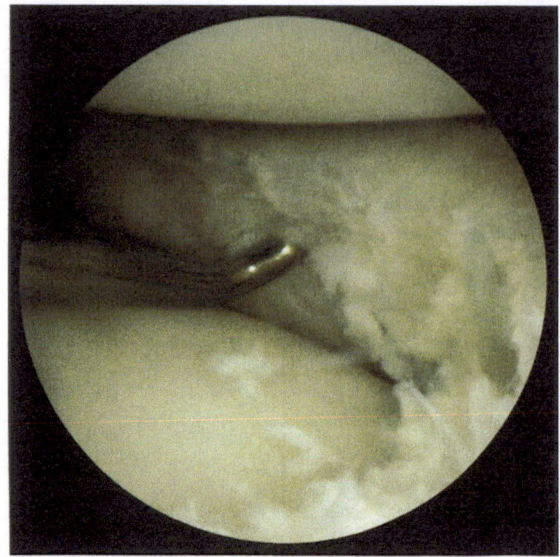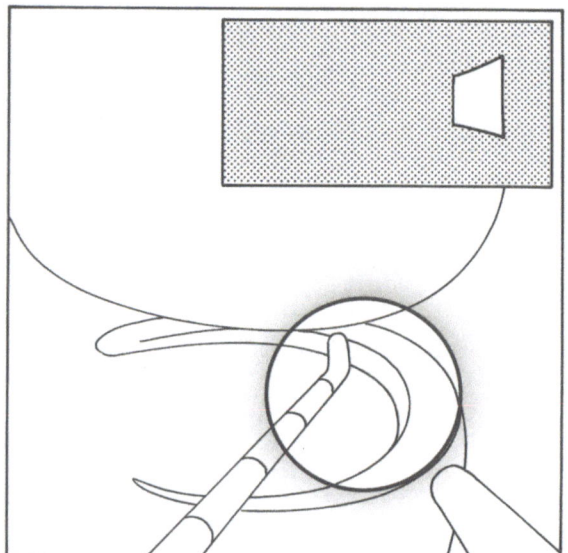

Fig. 163. Checking the base of the meniscus with the probe hook after resection of horizontal tear

19.6 Degenerative Lesions and Fraying

After the age of 30–40, almost every meniscus exhibits degenerative histologic changes, especially after strenuous sporting activity. Wear and tear phenomena and fraying which are visible grossly and at arthroscopy indicate grave damage to the meniscus though they do not always require its operative removal. They are usually found in conjunction with impairment, ragged detachment, fraying, and damage in the corresponding surface of the articular cartilage.

The first stage in this prearthrosis consists of fraying of the free edge of the meniscus to varying depths. In the later stages, this grinding down of the free edge extends into the body of the meniscus. The whole meniscus – in the medial meniscus, however, often only the entire posterior horn – is ground between the joint surfaces, is of softer consistency, is more slender, shows ragged tears and fissures and a change to a brownish-yellow color, and no longer fulfills the buffer function of a healthy meniscus (Fig. 164).

However, such menisci do not always constitute a clinical problem, and one must therefore be cautious when considering excision of any meniscus with degenerative changes. A careful history, precise clinical findings, and the X-ray picture must be available to the surgeon at the time of arthroscopic diagnosis, and all four factors must be taken into account when deciding whether further operative procedures are required. The greater the amount of meniscus tissue to be removed, the stronger the indications for resection must be. In other words there will be little hesitation in nibbling away a few frayed fibers at the free edge of the meniscus with the basket forceps, as it were in passing; against this, the decision of whether to subtotally resect a degeneratively altered meniscus when there is already marked articular cartilage damage is much more difficult, and the question the surgeon must always ask himself is whether this operation will significantly ameliorate the patient's condition, considerably relieve his symptoms, and favorably influence the prognosis for the joint.

Frayings longer than a few millimeters at the free edge of the meniscus may be of some clinical relevance and may constitute the starting point for further tearing and damage to the meniscus. They should therefore be nibbled away with basket forceps; the forceps should be angled for the anterior horn region and curved for the dorsally placed

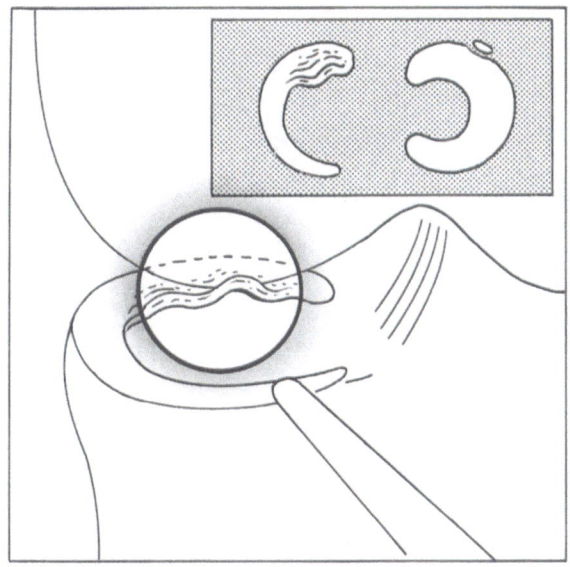 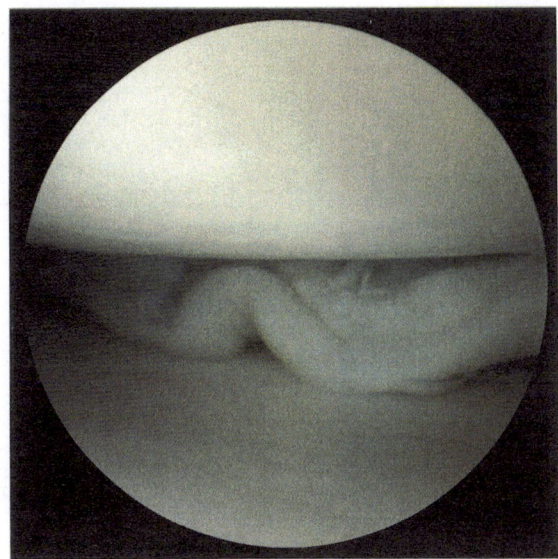

Fig. 164. Posterior horn of medial meniscus: marked wavy projections plus a tear at the base and degenerative changes

posterior horn. The free edge of the meniscus is then smoothed off.

Degenerative lesions of the medial meniscus requiring resection are situated almost exclusively at the posterior horn, which is subject to more biomechanical stress. Isolated anterior horn lesions, whether of a degenerative nature or some type of recent tear, are very rare.

Removal of a degenerate posterior horn of the medial meniscus is not altogether a simple arthroscopic operation, as there is no tear already present to facilitate the procedure; consequently, a circular incision must be made in the difficult-to-access posterior horn region (Fig. 165).

Essentially, the procedure resembles that described for circular (longitudinal) tears of the base of the posterior horn (see Sect. 19.2), but with the difference that not only must the still persistent bridging at the base be divided laterally and medially, but at each of stages 2 and 4 (posterior horn section and anterior horn section, respectively) half of the posterior horn must be sectioned off longitudinally at the base.

One difficulty here is that the two incisions must come together exactly in the middle and not bypass one another. The other awkwardness is the "problem zone" of the arthroscopic surgeon, i.e., the middle of the base of the posterior horn of the medial meniscus. As a rule, the lateral and medial thirds of the horn are fairly accessible to the arthroscopic surgeon with some experience, but the middle third is more or less concealed by the medial condyle and is difficult to reach with arthroscopic instruments from the anterior incisions. However, with practice, every surgeon should succeed without any problems in working away at the base of the meniscus from the intercondylar fossa and from the intermediate zone up to a bridge of about 1 cm in the middle. This is somewhat similar to the extended procedure for a longitudinal posterior horn tear. The methods available for the "critical last centimeter" are as follows. One works gradually from either the intercondylar fossa (with a curved basket forceps) or the intermediate zone (with a straight forceps), but continuously further forward, until only a quite narrow bridge remains. The meniscus is then seized very firmly with a grasping forceps to tear off the last remaining bridge and remove the posterior horn from the joint. If this does not succeed, palpation is carried out using the probe

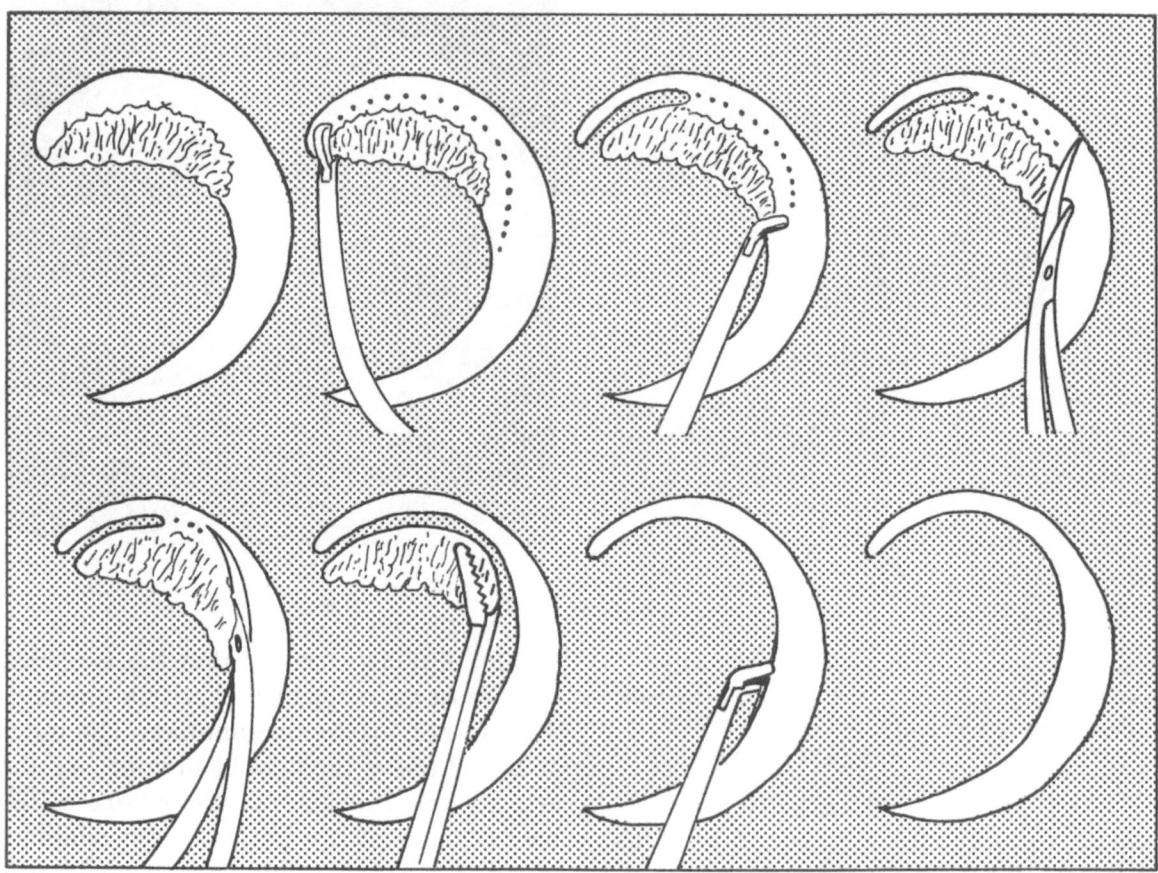

Fig. 165. Stages of operation in resection of posterior horn of medial meniscus with degenerative changes (see text)

hook to discover whether the residual bridging can be best divided from the intercondylar fossa or from the medial aspect.

The most favorable procedure having been determined by palpation, the posterior horn is then grasped with a slender forceps introduced through the medial incision, either from the intercondylar fossa or from the medial side. A graduated pull on the grasped posterior horn will then expose the residual bridging, and this can be divided either from the intercondylar fossa with a bent basket forceps, or from the medial aspect with a straight forceps likewise inserted through the medial incision (Fig. 149).

It is essential here that the meniscus be grasped firmly and the residual bridging

dragged under the condyle into the visual field, as it is more easily transected when taut.

In very obstinate cases and very narrow knee joints even this procedure is occasionally unsuccessful, so it becomes necessary to introduce the basket forceps via a further posteromedial incision behind the tibial collateral ligament. The almost completely divided posterior horn is seized firmly in the grasping forceps introduced anteromedially, put under tension, and the residual bridging transected with the basket forceps inserted dorsally.

If this procedure, too, fails to bring about the desired result, the posteromedial incision can be extended into a miniarthrotomy of 2–3 cm, the posterior recess and the base of the posterior horn can be well exposed with narrow joint hooks, and the meniscus partially resected. However, the experienced arthroscopist will find this necessary only in very rare and extreme cases.

19.7 Subtotal Medial Meniscectomy

A subtotal meniscectomy when a large part of the meniscus has not been avulsed is rarely justified in the authors' opinion. However, it is occasionally necessary to remove a very tattered meniscus exhibiting no major tear at the base. The aim of this standard intervention is to leave behind a base 2–3 mm wide to maintain stability, and to remove the rest of the meniscus up to its free margin.

Witz some practice, this intervention – formerly performed by arthrotomy for all types of meniscus lesion – can be carried out via the arthroscope from the standard anterolateral and anteromedial incisions. Making five or six incisions around the medial joint space for the performance of subtotal medial meniscectomy, as described in some of the literature, is unnecessary with the appropriate operative technique.

As with the open procedure, the most important instruments for subtotal arthroscopic resection are dissecting scissors slightly bent at the tip. The arthroscope is inserted through the lateral incision and the dissecting scissors via the medial. The aim of the subsequent operative procedure is to construct an artificial bucket-handle tear using the scissors (Fig. 166). Close to its base, the body of the meniscus is cut through using small cuts from above with the dissecting scissors until one blade of the scissors can be stuck through the small hole thus produced, and then the meniscus can be cut away from close to its base in the normal circular fashion.

A 5- to 8-mm bridge is left at the anterior horn for as long as possible. The base of the posterior horn is removed as far as possible from the intermediate zone.

Fig. 166. Stages of operation in subtotal medial meniscectomy (see text)

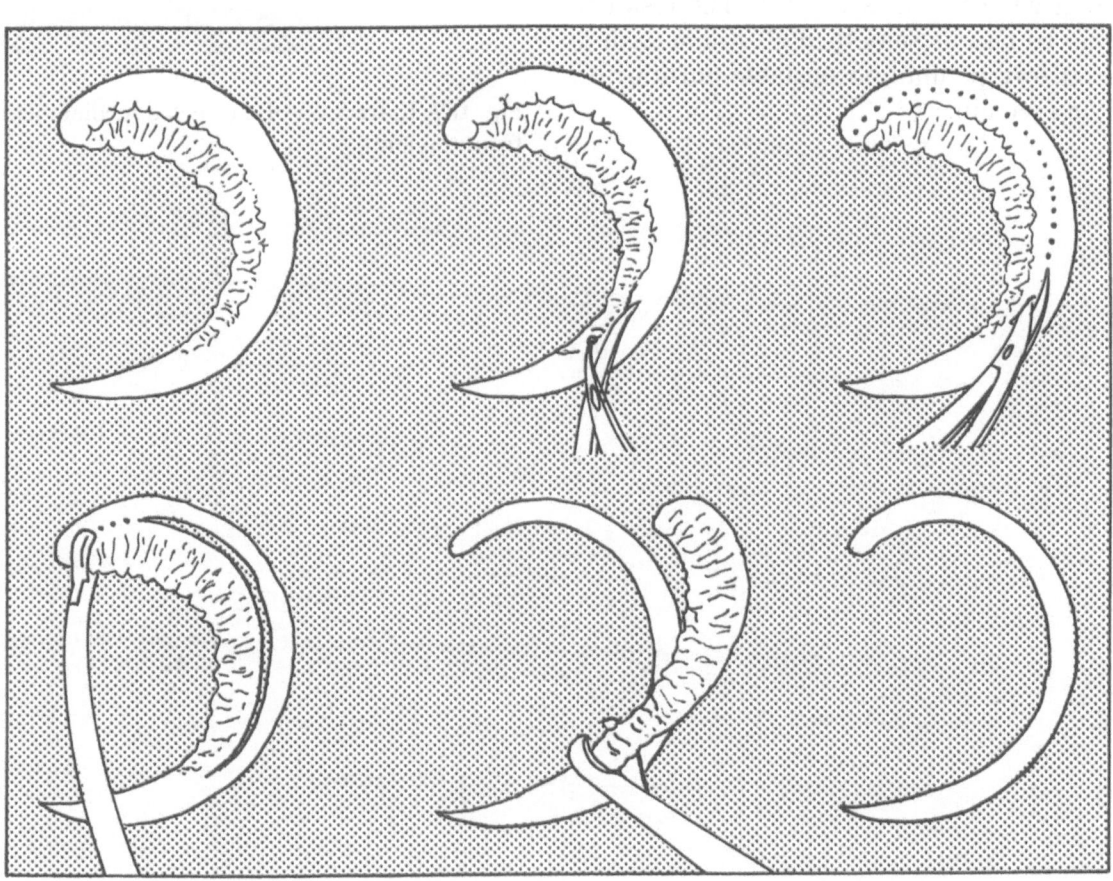

The next stage is the removal of the site of attachment from the intercondylar fossa with a curved basket forceps as far as possible, as previously described for resection of the posterior horn. If a bridge remains in the posterior part of the posterior horn, the procedure is a described in Sect. 19.6.

If vision is greatly obstructed because the meniscus still forms a bridge at the anterior horn and therefore cannot be completely displaced into the intercondylar fossa, one can begin by dividing the bridging at the anterior horn and then remove the last connection to the base in the central posterior horn region. However, it is usually possible to make a circular cut in the posterior horn at its base, to then displace the meniscus upwards into the medial recess like a bucket-handle lesion after posterior horn section, to transect the attachment to the base of the meniscus at the anterior horn, and finally to grasp the entire meniscus, now lying free in the joint, with grasping forceps and extract it from the joint (Fig. 167). This procedure corresponds to that described in Sect. 19.1. The residual meniscus base is smoothed all round with a basket forceps until no unstable portions or fraying remain.

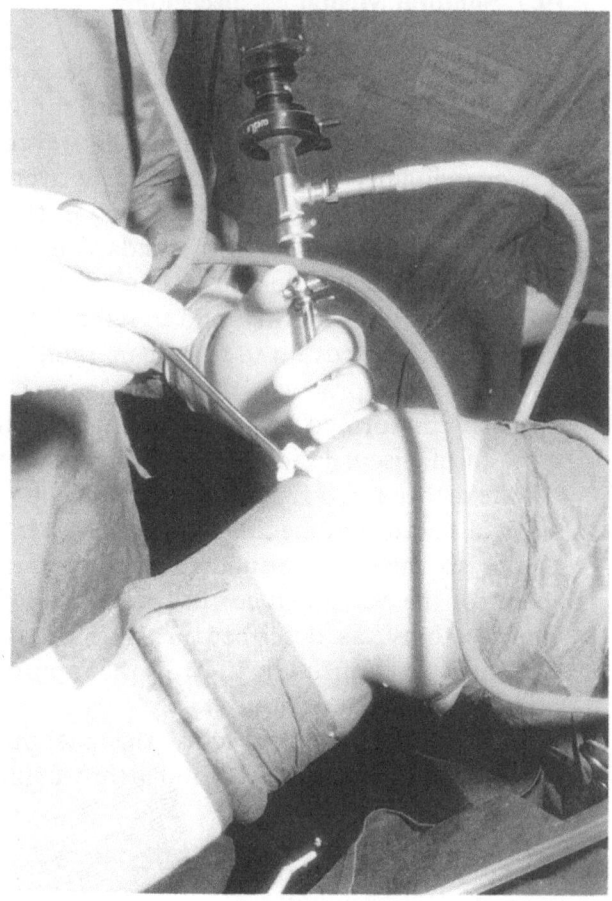

Fig. 167. Extraction of a resected medial meniscus from the joint

CHAPTER 20

Technique of Arthroscopic Lateral Meniscus Operations

Lesions of the lateral meniscus are more rarely observed than those of the medial meniscus; however, they are found more often than was previously supposed from clinical evidence. The clinical diagnosis of pathologic changes in the lateral meniscus is notably more difficult than for medial meniscus lesions. Therefore, it is not uncommon to be surprised by arthroscopic demonstration of a lateral meniscus lesion that has been causing atypical symptoms or has even been silent.

The incidence of tears, their sites, the form of the lesions, and resulting operative procedure differ in several ways between the lateral meniscus and the medial meniscus. Anatomic differences are responsible for this:

1. The rounder and narrower C-shape of the lateral meniscus, such that it makes three-quarters of a circle with a very much narrower radius than the medial meniscus
2. The markedly greater transverse extent of the body of the lateral meniscus
3. The greater thickness of the lateral meniscus at its base
4. The popliteus tendon at the transition from the middle to posterior thirds and the lack of attachment at the popliteal hiatus in the lateral meniscus
5. The greater mobility of the lateral meniscus at its attachment and its naturally greater instability

These anatomic differences result in a reduced tendency of the lateral meniscus to tear, a significantly higher incidence of transverse fissures, and a higher proportion of lesions in the region of the anterior half of the meniscus, and mean that a cautions operative approach is required in the region of the popliteal hiatus.

Arthroscopic inspection of the whole of the lateral meniscus – with varus stress, medial rotation of the lower leg and reduced flexion of the knee – is usually easier than inspection of the medial meniscus. The operative procedure for the majority of tears does not differ significantly from that previously described for the medial meniscus. Therefore, it is not necessary to discuss further every type of tear, as was done for the medial meniscus.

However, the following general advice may be given. In many situations at the lateral meniscus it may be very helpful to introduce the arthroscope from the anteromedial incision and to operate from the anterolateral. In particular, we shall describe in some detail resection of a bucket-handle tear, partial removal of the posterior horn with special attention to the popliteus tendon, partial anterior horn resection (virtually confined to the lateral meniscus), and removal of a discoid lateral meniscus.

20.1 Lateral Bucket-Handle Tear

The individual stages of resection of a bucket-handle tear of the lateral meniscus (Fig. 168) do not differ essentially from those for the same lesion of the medial meniscus.

Stage 1: Exposure, Repositioning

With the arthroscope in the lateral incision, the probe hook is used to investigate the exact extent of the tear from the medial incision, any displaced meniscus is replaced, and the line of incision at the posterior horn is established (Fig. 169).

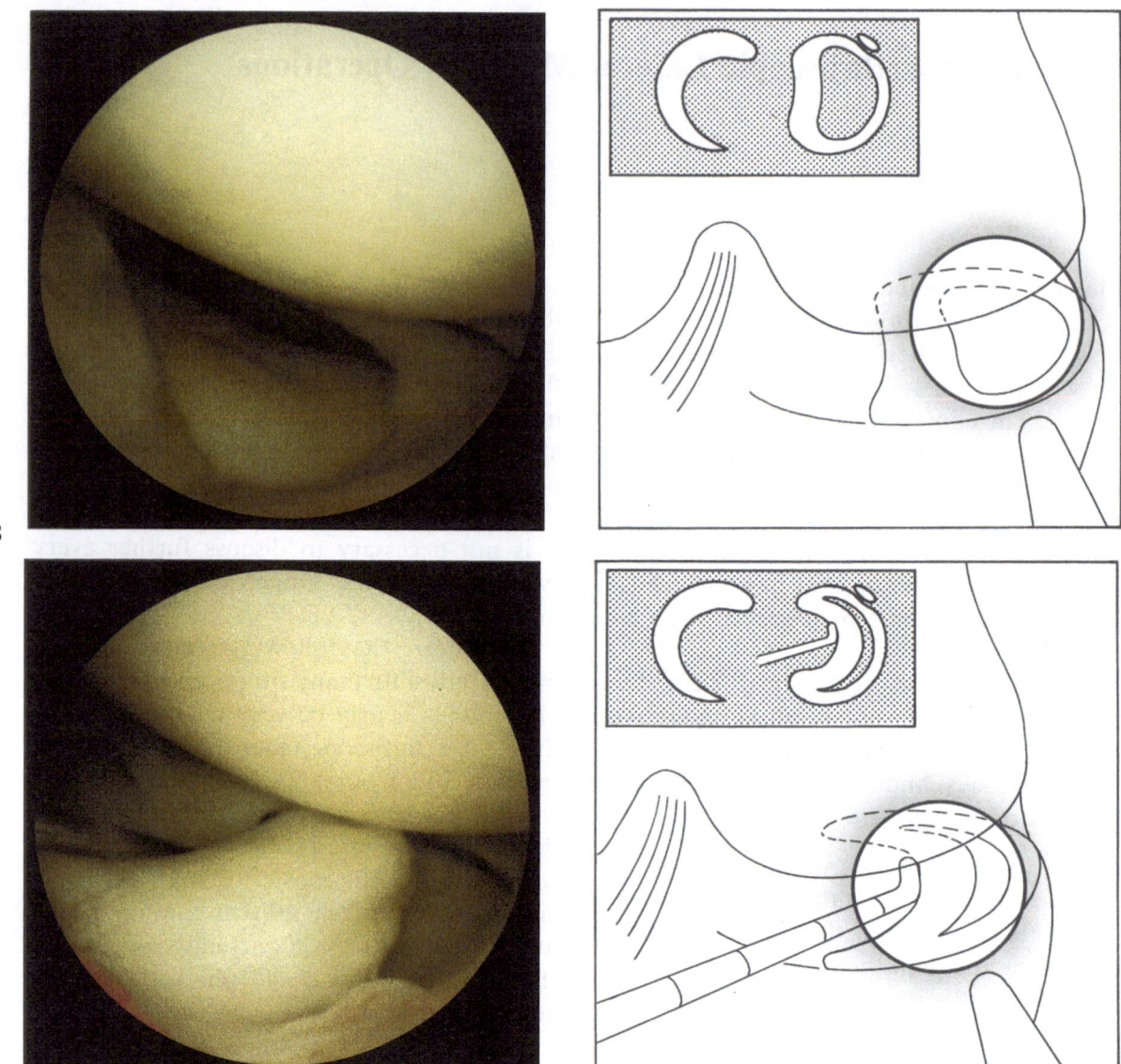

Fig. 168. Bucket-handle tear of lateral meniscus, with the bucket-handle portion displaced between the femoral condyles

Fig. 169. Reposition of the bucket-handle portion with the probe hook

Fig. 170. Beginning the resection of the lateral bucket-handle tear at the posterior horn with the basket forceps

Fig. 171. Transection of the connection to the base of the lateral bucket-handle portion at the posterior horn

Fig. 172. Resection of lateral bucket-handle portion: site of incision at posterior horn

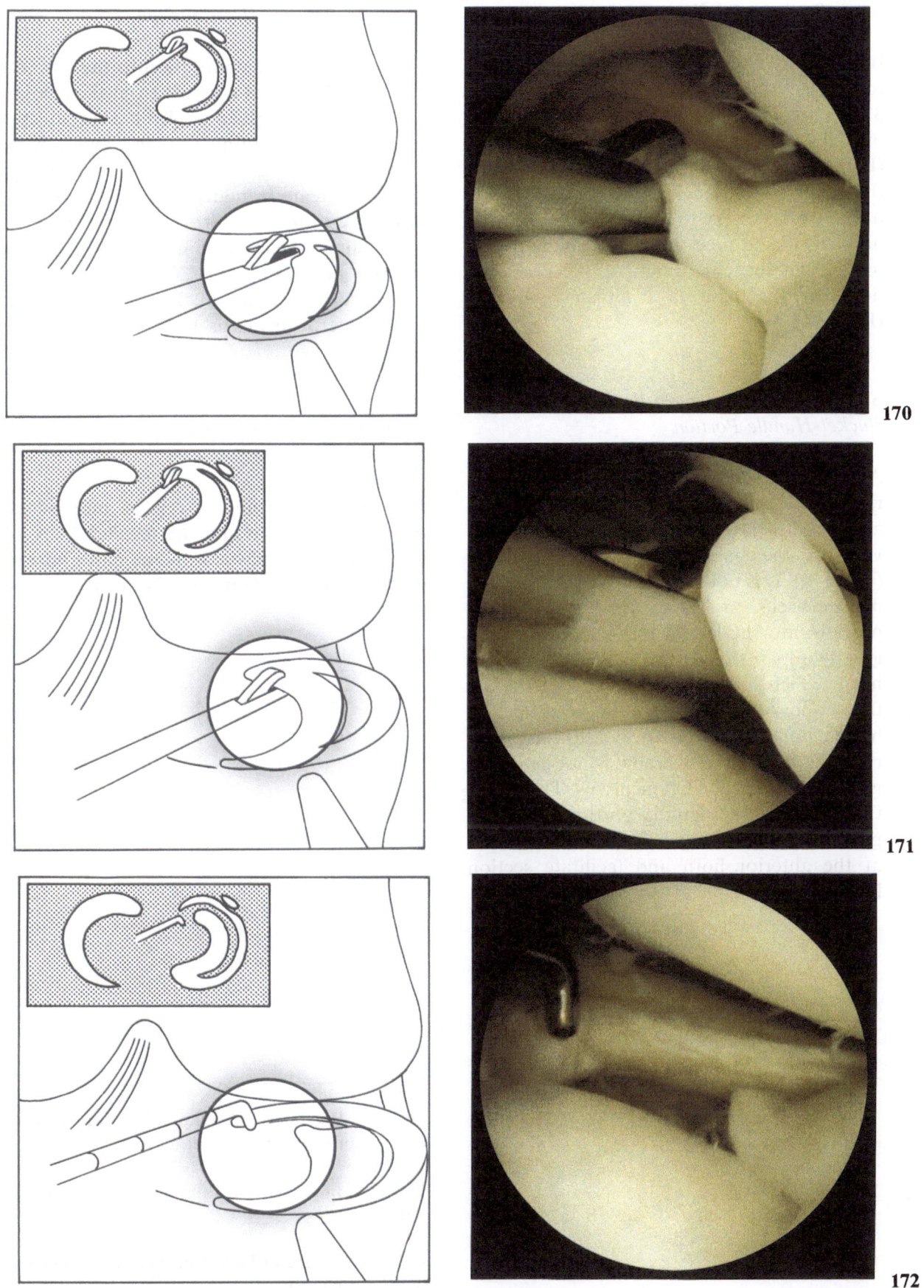

170

171

172

Stage 2: Posterior Horn Section

It is usually easy to transect the connection to the base at the posterior horn with a strong 3.4-mm basket forceps, working from the medial side through the intercondylar fossa (Fig. 170). To avoid too deep an incision into the body of the meniscus beyond the tear, it may be necessary to reintroduce the probe hook to locate precisely the position of the tear. Then the connection of the posterior horn to the base is completely divided (Fig. 171).

Stage 3: Displacement of the Bucket-Handle Portion

After completing the transection in the posterior horn region the bucket-handle portion can be dislocated laterally, giving a good view of the base of the posterior horn (Fig. 172). It is not necessary, as with the medial meniscus, to displace the bucket-handle portion into the lateral recess as this would greatly impair the view of the of the anterior horn, which lies directly in front of the arthroscope. Also, the risk of the freed bucket-handle portion floating away into the posterolateral recess irrecoverably is not nearly as great as with the medial meniscus. Therefore, the lateral bucket-handle portion is merely pulled slightly laterally to increase the tension at the anterior horn and facilitate section here.

Stage 4: Anterior Horn Section

Transection of the connection to the base at the anterior horn is effected from the medial incision, either with an angled basket forceps or with the dissecting scissors, and tapers from the free edge of the anterior horn towards the tear. In many cases it is easier to start by cutting away from the tear and end by dividing the connection to the base at the anterior horn (Fig. 173). When the transaction is completed the bucket-handle portion of the lateral meniscus lies free in the joint (Fig. 174).

Stage 5: Seizure and Extraction of the Bucket-Handle Portion

The slender grasping forceps is inserted at the second incision and the resected bucket-handle portion grasped at one end and extracted in its entirety from the joint (Fig. 175).

Fig. 173. Lateral bucket-handle portion: section ▷ of anterior horn with dissecting scissors

Fig. 174. Lateral bucket-handle portion free in joint

Fig. 175. Seizure of lateral bucket-handle portion with grasping forceps

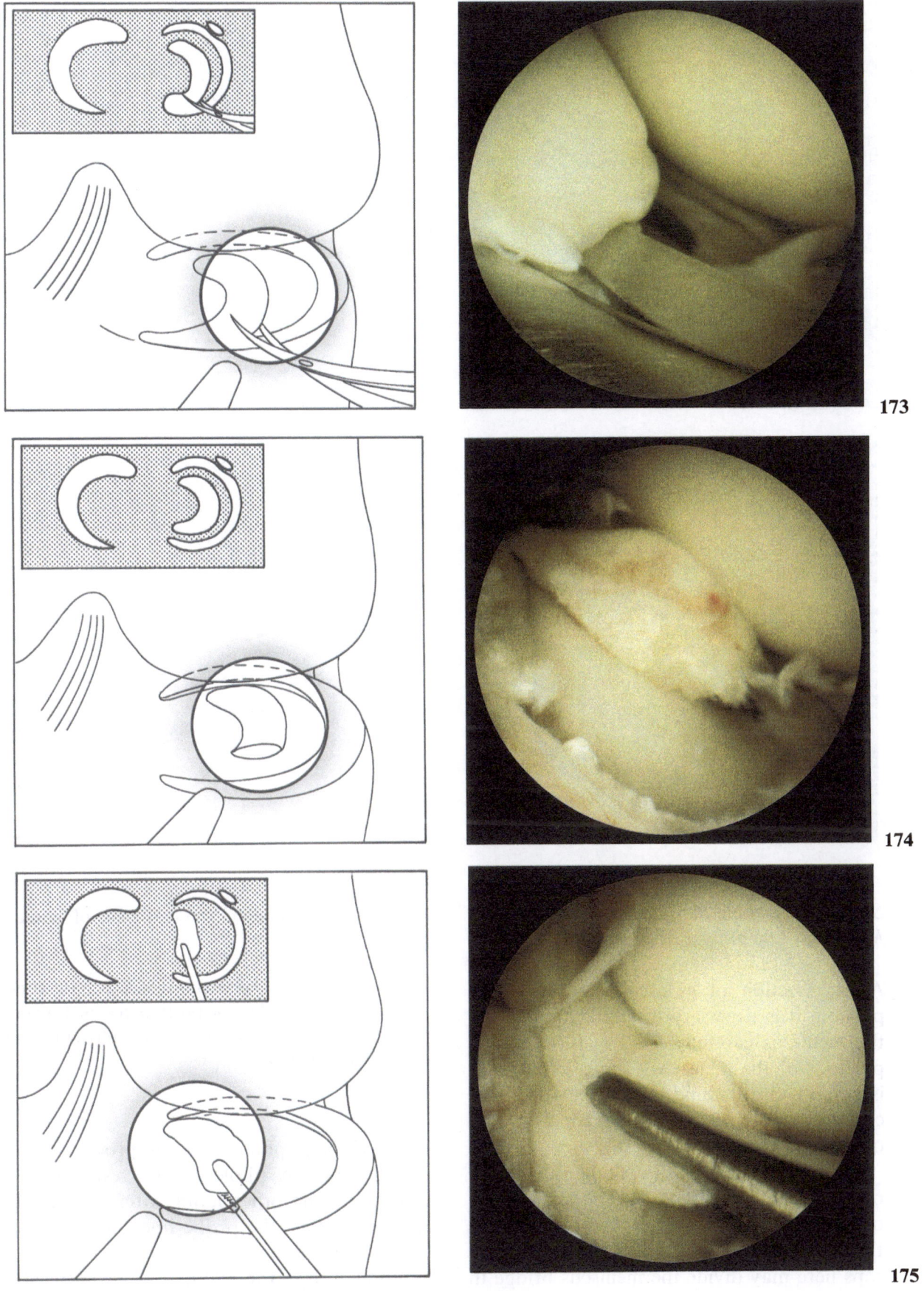

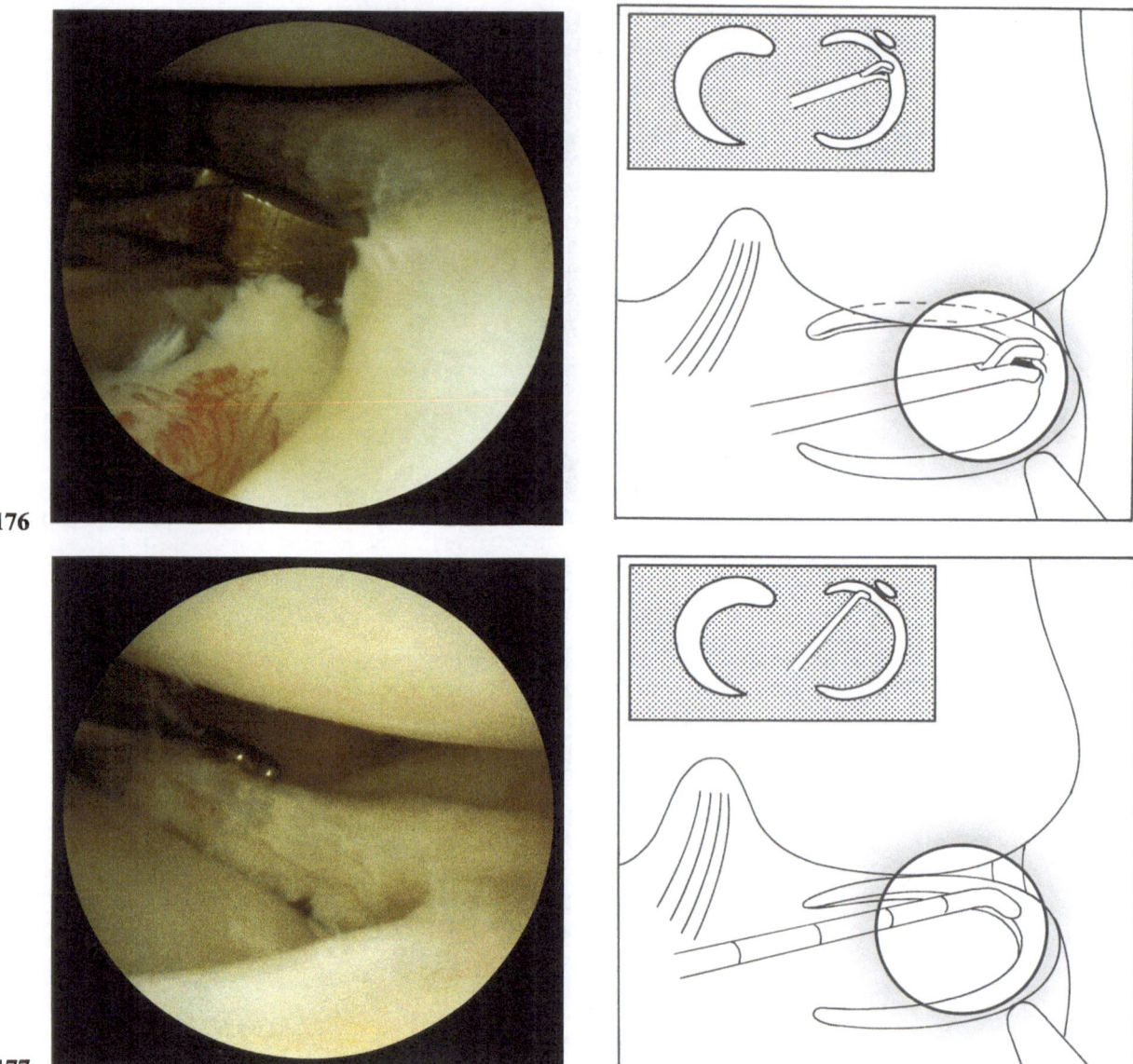

176

177

Stage 6: Checking the Base of the Meniscus, Smoothing, Afterresection

After resection of a lateral bucket-handle portion, it is necessary to check the base of the meniscus carefully for any further torn portions of the meniscus. The residual base is smoothed all round with the basket forceps, any frayings are removed, and any other tears resected (Fig. 176).

When trimming and touching up the base of the lateral meniscus, special care is required at the site of the popliteal hiatus. On the one hand, careless use of the basket forceps here may divide the meniscus bridge in

Fig. 176. Smoothing of residual base of lateral meniscus

Fig. 177. Checking the lateral meniscus base after resection of bucket-handle portion, testing for stability of the bridge in front of the popliteal hiatus with the probe hook

front of the popliteus tendon, producing instability of the whole of the residual meniscus; on the other hand, after smoothing has been done, the probe hook must be inserted into the hiatus to check carefully the residual bridge for stability (Fig. 177). The

146

base of the meniscus should always be preserved as a bridge in front of the popliteal hiatus if possible. However, if this bridge is too slender, unstable, or no longer functional it must be resected, though this simultaneously implies a subtotal resection of the lateral meniscus. It is often useful to change the arthroscope from the anterolateral to the anteromedial incision for some stages of the operation, or even for the entire operation, to improve vision and facilitate the operative procedure.

20.2 Lateral Posterior Horn Resection

Longitudinal basal tears, flap tears, transverse fissures, or degenerative fraying at the posterior horn of the lateral meniscus call for sparing resection so as not to imperil the stability of the meniscus and therefore of the knee joint.

Fig. 178. Lateral meniscus: posterior horn tear with degenerative changes in meniscus and articular cartilage surfaces

Fig. 179. Demonstration of displacement of posterior horn of lateral meniscus with probe hook

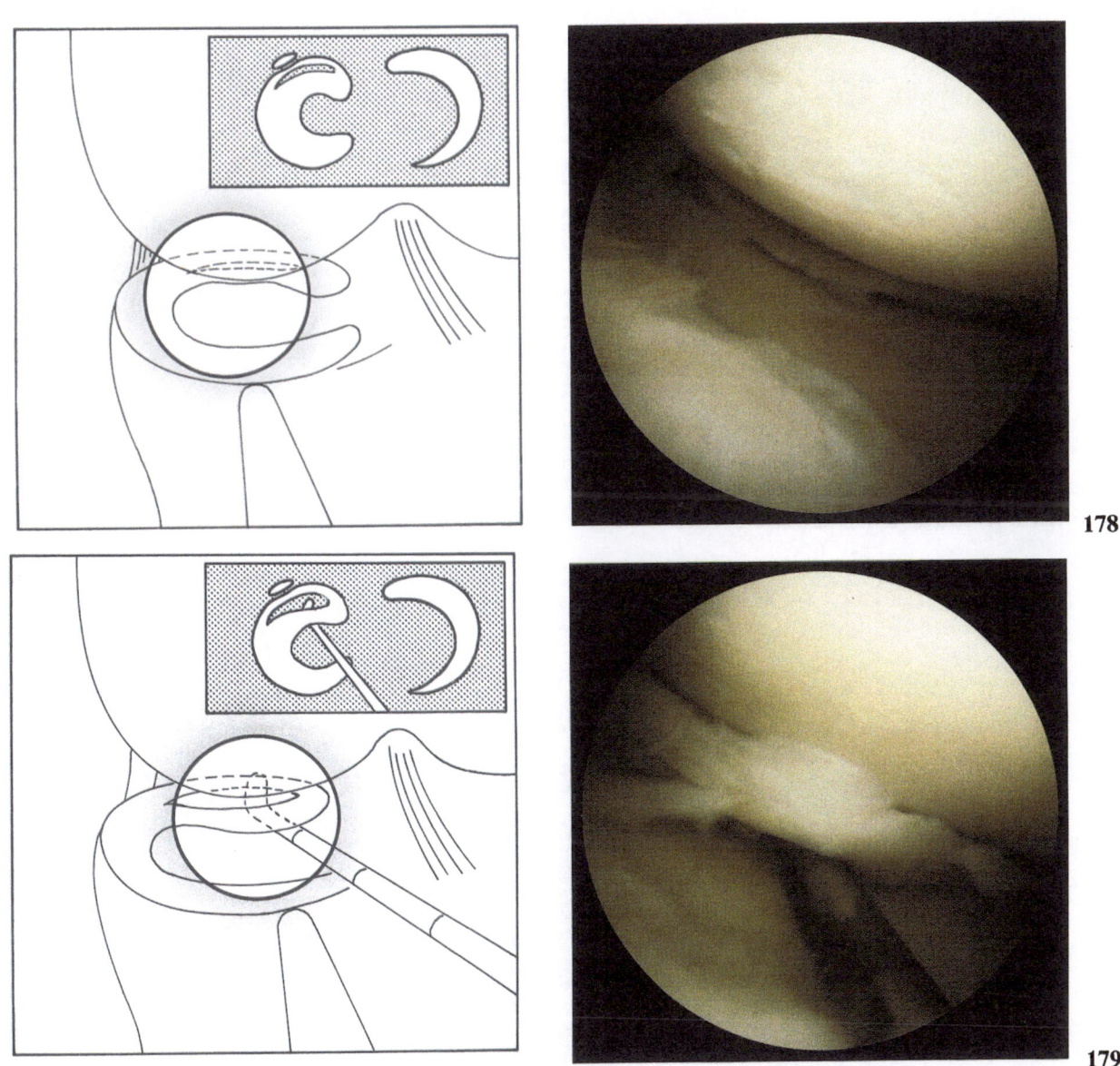

178

179

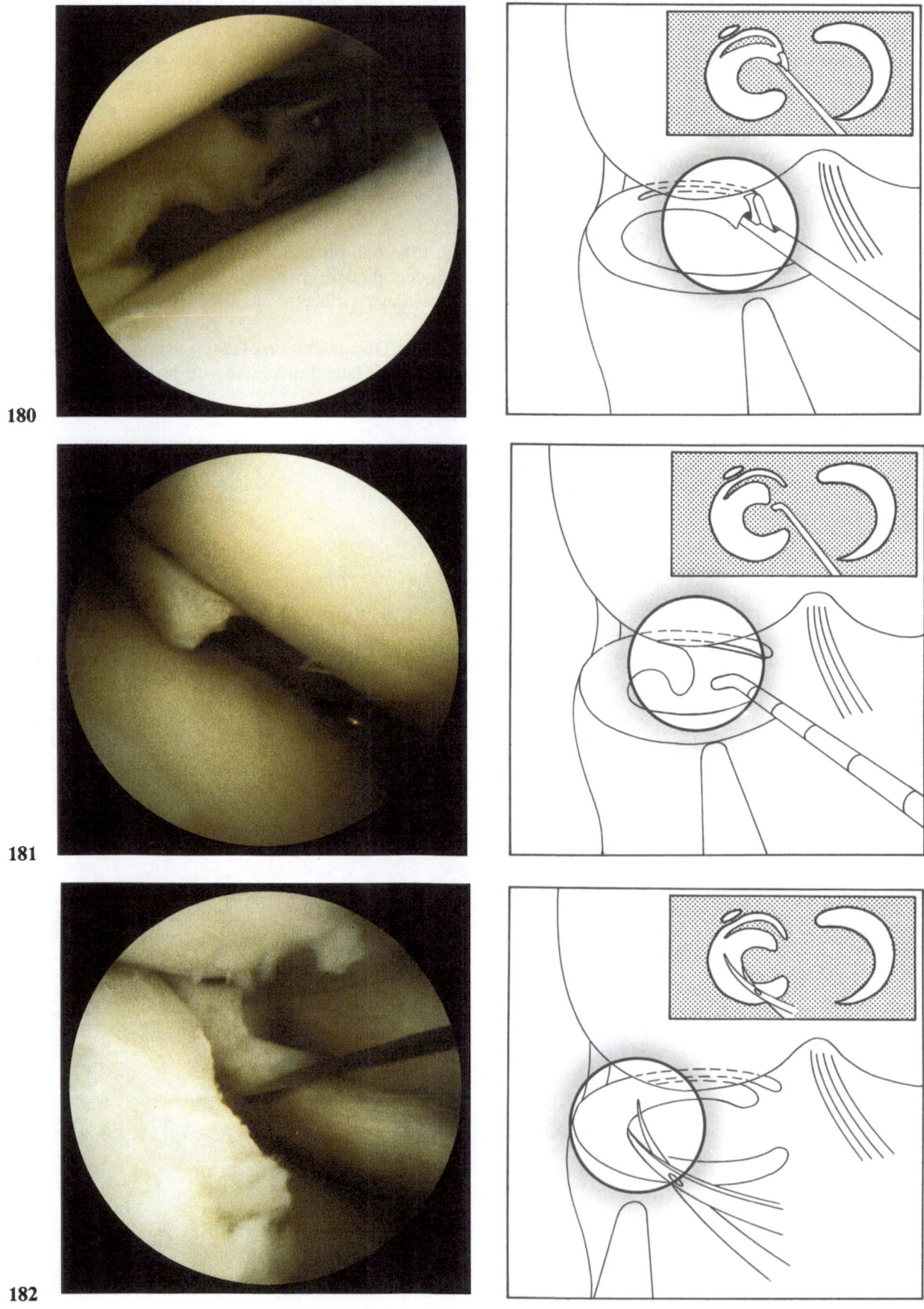

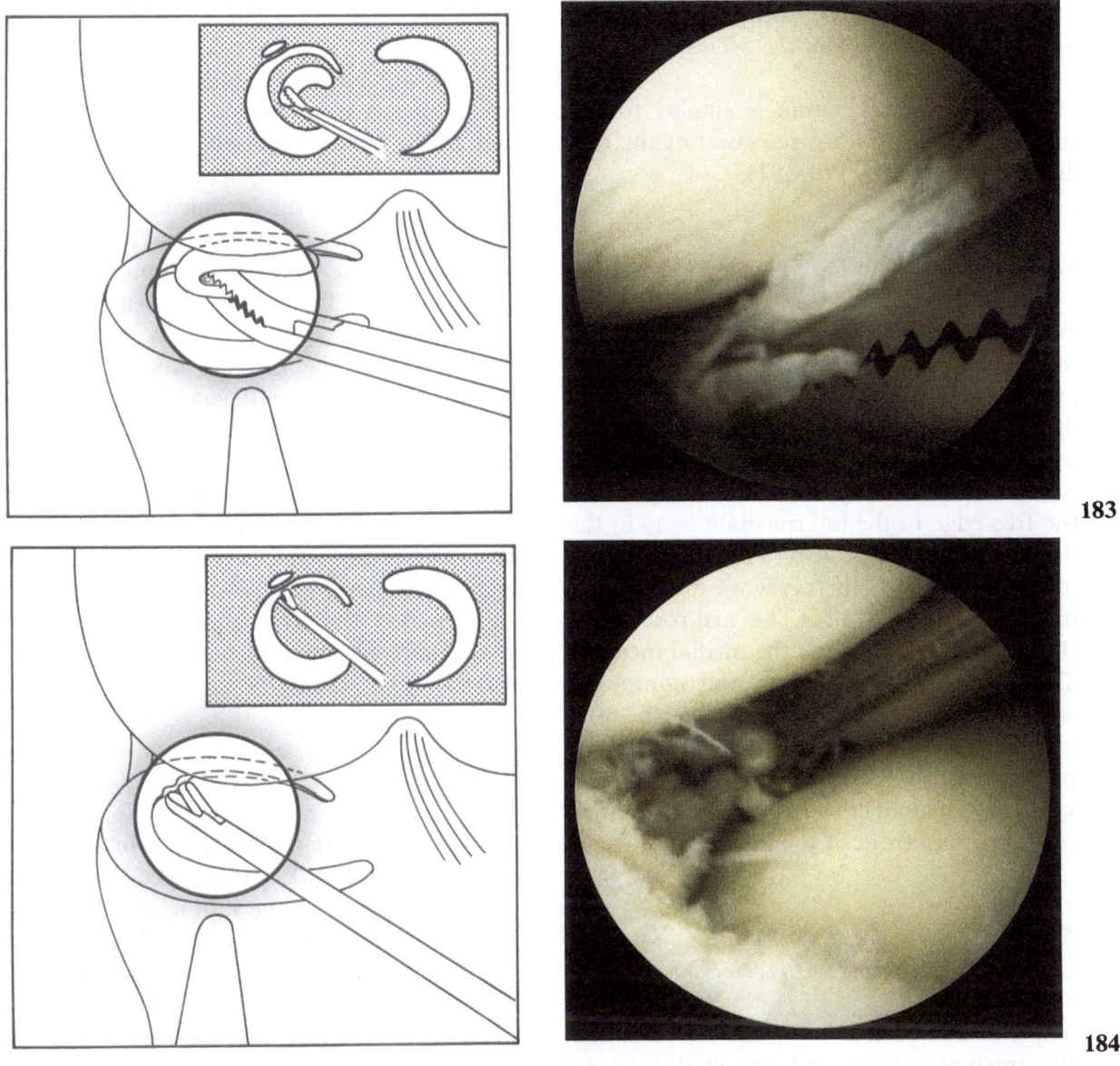

183

184

◁ **Fig. 180.** Beginning of resection of posterior horn of lateral meniscus from the intercondylar fossa with the basket forceps

Fig. 181. Posterior horn of lateral meniscus turned as a flap into the joint after division of connection to base

Fig. 182. Tapering resection in intermediate zone of lateral meniscus with dissecting scissors

Fig. 183. Seizure of separated posterior horn of lateral meniscus with grasping forceps

Fig. 184. Smoothing of residual base of lateral meniscus with basket forceps

Stages 1–3: Exposure, Posterior Horn Section, Repositioning of the Meniscus

Essentially, the procedure is similar to the stages in posterior horn resection of the medial meniscus (Figs. 178–181).

Stage 4: Division at the Intermediate Zone

With the arthroscope in the lateral incision, the extent of the tear is exposed with the probe hook from the medial aspect in the direction of the intermediate zone and the operative procedure then planned. Resection is begun with an angled basket forceps from the free edge in the intermediate zone in the direction of the tear. A notch is made in the meniscus to permit further work with dissecting scissors (Fig. 182). The arthroscope is then introduced through the medial incision. The resection is continued and completed with the dissecting scissors, from the previously made notch towards the tear at the posterior horn. Care must be taken to preserve an adequately broad bridge of the meniscus base in front of the popliteal tendon.

Stages 5–6: Seizure, Extraction, Checking, Smoothing, Afterresection

The freed meniscus fragment is seized with the grasping forceps and extracted in its entirety from the joint (Fig. 183). The residual base at the posterior horn is smoothed off from the medial incision (Fig. 184).

20.3 Lateral Anterior Horn Resection

The anterior horn or anterior half of the lateral meniscus are damaged much more often than in the medial meniscus.

Resection of this part of the meniscus constitutes one of the technically more difficult arthroscopic operations, as the affected part lies just in front of the optical system and the visual field is very often obscured by synovial fringes. In addition, the tangential impact of the instruments on the meniscus impairs their efficiency. The aim is a subtotal one-piece resection of the anterior horn with a tapering resection in the intermediate zone, leaving the entire posterior horn and without encroaching on the popliteal hiatus. Dissecting scissors prove very valuable here and are employed as in arthrotomy.

Provided the strict indications are met, as sparing a resection as possible is again performed in six stages:

Stage 1: Exposure

The entire extent of the tear is investigated with the probe hook, paying special attention to the extension of the lesion into the intermediate zone so as not to sacrifice unnecessarily too much of the meniscus (Fig. 185). Any existing vertical juxtabasal tears are displayed, so that they may be included in the incision.

Stage 2: Posterior Horn Section

The posterior horn remains untouched, provided it is intact. The site at the free edge in the intermediate zone at which the incision will later end is now notched (getting larger in the ventral direction) with an angled basket forceps (Fig. 186).

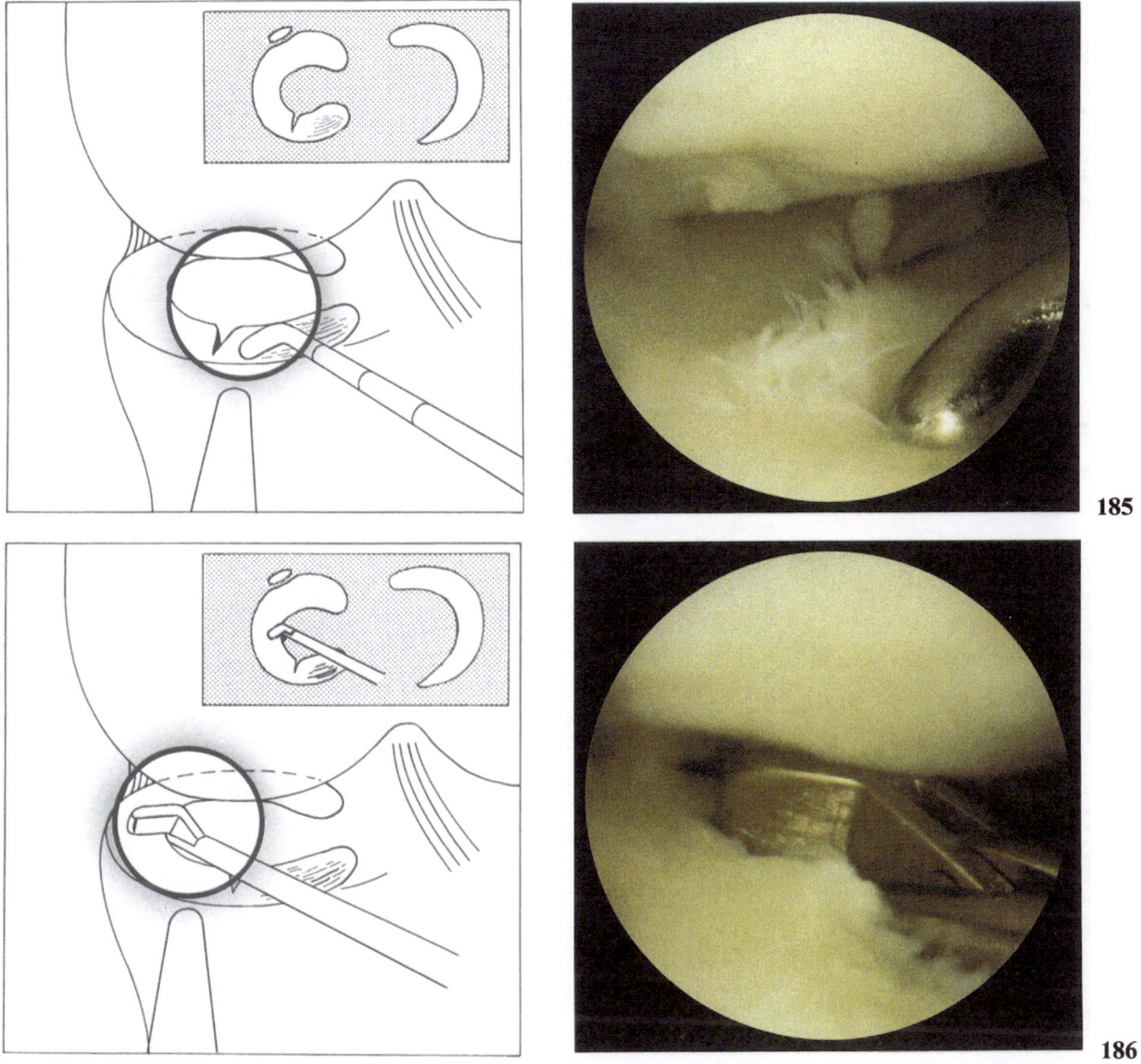

Fig. 185. Lateral meniscus: anterior horn lesion

Fig. 186. Tapering resection with angled basket forceps from intermediate zone to anterior horn

Stage 3: Repositioning

The anterior horn is again tested with the probe hook and the further procedure planned (Fig. 187).

Stage 4: Anterior Horn Section

The further operative procedure depends on the type of tear and the extent of the preexisting detachment of the anterior horn. Thus, if there is a longitudinal basal tear, a tapering cut can be made with dissecting scissors or

151

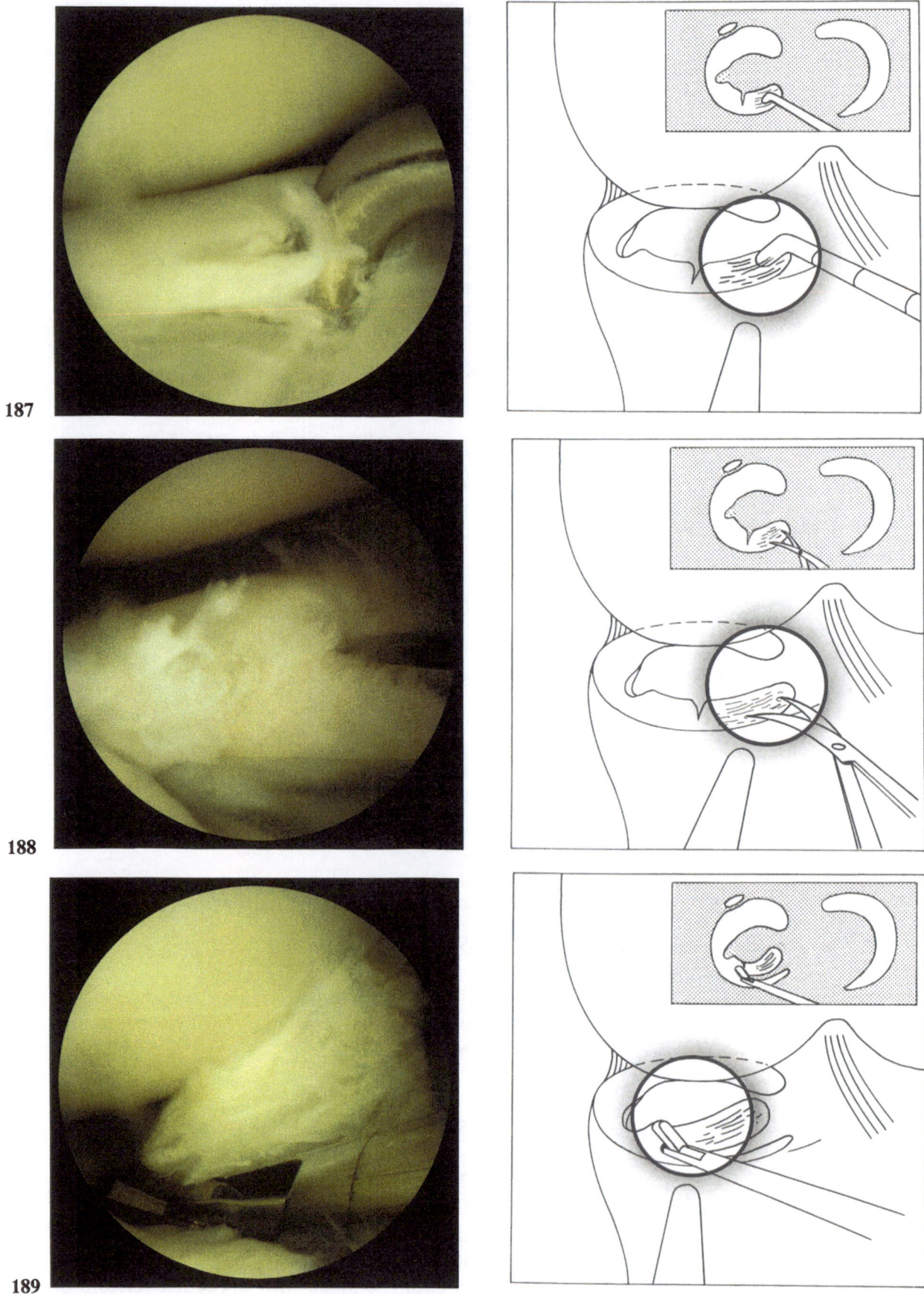

a straight basket forceps from the tear up to the prepared notch. For this, it is usually helpful to introduce the arthroscope from the medial side and the cutting instrument laterally.

If there is no juxtabasal vertical tear present from which to make a wider incision, the anterior horn is incised near its base from above with the dissecting scissors until one of the blades can be stuck through the "buttonhole." Then a cut is made, tapering up to the previously prepared notch, enabling the part of the meniscus to be resected to be safely demarcated from the part to be left.

This cut, once begun, is continued with the dissecting scissors along the base of the anterior horn in the direction of the distal attachment of the anterior cruciate ligament. In addition, the anterior horn is taken between the two blades of the scissors and the opened scissors are drawn ventrally so as to obtain a cut as close to the base as possible; the curve of the meniscus is cut following the anterior horn away from its base. The entire anterior horn to be resected, including any flaplike tears and transverse fissures, is now free in the joint.

Another possibility is to begin the resection from the distal attachment of the anterior cruciate ligament and to cut out the anterior horn longitudinally from there with the dissecting scissors (Fig. 188), the arthroscope being inserted at the anterolateral incision and the scissors anteromedially. There may be difficulties in obtaining a good view with this technique as the resection takes place immediately in front of the optical system. As described above, the line of incision is as close to the base as possible in order to obtain a subtotal resection in the usual manner. Normally, this can be done mainly with the dissecting scissors and the cut to the previously prepared notch is usually completed with a basket forceps (Fig. 189).

Stage 5: Seizure and Extraction

The anterior horn, now completely detached from the base, is seized with the narrow grasping forceps and extracted from the joint (Fig. 190). Floating off of the detached meniscus fragment into the lateral compartment is not nearly as much of a risk as at the me-

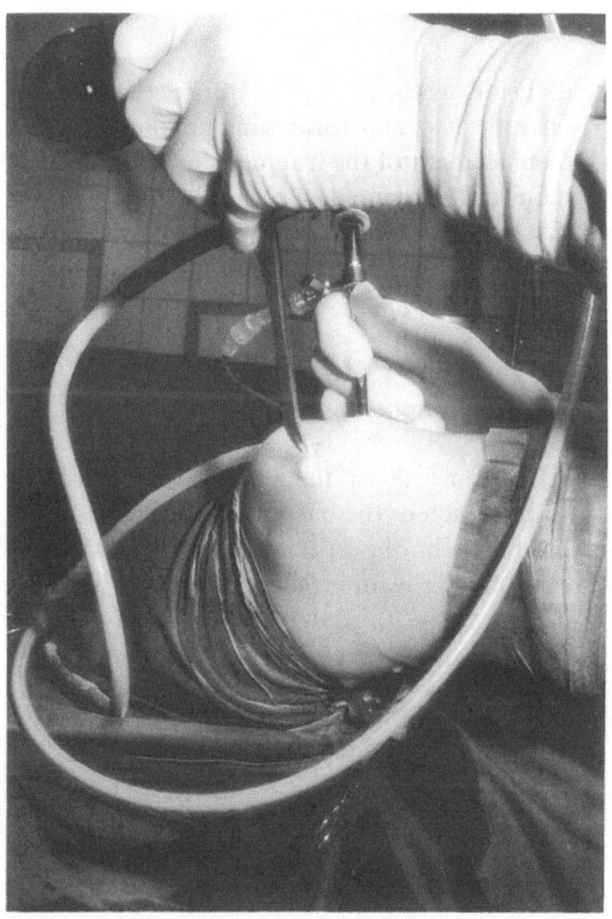

◁ **Fig. 187.** Palpating the damaged base of the anterior horn of the lateral meniscus with the probe hook

Fig. 188. Beginning of resection of lateral anterior horn with dissecting scissors

Fig. 189. Completion of resection of anterior horn of lateral meniscus with basket forceps

Fig. 190. Extraction of segment of meniscus from the joint

153

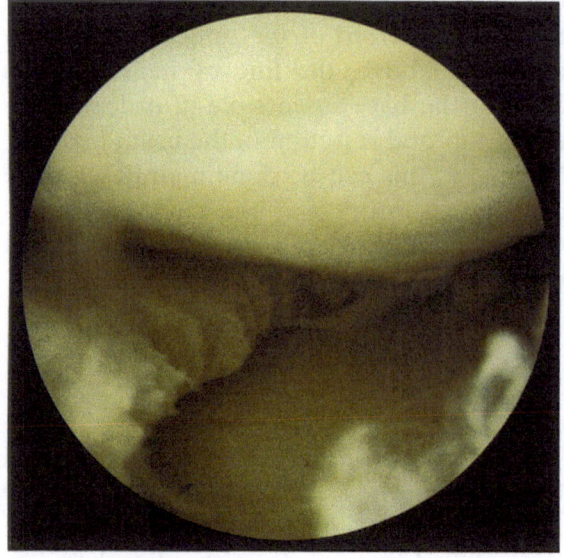

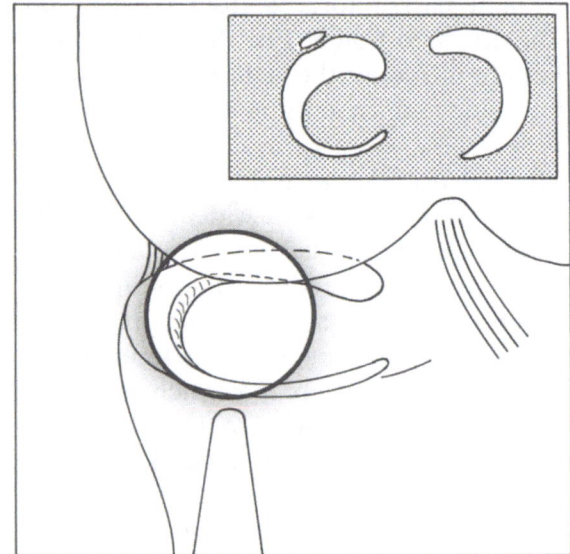

Fig. 191. Condition of lateral meniscus after partial resection of anterior horn

dial side, as the posterolateral recess does not have the saccular form which makes anterior displacement of the fragment so difficult. The meniscus fragment which has temporarily disappeared can be retrieved with the probe hook or the sucker into the anterior joint space.

Stage 6: Smoothing

After removal of the part of the meniscus to be resected, the base is again checked with the probe hook, especially at the tapering resection in the intermediate zone (Fig. 191). Any fraying, ragged tears, or other fissures are smoothed off with the basket forceps.

20.4 Discoid Lateral Meniscus

The diagnosis of this anatomic variant presents few difficulties as a rule. The free edge of the lateral meniscus does not present its typical half-moon appearance in the lateral joint compartment, but the entire compartment is seen to be occupied with meniscus tissue with the free edge in the intercondylar fossa (Fig. 192). The existence of a discoid meniscus is not in itself an indication for subtotal resection. However, the meniscus usually exhibits fissures or marked degenerative changes in its central portion which require subtotal resection. The subtotal removal of a lateral meniscus, even if it is the normal half-moon shape and particularly when it is discoid, is technically rather demanding and is performed in the following stages.

Stage 1: Exposure

The extent of the tear in the lateral meniscus and the planned line of resection are again exposed with the probe hook.

154

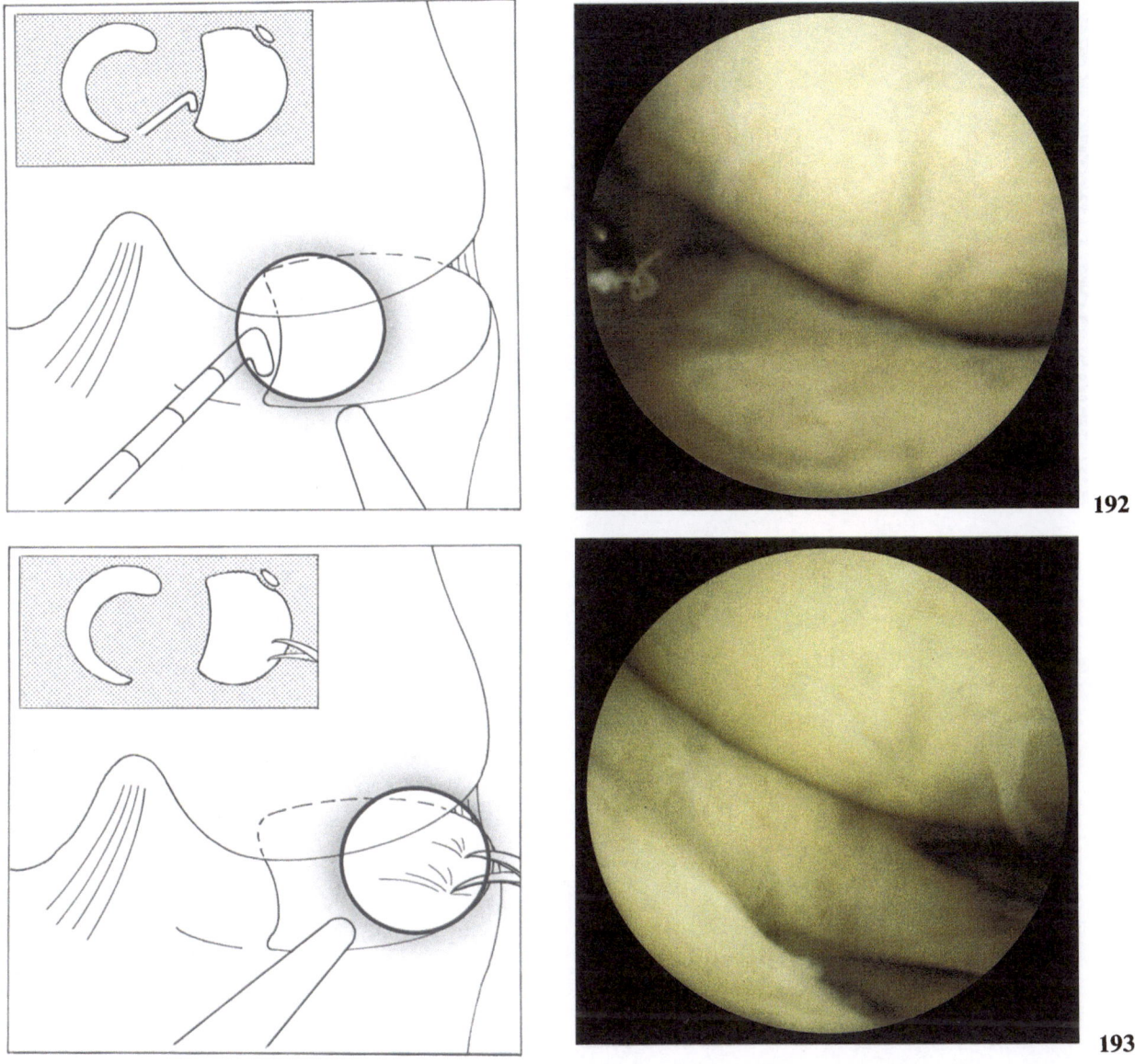

Fig. 192. Discoid lateral meniscus

Fig. 193. Beginning of resection of lateral discoid meniscus with dissecting scissors at intermediate basal zone

Stage 2: Anterior Horn Section

Especially with a discoid meniscus, it is not usually possible to begin the resection at the posterior horn as the joint space is occupied by the meniscus and a free view of the base of the posterior horn is not available. Therefore, a "buttonhole" is constructed close to the base of the meniscus at the transition from the anterior horn to the intermediate zone, using the dissecting scissors from the lateral incision and under observation from the medial side (Fig. 193). One blade of the scissors is stuck through the hole so created

155

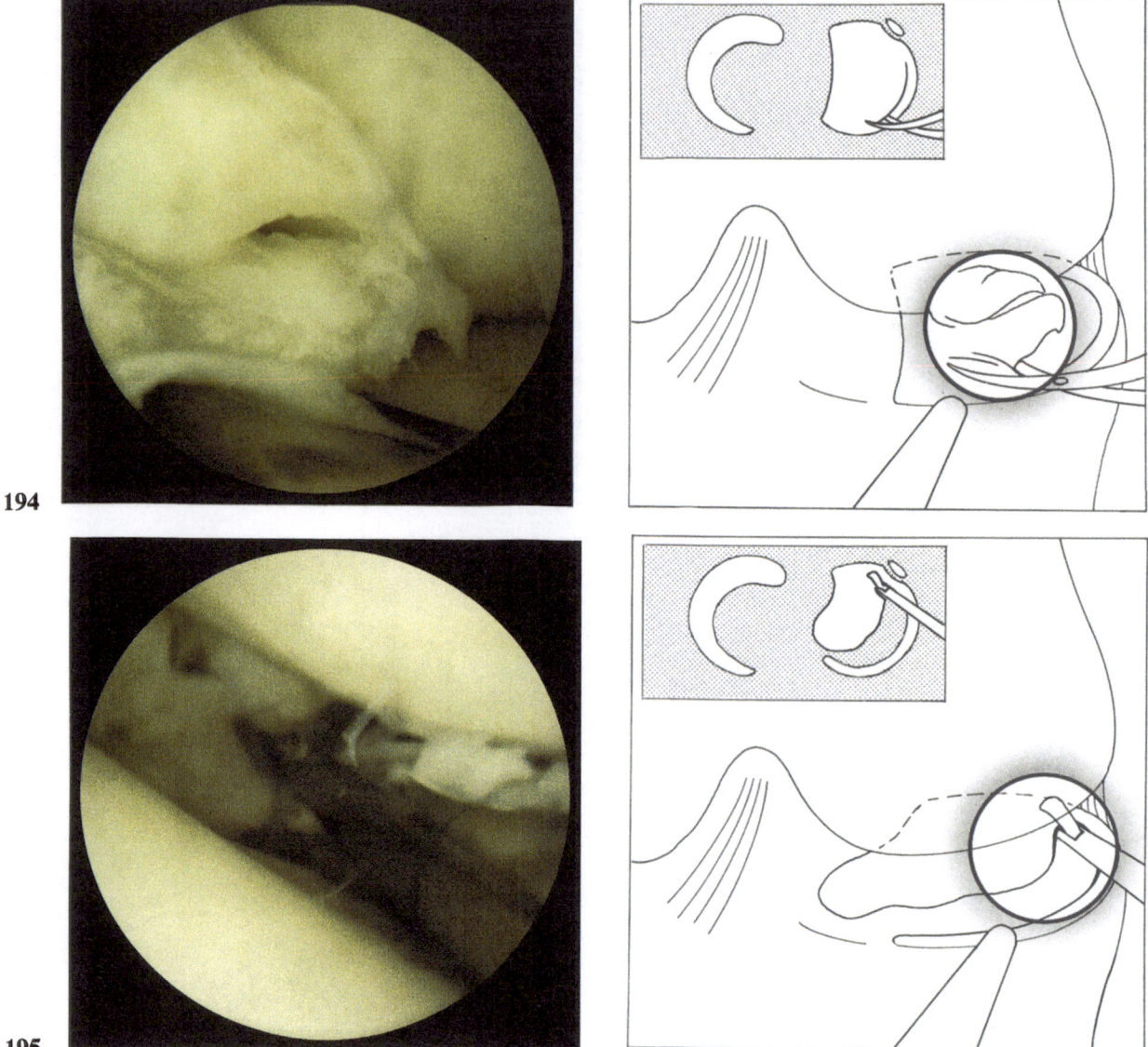

Fig. 194. Subtotal removal of discoid lateral meniscus at anterior horn

Fig. 195. Resection of posterior horn of discoid lateral meniscus with basket forceps

and the base subtotally divided along the anterior horn, in typical fashion (Fig. 194). The incision is carried up to the distal attachment of the anterior cruciate ligament. Then the scissors are switched dorsally from the primary incision and the initial incision at the base is pursued in the direction of the popliteal hiatus. Leaving as much of a meniscus bridge as possible in front of the hiatus, the surgeon cuts with the scissors or basket forceps up to the posterior horn insofar as the visual field and the curve of the condyle permit posterior horn section from here (Fig. 195).

Stage 3: Repositioning

The arthroscope is introduced from the lateral side, and from the medial side the lateral meniscus is drawn as far laterally as possible

156

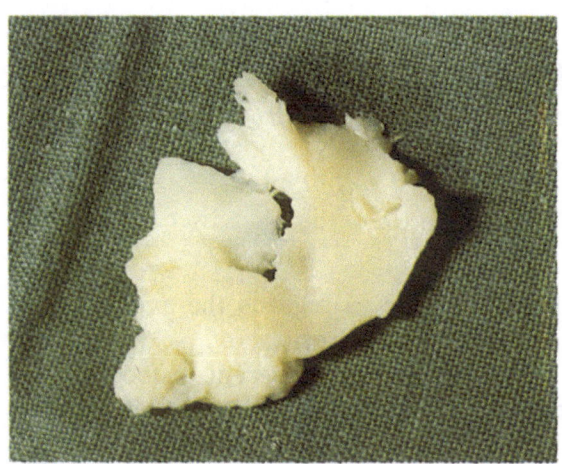

Fig. 196. Specimen: discoid lateral meniscus after subtotal arthroscopic resection

with the probe hook in order to expose the persisting base of the posterior horn from the intercondylar fossa.

Stage 4: Posterior Horn Section

The residual connection to the base at the posterior horn is then in turn divided with the straight basket forceps. Should exposure present difficulties, a narrow grasping forceps can be additionally introduced via the medial incision and used to seize the discoid

meniscus, now largely detached. Traction on the forceps will bring the residual bridge at the posterior horn more into the visual field, where it can be transected with the basket forceps.

Stage 5: Seizure and Extraction

The discoid meniscus, now lying quite free in the joint, is grasped with the forceps. If it proves difficult to extract the relatively large discoid meniscus in its entirety from the joint through the incision, it can be spread out with scissors and then removed as a whole (Fig. 196).

Stage 6: Smoothing

The residual meniscus base is again tidied up all round with the basket forceps. Cautious smoothing is indicated at the region of the popliteal hiatus so as to leave behind an adequately stable meniscus bridge. After completing the resection, the residual meniscus base is checked with the probe hook (Fig. 197).

Fig. 197. Operative result after subtotal lateral meniscectomy

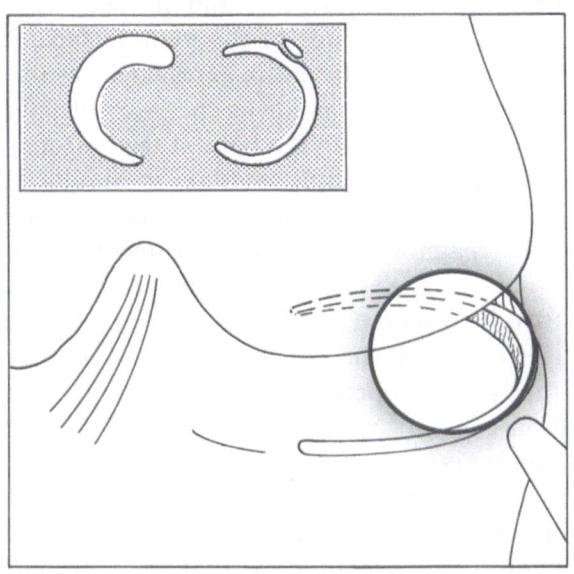

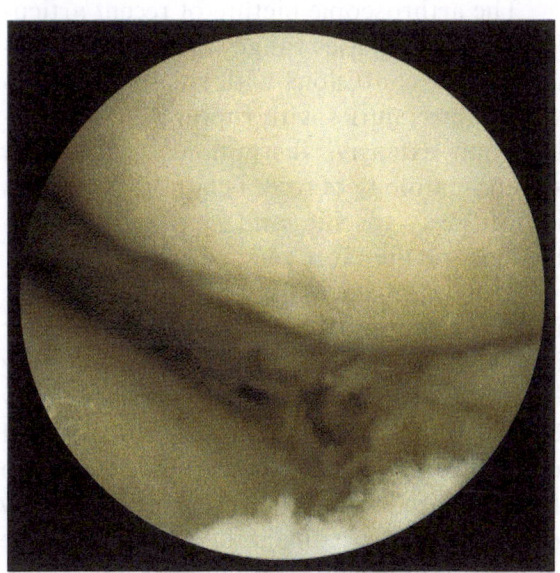

CHAPTER 21
Procedures on the Articular Cartilage

Neither clinical and radiologic investigation nor arthrography, nor even a small trial arthrotomy, can compare with arthroscopy in diagnosing the degree of damage to the articular surface of the knee joint. None of the other investigative techniques provide nearly as much and as reliable information on the state of the joint surface as arthroscopy. Assessment of the articular cartilage of the knee presents no major difficulties even to the less-experienced arthroscopist. All the cartilage surfaces – the back of the patella, the patellofemoral articular surfaces, the femoral condyles, the joint surfaces of the tibial head and the intercondylar region – are well visualized with arthroscopy. Under normal circumstances they show a completely smooth surface with a shiny gloss. Inspection alone of the articular cartilage is not enough; it is an essential part of the investigation to palpate the cartilage layer with the blunt probe hook to assess the consistency and elasticity of the cartilage. Healthy joint cartilage is slightly elastic; when the layer is damaged, the probe sinks into the softened cartilage.

The arthroscopic picture of recent articular cartilage injuries ranges from foci of softening and contusions with small fissures to very severe injuries with rupture of the cartilage and extensive disruption. The clinical symptomatology of recent chondral fractures is in no way specific, and most recent cartilage lesions therefore remain undetected.

The use of the arthroscope for diagnosis in recently injured joints, therefore, is of great importance. Any cartilage lesions that may be present can generally be diagnosed only by this means. Such lesions may be smoothed off arthroscopically and disrupted cartilage fragments removed from the joint. The early diagnosis and treatment of recent cartilage injuries with the arthroscope is of great pro-

phylactic value as regards the avoidance of posttraumatic arthrosis.

The diagnosis of recent osteochondral fractures is usually confirmed by the inevitable hemarthrosis and the radiologic demonstration of the displaced fragments. Here, the importance of arthroscopy lies in the exposure and inspection of the cartilage defect and the displaced fragments. Within the joint, the size of the displaced fragment, the cancellous component still present, and the site of the defect are to be assessed. These criteria are decisive in deciding whether the osteochondral fragment is to be replaced and reattached or simply removed.

A *chronic* cartilage lesion giving rise to no significant clinical or radiologic features is the commonest incidental finding on arthroscopic investigation of the knee joint. Arthroscopy is usually indicated on other grounds, such as intraarticular limitation of movement due to a meniscus injury or loose bodies. Very frequently, the arthroscopic image shows localized or extensive fraying at the femoral condyles, occasionally also at the tibial articular surfaces, and infractions or superficial abrasions of the joint surface. In advanced cases the entire cartilage layer may be ground down as far as the layer of sclerosed bone covering the base of the defect.

The arthroscopic picture is similar in chondromalacia patellae, which can be clinically diagnosed much more often than the other cartilage lesions. Apart from simple foci of softening, the commonest appearance is fraying of the cartilage layer, and more rarely burst-open areas of cartilage destruction which occasionally also extend down to the bone.

The arthroscopic treatment of cartilage lesions always presents a compromise. It should be perfectly clear that no instrument

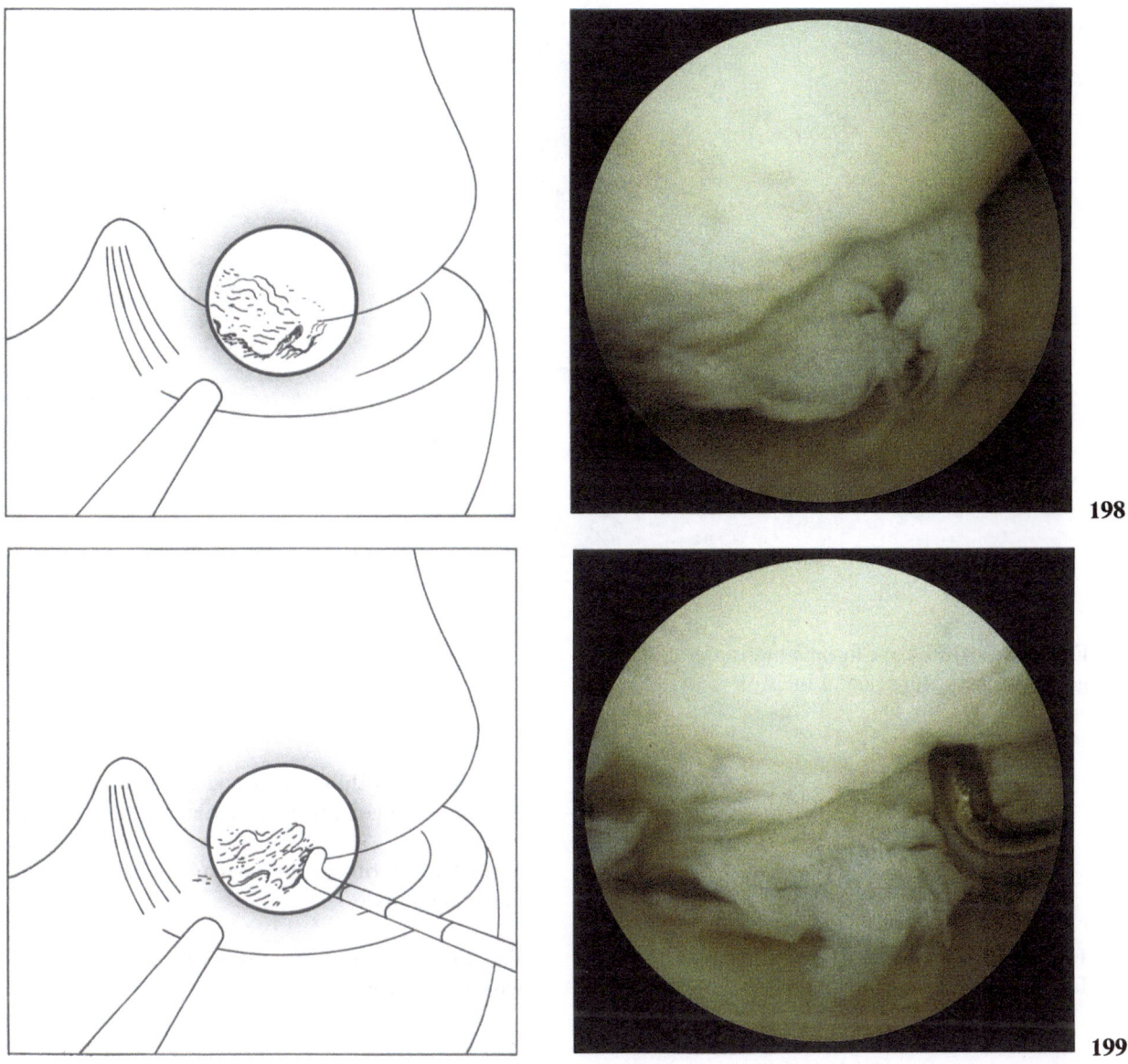

used via the arthroscope can achieve as precise, minimal, and yet tidy smoothing of the articular surface as can be obtained in an open procedure. However, the question is whether the only slightly better therapeutic result obtained by arthrotomy justifies the much greater operative expenditure, and whether the long-term prognosis for the knee is significantly improved thereby.

In the authors' opinion, limited soft foci and frayings can easily be tidied up arthroscopically. A small cartilage gouge is inserted through a second incision and the cartilage surface carefully smoothed (Figs. 198–204).

Fig. 198. Large cartilage defect at medial femoral condyle

Fig. 199. Demonstration of cartilage defect and its extent with probe hook

The turned-out margins of the defect can likewise be evened out with this gouge or with a basket forceps. It is also the authors' opinion that the motor-driven instruments of the different manufacturers, with their various smoothing, polishing, and resection heads, provide no significant improvement in

159

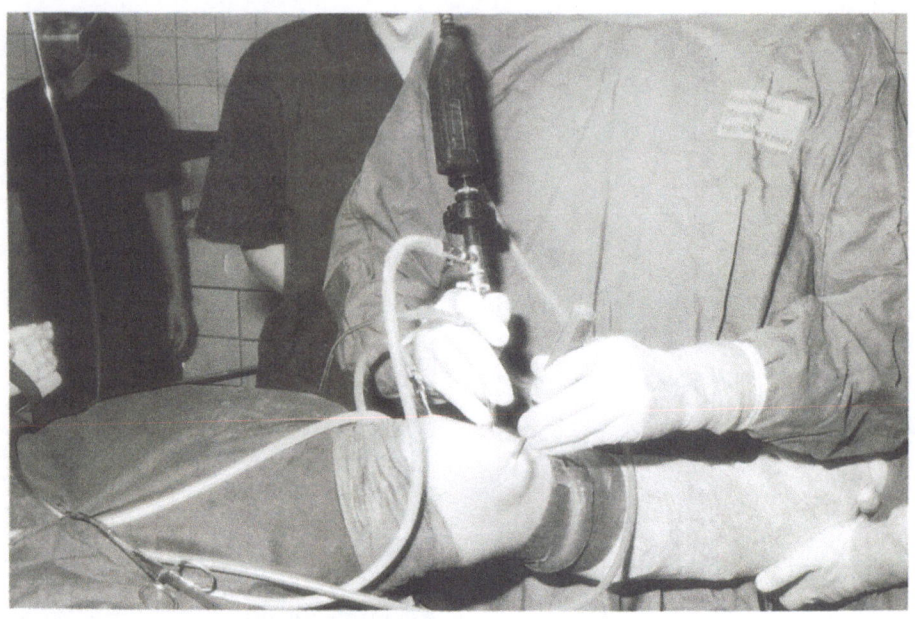

Fig. 200. Arthroscope in the anterolateral incision, gouge in the anteromedial incision

Fig. 202. Smoothing of turned-out margins of de- ▷ fect and softened areas of cartilage with the gouge

Fig. 203. Smoothed-out cartilage defect at medial femoral condyle

Fig. 201. Removal of degenerated flaps of cartilage at medial femoral condyle

Fig. 204. Resection of residual cartilage fringes with basket forceps

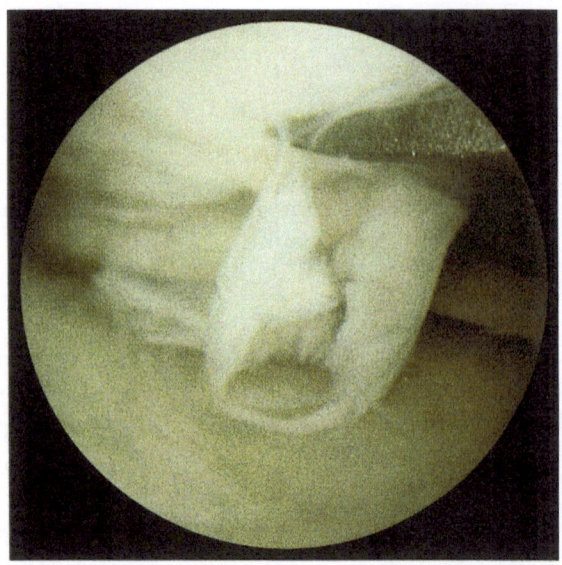

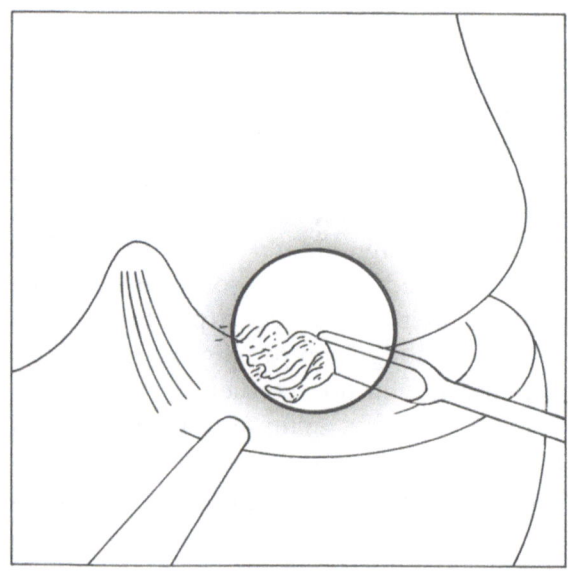

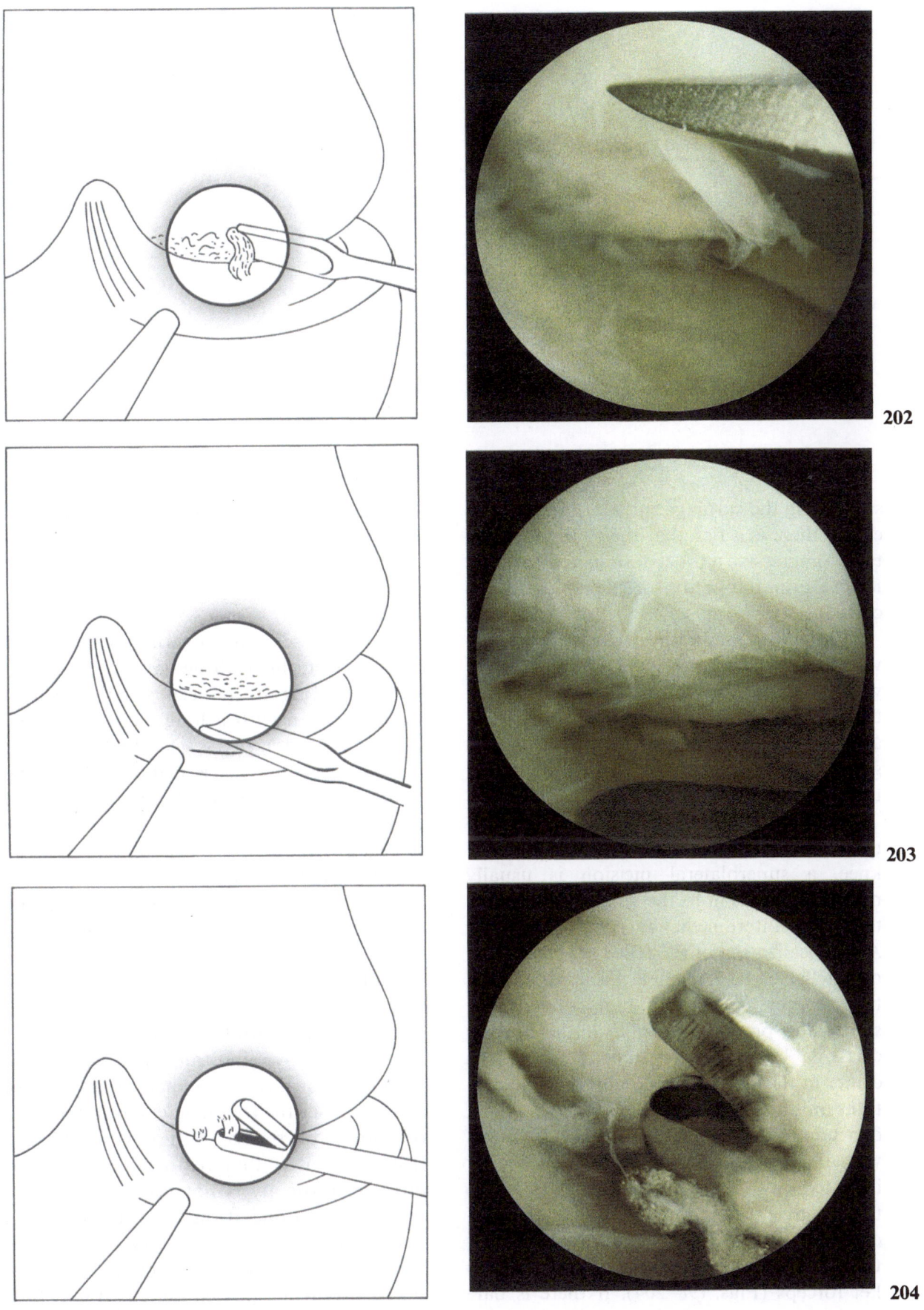

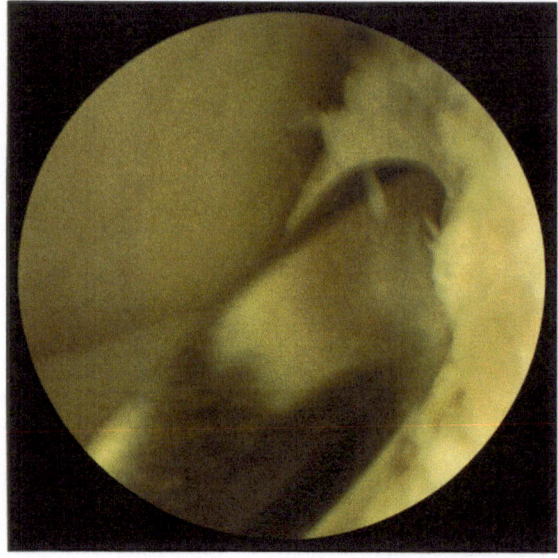

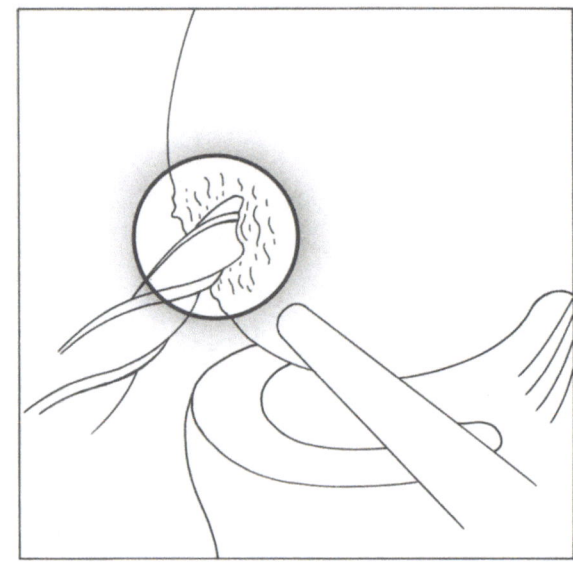

Fig. 205. Drilling of the sclerotic base of the cartilage defect

smoothing the cartilage surface, and to some extent there is a risk that their use may lead to too aggressive a procedure such as overextensive grinding or too deep planing of the cartilage layer.

In connection with extensive and advanced cartilage lesions one must also ask what therapeutic improvement can be obtained by arthrotomy in comparison with an arthroscopic procedure, and whether the progress of the existing arthrosis can be halted thereby.

For the smoothing of chondromalacia patellae, undertaken with hyperextension of the knee, a superolateral incision is usually needed in addition to the standard anterolateral and anteromedial incisions (Fig. 107). After localization of the focus at the posterior patellar surface, the defect is accessed with the sharpest possible 8-mm gouge. The smoothing process is begun at the healthy cartilage layer and continued toward the center of the defect; the chondromalacic portions are then shaved off with the gouge and, depending on their size, are either extracted with the grasping forceps or are sucked or irrigated out. A similar procedure applies to the relatively common defects at the condyles, in that shredded projections can for the most part be nibbled away with the basket forceps (Figs. 198–204). If there is bare

bone with a sclerotic covering at the center of the defect, this is drilled at several points, the drill being introduced via the arthroscopic incision with a long tissue-protective sheath (Fig. 205). If the sclerotic layer is not excessively hard, these drillholes into the spongiosa can also be made with a very small sharp curet. The drill debris is very carefully sucked away.

The very high magnification of the actual conditions in the arthroscopic image on the monitor, which renders every unevenness visible, and the far from perfect equipment for smoothing the cartilage are adverse factors that may leave the critical surgeon not altogether satisfied with his results.

Arthroscopy is indicated in osteochondritis dissecans only when there is any doubt as to whether the fragment can be reattached or should be removed. If it is established from the outset that reattachment is to be done, arthroscopy is not necessary; arthrotomy will be done at once and the fragment fixed with Kirschner wires. In doubtful cases arthroscopy can provide additional information as to further procedure, and it may then be that the fragment will be removed and the defect smoothed off.

Fixation of the fragment with special instruments and fine pins is very attractive at first sight. Obviously, the bed of the fragment can be touched up under arthroscopic vision, but processing of the fragment itself is not successful. Such processing is often necessary, however, to obtain an exact fit when the fragment has been detached for some time.

Advanced erosion and defects in the articular cartilage which have already led to radiologically demonstrable arthrotic changes do not enter the sphere of arthroscopy and arthroscopic treatment.

The authors have no long-term experience or recent results with the abrasion arthroplasty so strongly advocated by Johnson. With this technique the last cartilage remnants and the sclerotic bony layers are removed with motor-driven shavers after exposure of the bone. The worn-out hyaline cartilage is then replaced by fibrocartilage. The results of such radical treatment are still awaited.

Persistent intraarticular disorders of movement and especially recurrent attacks of locking such as occur in meniscus injuries cause severe mechanical cartilage damage which is often encountered at the medial side of the joint. This medial cartilage attrition then leads to a varus deformity.

Often, treatment is limited in a joint so damaged; when it is clear that the problem is one of locking, intraarticular obstructions to movement can be removed. However, the mainstay of treatment is usually osteotomy in the supracondylar area or at the upper end of the tibia to correct an established malposition and to transfer weight transmission to the still intact articular cartilage at the opposite side (Figs. 206–209).

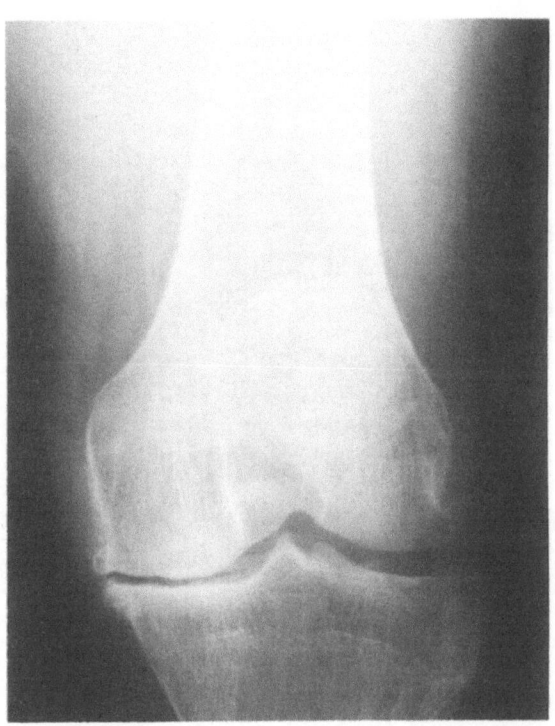

Fig. 206. Left knee with varus arthrosis and marked narrowing of the medial joint space

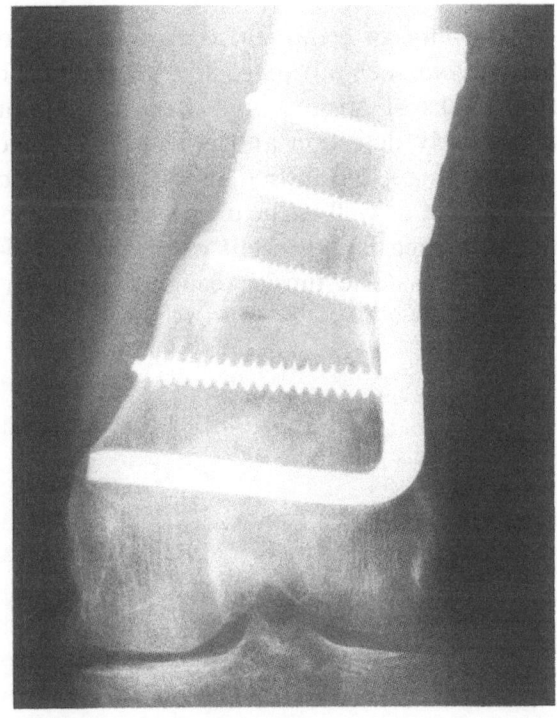

Fig. 207. The case shown in Fig. 206: result after corrective supracondylar osteotomy, restoration of medial joint space

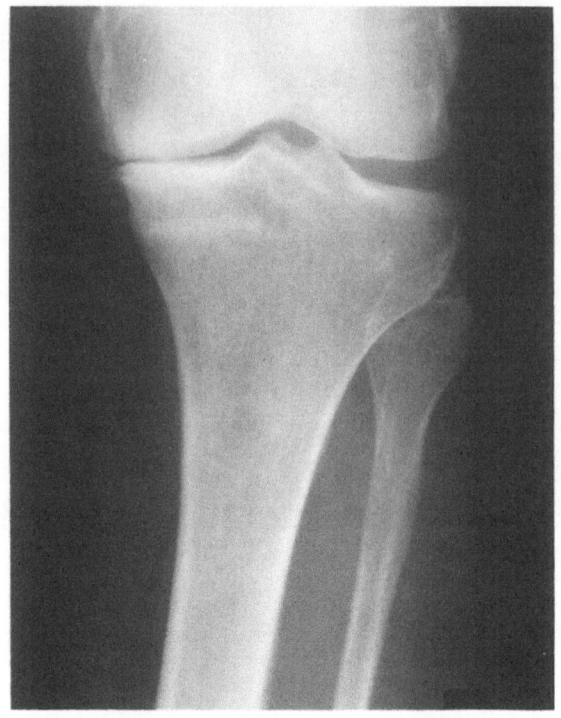 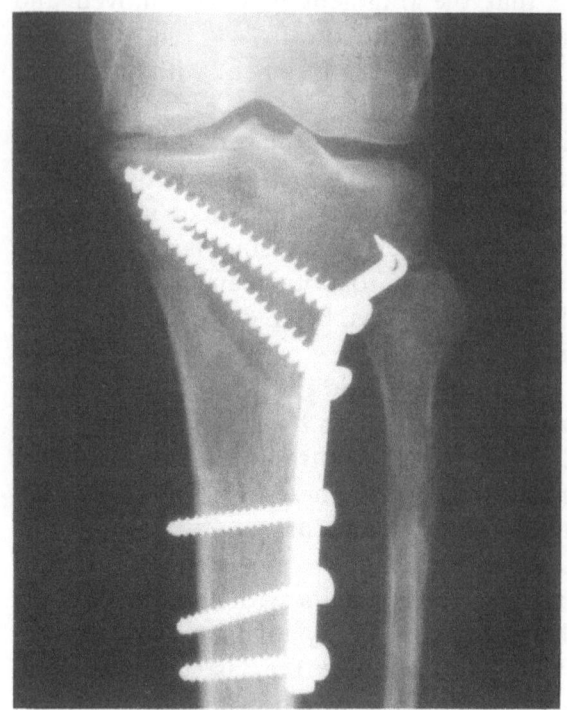

Fig. 208. Unstable varus arthrosis of the knee with marked narrowing of the medial joint space and deformity of the lower leg

Fig. 209. The same case as in Fig. 208: result after valgus osteotomy

The aim of treatment, however, should be to avoid such advanced states. One of the main tasks of arthroscopy of the knee joint is the early detection and prompt operative treatment of intraarticular obstruction to movement, as well as the diagnosis and treatment of preexisting recent or chronic cartilage lesions. The timely recognition of impaired movement within the joint and of the existence of cartilage lesions by means of arthroscopy allows early elimination of the functional disorder, either by arthroscopic operation or by arthrotomy. The prognosis for the joint is thereby significantly improved and the development of premature arthrosis avoided.

CHAPTER 22
Other Arthroscopic Operations

In addition to the commoner indications for arthroscopic operation listed above – removal of loose bodies, total or partial resection of the medial or lateral meniscus, and the smoothing of articular cartilage lesions – there are also less frequent indications for arthroscopic intervention.

22.1 Procedures on the Synovial Membrane

Inspection of the joint capsule and synovial membrane form part of routine arthroscopic diagnosis. Increased vascular injection and thickening of the villi are indicative of an irritative condition of the joint, often associated with formation of a serous effusion. More marked inflammatory changes with villous synovitis, especially if suggestive of rheumatoid disease or hyperuricemia, as well as changes in the synovial membrane typical of chondromatosis, are indications for synovial biopsy.

Under arthroscopic vision, the biopsy forceps is inserted through a second incision and a few small samples are taken from the synovial areas showing the greatest macroscopic changes. These are sent for histologic examination. Moreover, cordlike scarring or fibrous adhesions may be found, especially in the suprapatellar recess, for instance after a previous knee joint operation with subsequent prolonged immobilization. These synovial scars and adhesions in the suprapatellar recess can be divided and detached with a scissors, basket forceps, or diathermy electrode.

The hypertrophic synovial villi that are occasionally tucked into the joint and obstruct movement can also be removed arthroscopically; the base of the pedicle is divided with a basket forceps and the villus seized with a grasping forceps and removed from the joint. It may be easier to do this in many cases if the villus is first grasped with the forceps and gently tugged to exert tension on the pedicle.

In synovitis associated with marked villous hypertrophy, the enlarged villi sometimes greatly obstruct vision in the various joint compartments. If this is so, it may be necessary to remove part of the obstruction. Individual villi can be seized at their base with the large basket forceps and pulled off and removed from the joint. A motor-driven instrument can be very helpful here, as the obscuring hypertrophic villi of the inflamed synovial membrane can be successively resected with it and simultaneously sucked away.

Even the performance of the small-scale partial synovectomy described above will make it clear to the surgeon how tiresome an arthroscopic synovectomy is bound to be. Some authors report on arthroscopic synovectomy in the English-language literature, but with considerable reservations. Its biggest disadvantages are that it cannot be really radical and that it takes up a great deal of time. Therefore, it is the authors' opinion that synovectomy is best done using an open procedure and is too demanding for arthroscopy.

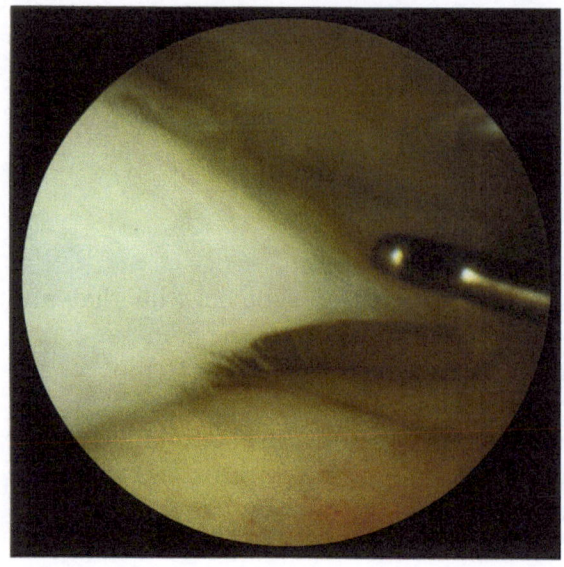

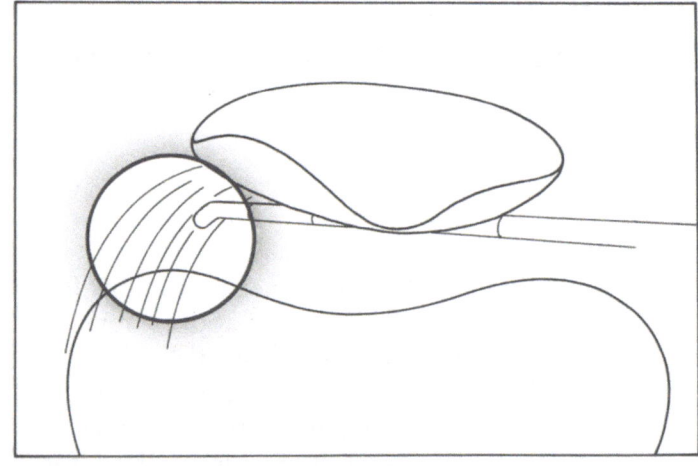

Fig. 210. Large hypertrophied medial parapatellar plica demonstrated by probe hook

22.2 Resection of a Hypertrophied Medial Plica

Synovial folds of greatly varying size extending out from the synovial membrane are well known. Clinically, only the medial patellar plica (alar fold) is relevant, and then only when it is hypertrophied as a wide bandlike structure, bulging into the joint like a sail. This synovial fold, with a varying degree of fibrosis, runs from the joint capsule at the superomedial margin of the patella, broadening like a sail distally to the infrapatellar fat pad.

A plica is of pathologic importance only when it causes symptoms, and these are similar to those of a meniscus lesion, i.e., pain more marked at the inner side of the knee, localized medial parapatellar tenderness, a clicking or snapping obstruction to movement over the medial joint space, and occasional transient locking.

The arthroscopic appearance is unmistakable. A saillike structure stretches between the inner side of the back of the patella and the medial condyle (Fig. 120). There may occasionally be difficulties in penetrating the medial compartment with the arthroscope between the hypertrophied medial plica and the condyle. Sometimes there are already

changes in the articular cartilage of the condyle due to continued friction with the plica.

The existence of clinical symptoms and the arthroscopic finding of a structural cause for these in the hypertrophied medial plica constitute an indication for operative resection. This arthroscopic procedure presents no very great difficulties. With the instrument in the anterolateral incision, and using a straight optical system, there is an excellent view of the entire plica. The puncture site at the superolateral margin of the patella is extended into an incision and the hypertrophied plica is nibbled away all round from its free edge to its base (Figs. 211–213). The resulting fragments are sucked and irrigated out.

Fig. 211. Beginning of plica resection with large ▷ basket forceps, introduced from superolateral incision

Fig. 212. Progressive nibbling resection of broadened saillike medial plica

Fig. 213. Result after resection of medial parapatellar plica

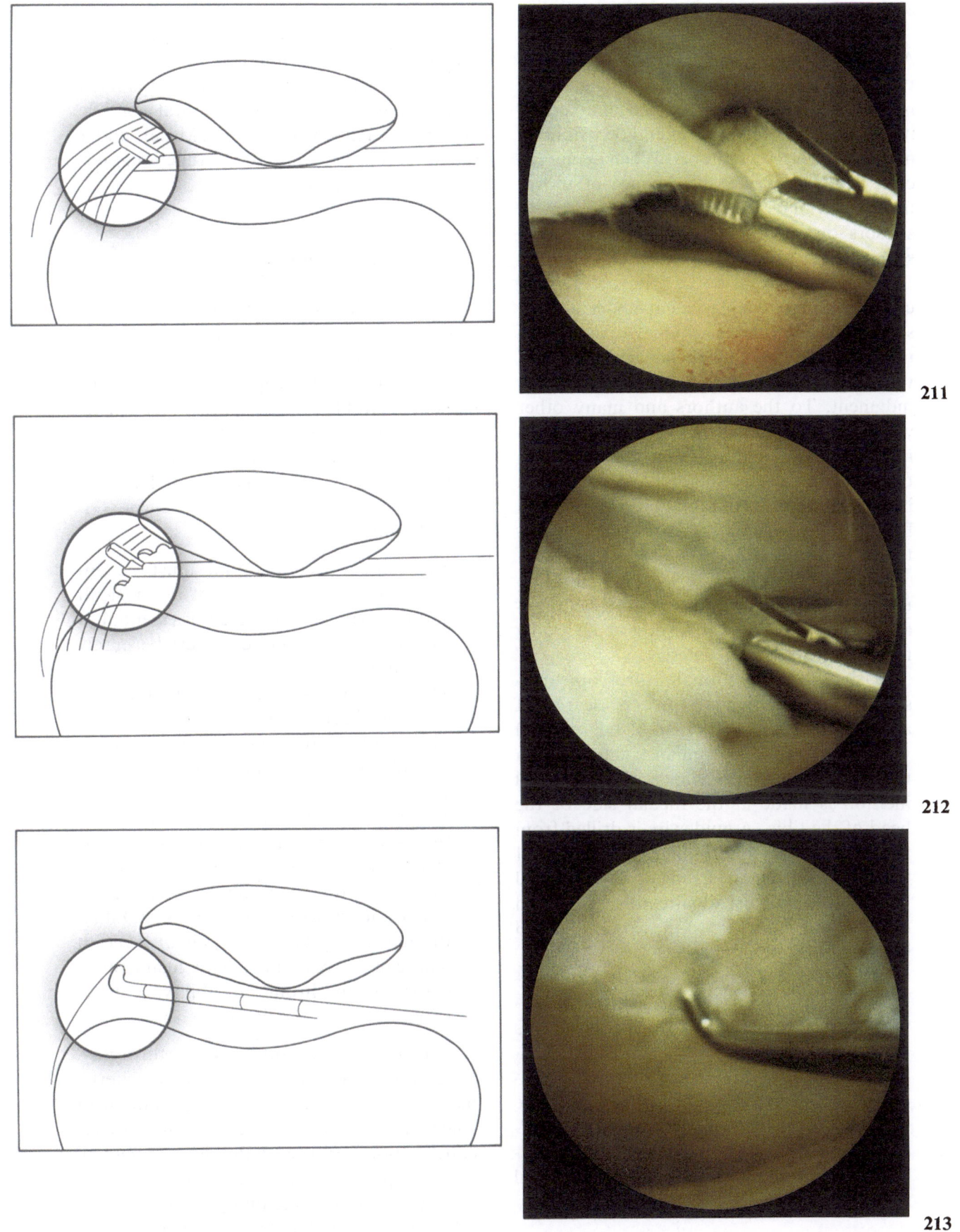

211

212

213

22.3 Cruciate Ligament Procedures

After long-standing partial or complete ruptures of the anterior cruciate ligament, rounded residual stumps may become turned in between the joint surfaces and occasionally may give rise to symptoms. When such cruciate remnants cause disturbance of movement they can be removed from the joint with scissors or a basket forceps under arthroscopic monitoring.

Recently, several authors have described cruciate ligament replacement under arthroscopic control. The traditional open operation to repair the cruciate ligament using autogenous tissue is itself a matter for careful judgment. To the authors and many other workers the implantation of an artificial ligament appears even more problematic. Besides the many other imponderables, the tolerance in the joint and the durability of the artificial ligament have not yet been thoroughly investigated.

The technical procedure for implantation under arthroscopic control is not exceptionally complicated and will be described, if only for the sake of completeness.

Using the conventional arthroscopic incisions, the intercondylar fossa is cleared of all cruciate ligament remnants and synovial villi with a motor-driven instrument. With the aid of a guide appliance, an additional incision is made at the medial side of the head of the tibia. A guidewire is drilled from the distal end at the original attachment of the anterior cruciate ligament to the tibial head and the medial tibial condyle is drilled out over this guidewire to the extent required by the size of the implant.

At the lateral femoral condyle an analogous procedure is carried out from the proximal end in such a way that the channel comes to lie as far dorsal as possible in the intercondylar fossa, so imitating the original biomechanics of the anterior cruciate ligament. The sharp edges of the drillholes inside and outside the joint must be rubbed down to prevent friction of the implant at these critical sites.

The artificial ligament is then introduced into the joint from the proximal end and drawn through the drillhole in the tibial head with a grasping forceps. The implant is fixed with staples to the lateral femoral condyle and the medial side of the tibial head, under the tension appropriate to the functional position of the knee joint.

22.4 Meniscus Suture

In certain meniscus lesions partial resection can be avoided and the avulsed portion of meniscus can be sutured back into place. Only a very small proportion of meniscus tears are suitable for this type of reconstruction. The success of meniscus suture depends greatly on the correctness of the indications. In general, if there is to be a real chance of restoration of the meniscus the following criteria should be satisfied:

1. The patient's cooperation must be ensured, as an appreciation of the difficult and tiresome aftertreatment is essential
2. The tear in the meniscus must be purely longitudinal
3. The tear should be as close to the base of the meniscus as possible
4. The avulsed portion of the meniscus should exhibit no significant degenerative changes
5. The meniscus tear should not be old since the more recent the tear, the greater the chances of success of suture
6. Meniscus suture can only be attempted in a knee joint with ligamentous stability, though it may be that repair of a recent tear can be combined with ligamentous suture or, in chronic instability, with reconstruction of the ligaments

Open meniscus suture by arthrotomy, long performed according to these criteria, has now been superseded in the opinion of some authors by arthroscopic meniscus reconstruction because of the development of special equipment. The newly developed instruments consist essentially of double-barreled guide cannulae, available with various tip angles, through which the individual sutures are placed.

The operative technique of arthroscopic meniscus suture is very demanding. The first essential step is smoothing of the site of tear with a basket forceps, both at the base and in the avulsed portion. For the suture of a lateral meniscus tear a knee position of about 45° flexion is advised, while a medial meniscus tear is dealt with in maximum extension. The angle at the tip of the double-barrelled guide cannula is chosen to correspond to the nature of the tear and the ease of access, and the instrument is inserted into the knee from the opposite side.

After repositioning the meniscus portion to be sutured, the guide cannula is approximated to the avulsed portion of the meniscus. The two threaded needles are thrust outwards through this double-barrelled cannula, through the avulsed portion of meniscus and the base of the meniscus, and then through the other soft parts and the skin. In doing so, care should be taken to ensure that the ruptured portion of meniscus is adjusted as well as possible to the base. One or more mattress sutures will be placed, depending on the length of the tear.

Finally, the outwardly drawn sutures are tightened and exact repositioning and the result of the suture checked with the probe hook. A skin incision is made at the site of emergence of the separate sutures, which are tied over the deep fascia. Different authors then recommend either functional aftertreatment or a period of immobilization of between 3 and 6 weeks without bearing weight on the leg.

The uncertainties of open meniscus suture have been made clear already by the tight restrictions listed above. In the authors' opinion, in the light of the currently available equipment and present techniques, the results of arthroscopic suture come nowhere near comparison with those of arthrotomy. Repositioning of the avulsed portion of meniscus cannot be as precise as in the open procedure; the sutures placed by means of the arthroscope fix markedly smaller surfaces than in open reconstruction. And at certain sites of predilection for meniscus tears, such as at the center of the posterior horn of the medial meniscus, no suture can be inserted at the meniscus base under arthroscopic control because the view is so limited. Blind tying in a small incision "somewhere in the depths" does not lead to reliable stabilization.

The complication rate of arthroscopic meniscus suture is greater than in the conventional open procedure. All the limiting factors, the considerably higher complication rate, the very demanding operative technique, and the other serious disadvantages mean that only very few situations exist where arthroscopic operation is appropriate.

22.5 Lateral Release

Transection of the lateral patellar retinaculum from the tibial head to the beginning of the muscular portion of the vastus lateralis is a measure intended to alter the biomechanics of guiding the patella in the patella articular surface of the femur. Lateralization of the patella due to increased tension and shortening of the lateral retinaculum are indications for this procedure. This lateralization, which may lead to subluxation of the patella, causes localized pressure loading on the lateral patellar facet during flexion of the knee. The consequence of this is degeneration, softening, fibrillation, and increased friction of the cartilage layer at the loaded zones of the patellar articular surface and the lateral femoral condyle.

No extensive inspection of the joint is necessary for division of the lateral retinaculum; it is enough to section the joint capsule and fascial layer from the tibial head to the start of the musculature of the vastus lateralis under arthroscopic control, leaving only the subcutaneous layer and skin lateral to the patella. Using the anterolateral incision, the joint capsule and fascial layer are first cut with small dissecting scissors, moving distally to their attachment to the tibial head. A subcutaneous tunnel is created between the subcutaneous layer and fascia by spreading the scissors as the first step. The capsule and fascia are then taken between the scissor blades and divided progressively up to the bony attachment (Fig. 214). The procedure can also be carried out in a proximal direction, a lateral parapatellar tunnel being driven to the suprapatellar incision and the capsular and fascial layers being again taken between the scissor blades and completely divided (Fig. 215).

Subsequently, the arthroscope is introduced from the anterolateral incision, dissecting or large hooked scissors inserted in the superolateral incision, and the cut extended proximally until muscle tissue of the vastus lateralis is clearly visible (Figs. 216–218). The entire length of the completed transection of the lateral retinaculum and joint capsule is then checked with the arthroscope from the anteromedial side. Performed correctly and for the right indications, the capsular and fascial margins gape apart by at least 1–1.5 cm due to the relief of tension. Appropriate smoothing of articular cartilage defects at the back of the patella and on the lateral femoral condyle are also usually necessary.

The movement of the patella along the patellar articular surface of the femur during flexion of the knee is now rechecked. This should show that after transection of the lateral retinaculum there is relief of pressure at the lateral patellar facet, medial transfer of the patella, and better movement of the patella (Figs. 219, 220).

As with other arthroscopic operations, hemarthrosis after lateral release is prevented by the postoperative application of a pressure

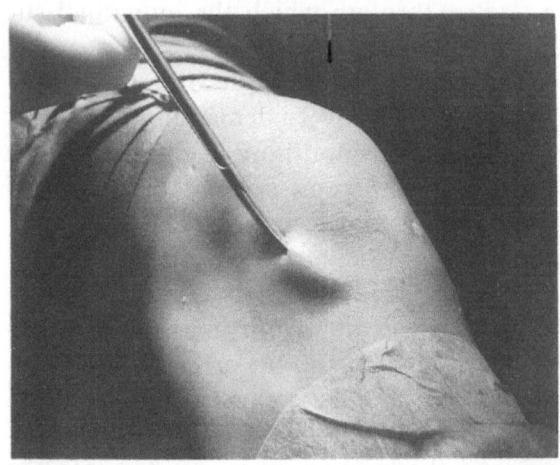

Fig. 214. Section of lateral retinaculum progressing distally from the anterolateral incision

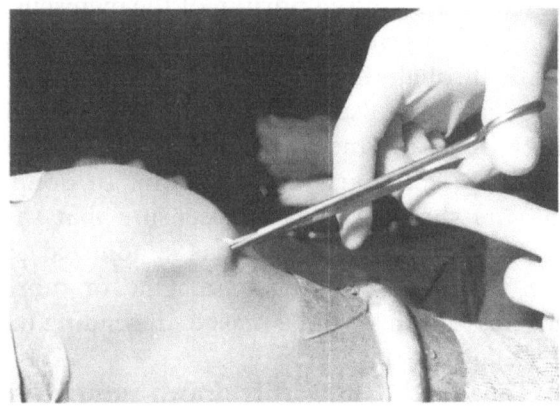

Fig. 215. Section of the lateral retinaculum progressing proximally from the anterolateral incision

Fig. 216. Section of the lateral retinaculum with ▷ dissecting scissors from the superolateral incision, progressing proximally

Fig. 217. Section of lateral retinaculum with dissecting scissors continued up to musculature of vastus lateralis

Fig. 218. Wide gaping of margins of incision after section of lateral retinaculum

170

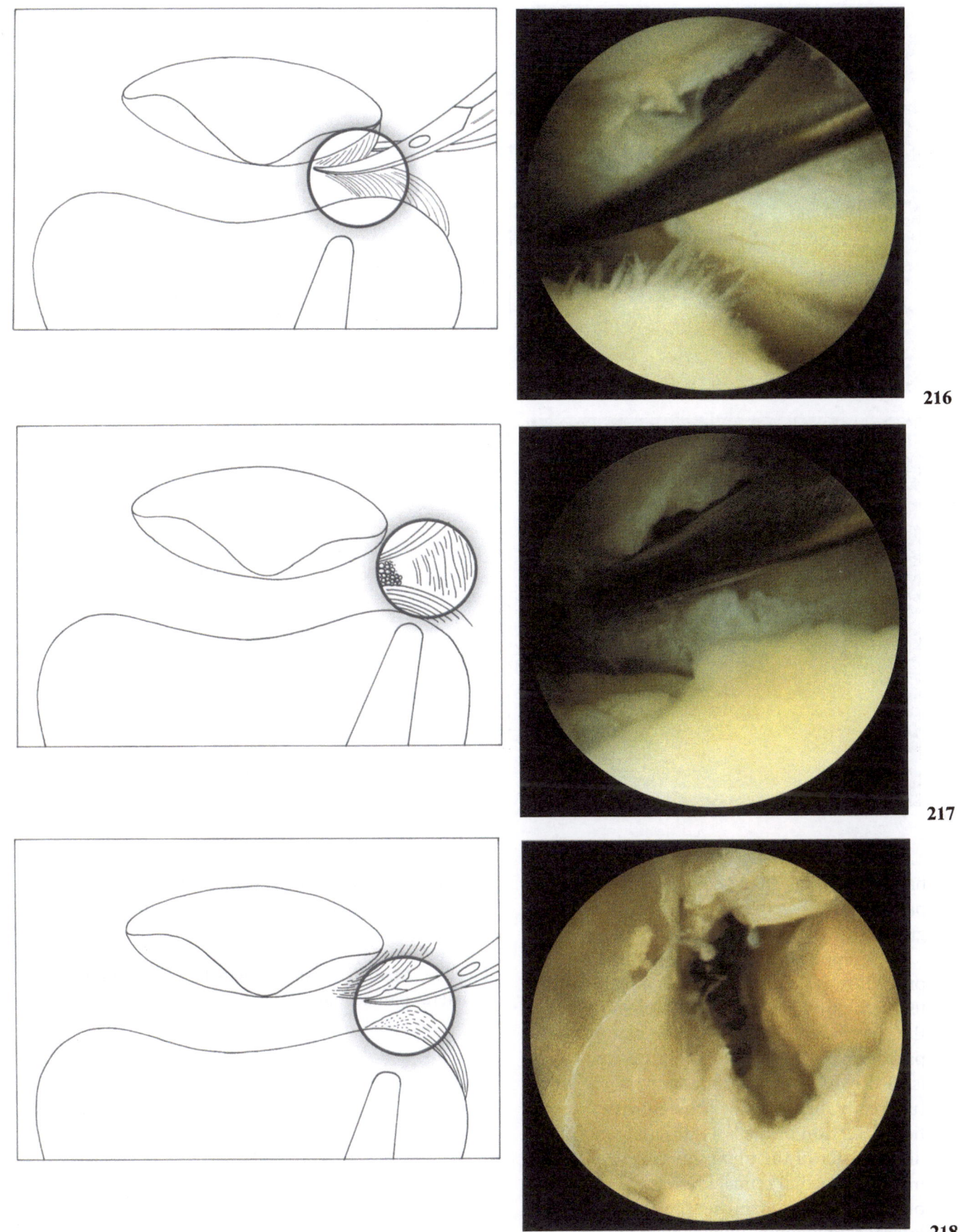

216

217

218

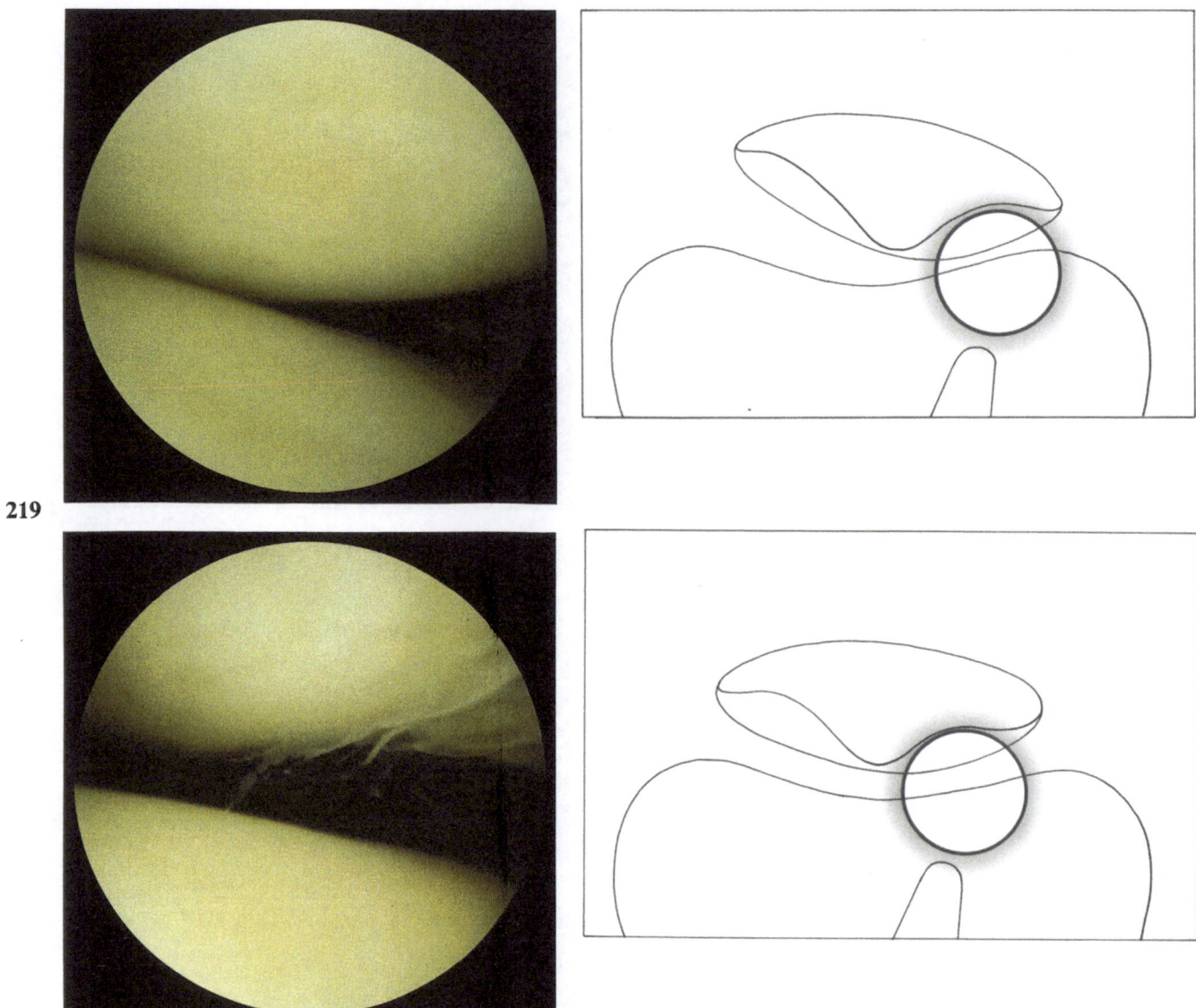

219

220

bandage around the knee using several rolled pads. Bearing weight on the knee is allowed gradually, as after a meniscus operation.

The application of this type of operative procedure is determined by the degree of lateralization. The technique is unsuitable for the treatment of habitual subluxation of the patella. With very severe lateralization, which is also caused by lateralization of the tibial tuberosity, medial joint revision with transarticular section of the lateral retinaculum, medial transfer of the tibial tuberosity, and reefing of the medial retinaculum is the technique of choice since arthroscopic section of the lateral retinaculum alone is inadequate.

Fig. 219. Lateralized patella with focal contact between lateral patellar facet and lateral femoral condyle

Fig. 220. Medial transfer of patella after section of lateral retinaculum

172

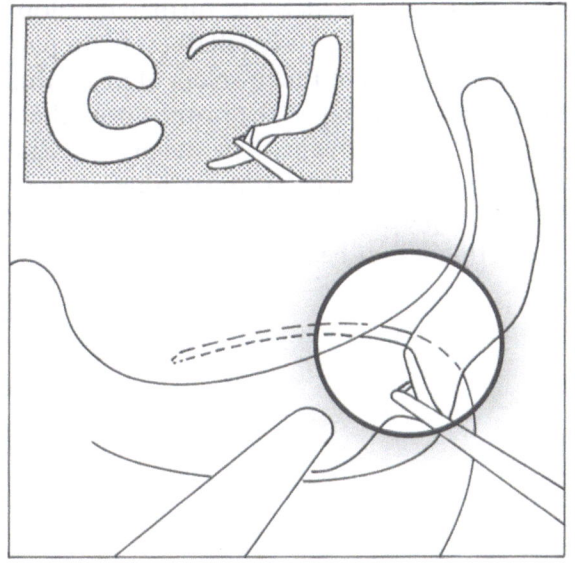

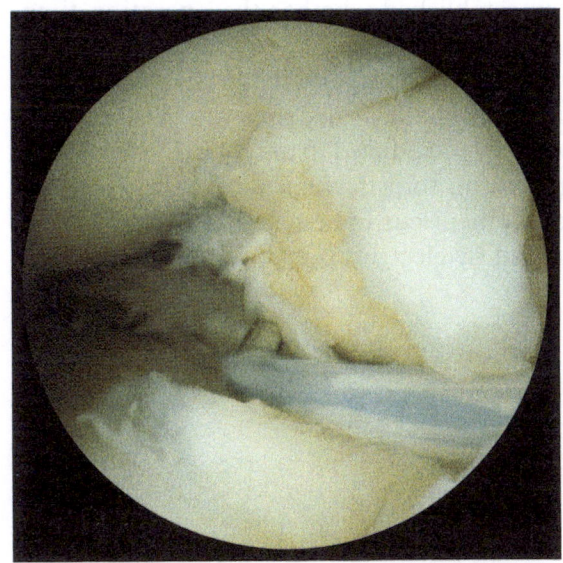

22.6 Removal of Metal and Foreign Bodies

Osteosynthesis material introduced into the joint, e.g., screws for fixation of the fragment of osteochondritis dissecans or of an osteochondral shearing fracture, can be removed by means of the arthroscope without the need for further arthrotomy. Special care must be taken to position the second incision to allow an exactly perpendicular approach of the screwdriver to the screwhead. Withdrawal of the screw is done in the usual manner, and, if a screw longer than 4 cm was selected at the first operation, there is the advantage that the risk of the screw slipping away into the joint cavity is minimal. Embedded foreign bodies or portions of broken instruments (further discussed in Chap. 24) are seized with the grasping forceps from the second incision like loose bodies and extracted from the joint.

Fig. 221. Diathermy division of a medial bucket-handle tear at its connection to the base at the posterior horn

22.7 Diathermy

Partial meniscectomy, plica resection, lateral retinacular section, and the freeing of scarred adhesions can also be performed arthroscopically with a diathermy, electrode using recently developed appliances and instruments. For this, a nonconducting electrolyte-free solution is necessary as an irrigation medium. A probe hook, insulated up to its angle, is used for cutting. Diathermy surgery within the joint is still in the developmental stage. The various probe hooks and cutting wires are still not altogether satisfactory. A probe hook that is not insulated to its tip is dangerous, and it is very easy to damage the articular surface of the tibial head during division of the meniscus. The cut surfaces are no smoother than after a clean cut with scissors or after careful resection using basket forceps, and show blackish deposits.

Because of the simultaneous coagulation caused in the synovial vessels, the tendency to hemorrhage after section of the lateral retinaculum or plica is reduced. It has not yet been established whether the operation time may be shorter using diathermy.

Diathermy surgery requires considerable use of mechanical instruments. The arthroscope is introduced from one incision and the cutting tool through a second. The portion of meniscus to be resected is successively divided by electrosurgery (Fig. 221).

If there is considerable further development of the equipment for diathermy, in particular a solution to the problem of insulating the tip and the front of the probe hook, there may be future advances in the use of diathermy resection; for instance, in tapering or divergent partial resections it may allow a "smooth cut" to be made.

CHAPTER 23
Completion of Operation and Aftertreatment

Careful irrigation of the knee joint is necessary after completion of the arthroscopic operation, despite intermittent suction of the detached fragments of meniscus or articular cartilage, to wash out residual fragments under pressure. For this, 60–80 ml of normal saline or Ringer solution is injected under pressure through the outer tube of the arthroscope using a 100-ml syringe with a conical attachment and is then discharged through the same tube into a vessel (Fig. 222).

In this way the residual fragments are irrigated from the knee joint, and the process is repeated until no further particles appear. The small punctures are then each closed with a single suture (Fig. 223).

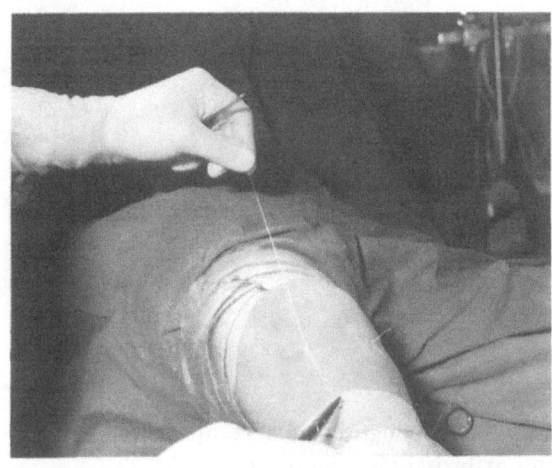

Fig. 223. Suture of arthroscopic skin incision

A sterile dressing and a compression bandage in the form of an elastic bandage are then applied and the tourniquet released (Fig. 224). The leg is kept raised in a foam splint. The patient may stand from the first postoperative day onwards and can take

Fig. 222. Postoperative irrigation of the knee joint through the arthroscope

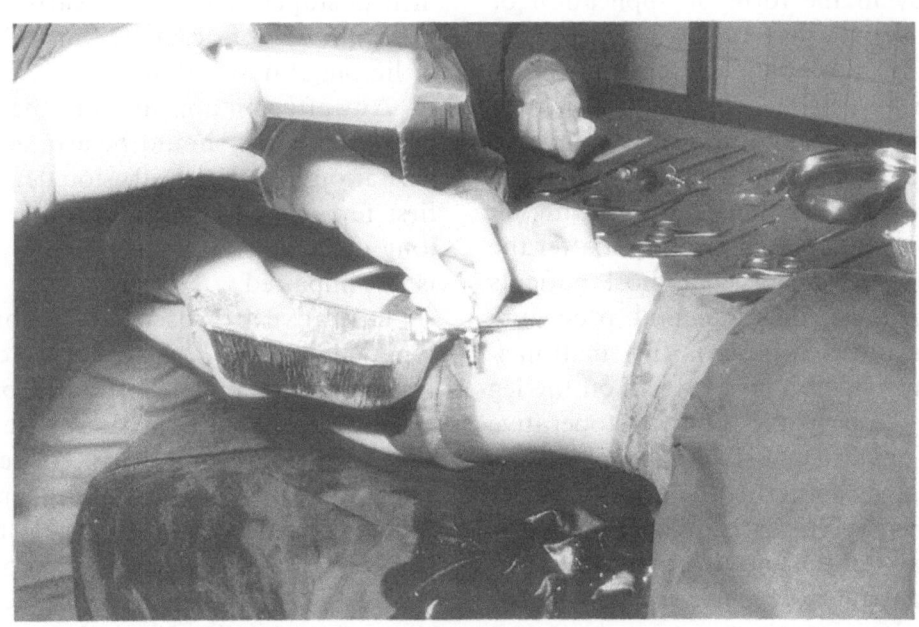

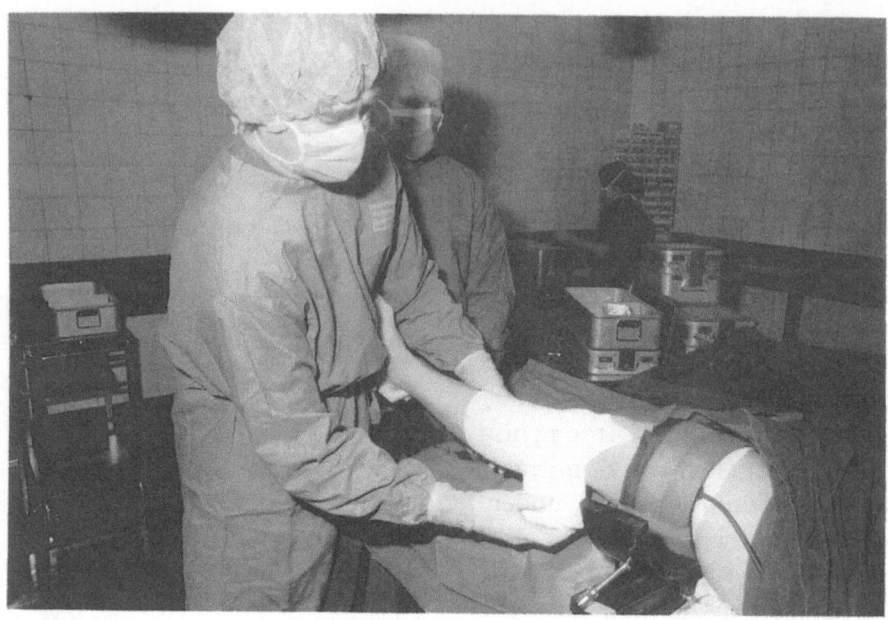

Fig. 224. Application of a compression bandage after arthroscopic operation

some 10–15 kg weight on the leg with the aid of elbow-crutches, as instructed by the physiotherapist before the operation.

Isometric quadriceps training is begun after recovery from anesthesia and continued throughout the entire postoperative period, both while in hospital and afterwards. Cryotherapy in the form of application of ice-packs over the bandage 3–5 times daily minimizes the postoperative reactive condition in the knee joint. The bandage is first changed on the second postoperative day and elastic bandaging is continued subsequently.

Our experience is that pain following an arthroscopic operation is very slight after the first postoperative day, and most patients tend to underestimate the joint procedure that has been carried out via the small incisions and to take too much strain on the leg too soon. During the first postoperative phase, the main task of the surgeon and the physiotherapist concerned in aftertreatment may even be to restrain the patient's activity. Full extension of the knee from the first postoperative day on is very important, whereas forced flexion exercises are unnecessary.

From the second postoperative day the knee may be flexed actively 2–3 times daily, each time as often as the limits of discomfort permit; thereby virtually free flexion to about 130°–140° is attained within the first few days.

The leg can start to bear weight at an early stage, depending on the degree of swelling or effusion in the joint. It is usual to be able to take half the body-weight and walk with elbow-crutches between the third and fifth postoperative days. Nearly all patients can walk without crutches and without pain or limping after 5–10 days.

Any effusion appearing in the early postoperative phase should be aspirated without hesitation. If such an effusion develops in the first few days aspiration should also not be long delayed, so that postoperative recovery is not impaired.

Operative arthroscopy is performed as an inpatient procedure as a matter of self-protection for the patient. But arthroscopic surgery can quite easily be done without admission if the patient is very cooperative and understanding. However, in general, it is more acceptable for both surgeon and patient for management over the few postoperative days to be on an inpatient basis. The duration of hospitalization is between 3 and 7 days, depending on the patient's collaboration and the condition of the knee joint.

The first outpatient follow-up visit is between the 10th and 14th postoperative days, at which time the stitches can be removed from the incisions. Subsequently, isometric quadriceps training, active exercises, and cryotherapy are performed both independently and under the eye of the physiotherapist. The final visit is at 4 weeks after operation. Follow-up after 6 months is advised, though unfortunately compliance is poor in many patients whose recovery follows a trouble-free course. The duration of incapacity for work depends on the physical strenuousness of the occupation, the individual patient's will to work, and the length of the general practitioner's sickness certificate.

Thus, office workers can return to work some 10–14 days after operation while heavy manual laborers usually require 3–4 weeks. Only rough guidelines can be laid down for sporting activities, e.g., swimming and bicycling at 2 weeks postoperatively; running on soft ground, weight-training, cross-country skiing, at 4 weeks; football, tennis, alpine skiing at 6–8 weeks. These rough guidelines are naturally to be individually interpreted taking into account the extent of the damage to the knee joint and the course of postoperative recovery as training is cautiously increased.

The patient can be given two very simple criteria as regards exertion:

it should not hurt, and the knee should not become swollen.

CHAPTER 24
Complications, Problems, and Hazards of Operative Arthroscopy

The greatest fear of every arthroscopic surgeon is infection – empyema of the knee joint. Fortunately, this complication is extremely rarely reported in the literature; in our own series of over 2500 arthroscopic knee operations not a single case of infection has occurred.

Nevertheless, this very favorable infection rate must not lead to neglect of sterility. Arthroscopy and arthroscopic operations are and will remain procedures on joints which call for scrupulous assessment of indications, careful preparation, sterile draping, and the least possible trauma.

Intraoperative care must be supplemented and continued by correspondingly cautious aftertreatment and close follow-up, with early aspiration of effusion and subsequent immobilization. This is the only way of perpetuating the present very favorable statistics.

A further undesirable complication is breakage of the very fine instruments during operation and consequent penetration of small foreign bodies into the joint. With careful supervision and inspection of instruments and sensitive handling, breakages within the joint should remain a rarity. However, this does not exclude the possibility of a blade of one of the fine cutting instruments breaking off against a firm sclerosed meniscus. It is then very important to maintain immobility to keep the broken part of the instrument in the visual field if at all possible, and to remove it from the joint with a grasping forceps as one would a loose body. Besides these risks specific to arthroscopic operations, there naturally remain the general risks of any operation – anesthetic accidents, anaphylactic shock, reduced cerebral circulation, cardiac arrest, thrombosis, and embolism.

A further specific complication of arthroscopy, though also rare, is the emergence of fluid or gas from the joint cavity into the tissues, the fluid giving rise to edematous swelling and the gas to the familiar emphysema. These extravasations are usually reabsorbed without complication and no longer demonstrable on the day after operation.

Special problems arise as regards vision during an arthroscopic operation. The surgeon's visual field may be particularly impaired if there has been hemarthrosis preoperatively or if there is hemorrhage during operation. Hypertrophic villi due to synovitis may also float repeatedly in front of the arthroscope, and likewise a very thickened infrapatellar fat pad may greatly hamper inspection of the various joint compartments. These may be relieved by forceful irrigation for hemarthrosis and hemorrhage, resection of individual villi, increasing the intraarticular hydrostatic pressure by raising the height of the infusion bottle, and displacing the fat pad or other hindrances to vision with the arthroscope or the probe hook.

In knee joints with very tight ligaments arthroscopic operations can be very difficult, especially in the posterior joint compartments, and in a few cases even impossible. In such cases an arthroscopic procedure should under no circumstances be forced, for this will do more harm than good to the patient. The less-practiced arthroscopic surgeon is particularly likely more than once to come up against the situation where an operation under arthroscopic monitoring, once begun, cannot be completed, except by taking an excessive amount of time or by incurring articular cartilage damage. In these cases, and when the operative outcome is uncertain, the arthroscopic operation must be abandoned and the procedure completed by arthrotomy.

178

As with open joint operations, the post-operative course may be complicated by effusion – hemarthrosis or serous synovitis – requiring aspiration. Persistent knee joint problems or repeated effusions are sometimes attributed to the "new" operative technique, but it should be remembered that these post-operative problems may develop even after arthrotomy; and in the authors' experience they occur less often after arthroscopic operation than after open arthrotomy.

The greatest danger of arthroscopic operations, especially with the inexperienced surgeon, is that the highly sensitive articular cartilage layer may suffer additional damage from incautious manipulation of the arthroscope or ther instruments. The desquamation of small flakes of cartilage, visible mainly by the "aquarium effect" in fluid irrigation, is of no clinical importance. However, the number of cartilage "flaws" that are bound to occur over and again initially should diminish with increasing practice and experience. However, even the beginner may minimize cartilage damage by cautious manipulation of the arthroscope within the knee joint, the use of blunt-ended accessory instruments, proceeding only under visual control, and using blunt penetration of the synovial membrane. A poor surgeon, even if experienced, can cause more damage at arthrotomy than a good and cautious operator with an arthroscope. With more or less appropriate manipulation, injury to other intraarticular structures such as the menisci or cruciate ligaments is almost impossible. However, special care should be taken in the posterior joint compartments to avoid injury to the vessels or nerves in the popliteal fossa from sudden slipping of the instrument.

A further risk factor in operative arthroscopy is that many surgeons are not sufficiently self-critical and overestimate their capacity and technical capability. There are many surgeons who, after a two-day seminar, consider they have learned this technique and can employ it as elegantly as the instructor. Without a careful history, clinical examination, and radiologic clarification, arthroscopy and "poking about" in the knee may be used for atypical knee pain, so bringing this promising method into disrepute.

CHAPTER 25
Practice of Operative Arthroscopy

The applications of arthroscopic operation are limited. Nevertheless, it involves a technically difficult procedure which calls for great experience in addition to manual skill and operative delicacy. Reliable assessment of the findings is guaranteed only in the hands of an experienced surgeon, and only with constant practice can the procedure be carried out carefully enough to bring the full the advantages of arthroscopic operation.

In the hands of a beginner, the time taken for an operative procedure may be 2–3 times as long as for arthrotomy. However, with patience and persistence any moderately capable surgeon with a capacity for stereoscopic appreciation can succeed, after initial difficulties, in gaining the practice and experience required to achieve arthrotomy operation times and later to take considerably less time. The minimization of the operative procedure, the ensuing significantly reduced trauma to the joint, the smaller time-lapse, and a therapeutic outcome comparable to that of arthrotomy, together with a much wider and comprehensive diagnosis of the entire knee joint in the hands of the practiced endoscopic operator – these are the principal advances in knee joint surgery achieved through operative arthroscopy.

CHAPTER 26
Arthroscopic Operations with Gas Filling of the Knee Joint

Arthroscopic operation with gas filling of the knee joint is possible and may be superior to the irrigation technique in certain cases. Our operative technique has certain features which we would like to elucidate, showing the advantages and disadvantages compared with the conventional fluid technique.

I am convinced that arthroscopic operation is only really superior to arthrotomy as a routine if it is associated with all the advantages of arthroscopy. Therefore, it should be carried out using local anesthesia and the results of operation should be equal to or better than those of arthrotomy. Hence, it is indisputable that a cleanly and rapidly performed partial meniscectomy under local anesthesia with gas filling is superior to an operative procedure under general anesthesia with fluid distension. The limited duration of local anesthesia obliges the surgeon to be self-disciplined and to fulfill his operation plan. With local anesthesia and gas distension, only some 30 min at most of excellent visual conditions are available to the surgeon; thereafter, vision is often impaired by bleeding from the intermittently damaged synovial membrane. If, therefore, the injured structure can be exposed, resected, and removed within the space of a few minutes, this method is superior to all others.

It is only a minor problem to maintain adequate gas pressure in the knee during the first 30 min. As already described, a pressure of between 20 and 30 mmHg is all that is required to distend the knee cavity adequately. If the instruments are inserted through trocars that fit them closely, the pressure can even be increased and maintained constant.

The disadvantage of the trocar technique is that at the moment there is no trocar available that is sufficiently flexible and capable of being anchored in position in such a way as to completely block off the entry sites in the synovium and that also allows the insertion of bent scissors and basket forceps into the knee cavity. But even without this trocar technology, it is always possible, within the first half hour, to expose the knee cavity very well under gas distension at low pressure and to conduct the operation even with bent instruments.

The problems of operation with gas filling and local anesthesia are, as stated, the limited time available and, less serious, the wearing-off of the anesthetic effect; more important, especially in women, is the development of gas emphysema around the site of insertion of the arthroscope after some 30–45 min. The tendency to bleeding is also increased and leads to impairment of vision. It is now possible under local anesthesia to change to irrigation and subsequent fluid distension, the operation continuing under constant fluid input via a suprapatellar cannula (see Sect. 16.1).

The use of diathermy for resection of portions of the menisci is also possible with gas distension. With the required adjustment of the current a hazy image develops during the cutting procedure, though the outlines remain quite recognizable. Moreover, gas can be exchanged by appropriate techniques in seconds, so excision of large parts of the menisci creates no problems. The same considerations regarding timing apply here under local anesthesia as for other operative procedures.

CHAPTER 27

Miniarthrotomy under Local Anesthesia

It has been known for years that diagnostic arthroscopy is capable of clarifying even clinically concealed meniscus lesions. After learning the diagnostic technique many workers have sought to exchange the inserted small hook for the scissors or basket forceps and to undertake arthroscopic operations. In many cases the operation has proved difficult and time-consuming. In operational management this makes the exact planning of a large operating program impossible. If diagnostic arthroscopy is being performed under local anesthesia, any operative procedure need not and should not take longer than 1 h. For these reasons, Gächter has advised miniarthrotomy under arthroscopic monitoring, which constitutes a compromise for the beginner. The diagnosis is established arthroscopically. The arthroscope is removed and a longitudinal 2- to 2.5-cm incision is made over the defective meniscus under general or local anesthesia. The capsule and synovial membrane are retracted with special flat (Langenbeck) retractors and the joint cavity exposed. As the surgeon already has precise information about the meniscus lesion and the course of the tear, the appropriate cuts with a Smillie knife can be made very rapidly under direct vision, especially with flap or bucket-handle tears (Fig. 225).

We have already found this "emergency solution" useful in many cases. We always use this technique if, because of severe synovitis or some other problem obscuring vision, the arthroscopic operation has proved difficult from the outset. The drawback of this type of operation, as with arthrotomy, is that it is difficult to judge the ultimate site of section at the posterior horn, whether this is for a flap tear or for a bucket-handle tear that is to be sectioned in a dorsal direction. Also, the possibility of further arthroscopic

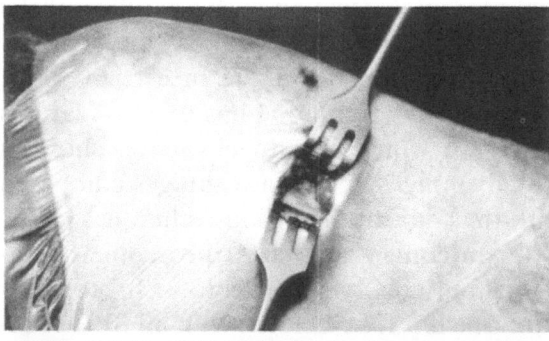
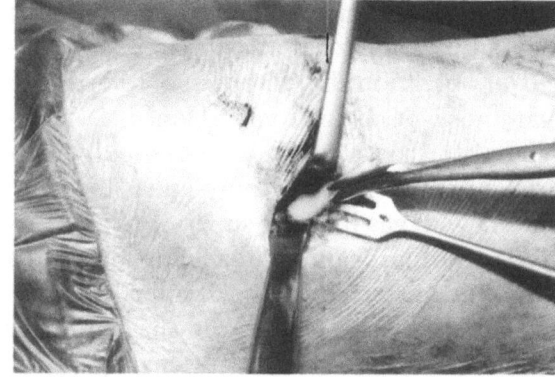

Fig. 225a, b. Miniarthrotomy under local anesthesia. **a** Longitudinal incision of retinaculum, **b** removal of bucket-handle tear

monitoring at the end of the operation is almost nonexistent, as the miniarthrotomy involves too large an exit orifice for fluid and far too large an exit for gas filling. Tidy posterior horn resection is therefore occasionally not guaranteed.

The technique of miniarthrotomy can also be used with outpatients. If a suction drain has been placed in the joint we recommend inpatient treatment for 2 days. Total replacement of arthroscopic operation by miniarthrotomy is certainly not justified. In our view, this method is to be considered only as a "good emergency solution" when a difficult endoscopic procedure threatens to become interminable.

CHAPTER 28
Perspectives

Arthroscopy of the knee joint is now fully established in the realm of diagnosis. Its techniques are standardized and its validity undisputed. It has replaced and rendered obsolete trial arthrotomy of the knee. In the future, diagnostic arthroscopy will have to compete with other imaging techniques such as computed tomography (CT) and magnetic resonance imaging (MRI). It is not yet possible to say whether ultrasonography will ever be able to provide noninvasive diagnosis of knee joint problems.

Endoscopic operative techniques in the knee are still in a state of development and expansion, and considerable progress has been made in recent years through the use of video techniques. In particular, the use of video techniques enables arthroscopy to be from a transformed so-called semisterile procedure into one that is completely sterile. Instrumentation for operations has also been considerably improved in recent years, though there is still room for further improvement.

Also, the standardization of the various operative techniques is in no way complete. It will certainly be some years yet before specific methods are taught didactically. Endoscopic procedures are becoming increasingly demanding technically. The coming years will

show whether meniscus suture, so elegant a procedure when seen endoscopically, will prove a real advance in treatment. The possibility may well emerge of improving cruciate ligament surgery, perhaps even using endoprostheses to replace the ligaments under arthroscopic control, with long-term success. Hitherto insoluble problems related to articular cartilage disorders may prove amenable to arthroscopic treatment and control. It is quite conceivable that cartilage-cementing substances might be developed which could be injected into deep cartilage fissures under arthroscopic control to produce better healing of cartilage tears. Moreover, why should it not be possible to fill up ulcers and punched-out cartilage defects with such substances to prevent the chronic irritative states that usually arise from these lesions?

Arthroscopic investigation of the other large joints – and possibly even small joints – presents an entirely new dimension in diagnosis and treatment. Especially in the shoulder joint, we may be fairly sure that the coming years will se diagnostic arthroscopy contributing to the understanding and treatment of pain. As for the other joints, as far as diagnosis and especially treatment are concerned, we are only at the beginning of developments that are as yet unpredictable.

References

Alm A (1974) The diagnostic value of arthroscopy of the knee-joint. Injury 5/4:319–324

Andersen RB, Rossel I (1973) Arthroscopy of the knee-joint in rheumatic diseases. Ugeskr Læger 135:71

Berner W (1983) Die arthroskopische Meniskusresektion. Unfallheilkunde 86:241

Bircher E (1921) Die Arthroendoskopie. Zentralbl Chir 48:1460–1461

Bircher E (1922) Beitrag zur Pathologie und Diagnose der Meniscus-Verletzungen. Bruns' Beitr Klin Chir 127:239–250

Brühlmann-Keller H et al. (1986) Arthrographie und Arthroskopie in der Meniscusdiagnostik. Unfallchirurgie 89:547–550

Burman MS (1931) Arthroscopy or the direct visualisation of joints. An experimental cadaver study. J Bone Joint Surg 13:669–695

Burman MS, Mayer L (1936) Arthroscopic examination of the knee-joint. Arch Surg 32:846

Burman MS, Finkelstein H, Mayer L (1934) Arthroscopy of the knee-joint. J Bone Joint Surg 16:255–268

Casscells W (1971) Arthroscopy of the knee-joint. J Bone Joint Surg [Am] 53:287–298

Dandy DJ (1982a) Arthroscopy and the management of the ruptured anterior cruciate ligament. Clin Orthop 167:43–49

Dandy DJ (1982b) The bucket handle meniscal tear: A technique detaching the posterior segment first. Orthop Clin North Am 13:369–385

Dandy DJ (1984) The arthroscopy of the knee. Gower, London

Dandy DJ, Jackson RW (1975a) The impact of arthroscopy on the management of disorders of the knee. J Bone Joint Surg [Br] 58/3:346–348

Dandy DJ, Jackson RW (1975b) The diagnosis of problems after meniscectomy. J Bone Joint Surg [Br] 58/3:349–352

Delbarre F, Aignan M, Ghozlan R (1975) L'Arthroscopie du genou. Institut de Rhumatologie et la Faculté de Médicine de Paris-Cochin

Dorfmann H, Dreyfus P (1971a) Arthroscopy of the knee (methods and results). Cah Sociol Demogr Med 12:561

Dorfmann H, Dreyfus P (1971b) Arthroscopy of the knee (methods and results). Minerva Med 62:2621

Dorfmann H, Seze S de (1972) Nouvelles observations sur l'arthroscopie du genou. Résultat d'une expérience personnelle. Sem Hôp Paris 48:3011–3019

Dorfmann H, Dreyfus P, Justin-Besancon L (1970) Arthroscopy of the knee-joint. Current status of the question. Sem Hôp Paris 46:3442–3450

Edgar MA, Lowy M (1973) Arthroscopy of the knee. Proc R Soc Med 66:512–515

Eickelaar HR (1975) Arthroscopy of the knee. Royal United Printers Hoitsema B.V.

Finkelstein H, Mayer L (1931) The arthroscopy, a new method of examining joints. J Bone Joint Surg 13:583–588

Fujimoto K (1949) Arthroscopic findings of the experimental arthritis caused by intra-articular injection of various disinfectant medicaments. J Jap Orthop Assoc 22:60

Gächter A (1986) Meniscectomy by mini arthrotomy in local anesthesia. In: Trickey, Hertel P (eds) Surgery and arthroscopy of the knee. Springer, Berlin Heidelberg New York Tokyo, p 113

Gallannaugh S (1973) Arthroscopy of the knee-joint. Br Med J III (5874):285–286

Geist EW (1926) Arthroscopy. Preliminary report. Lancet 46:306–307

Gillquist J, Hagberg G (1976) A new modification of the technic of the arthroscopy of the knee-joint. Acta Chir Scand 142:123–130

Gillquist J, Karpf PM (1982) Arthroskopische Operationen am Knie. Fortschr Med 3:51

Gillquist J, Oretorp N (1982) Arthroscopic partial meniscectomy technique and long-term results. Clin Orthop 167:29–33

Gillquist J, Hagberg G, Oretorp N (1977) Arthroscopy in acute injuries of the knee-joint. Acta Orthop Scand 48:190–196

Glinz W (1973) Arthroscopy in trauma of the knee-joint. International Congress on the knee-joint, Rotterdam

Glinz W (1974) Diagnostische Bedeutung der Arthroskopie bei Präarthrosen des Kniegelenkes. Unfallmed Berufskr 4:260–265

Glinz W (1976a) Die Arthroskopie bei Meniscusverletzungen. Unfallmed Berufskr 3/4:106–115

Glinz W (1976b) Arthroskopie beim Knorpelschaden des Kniegelenkes. Hefte Unfallheilkd 127:46–57

Glinz W (1977) Arthroskopische Diagnostik der traumatischen Knorpelläsion am Kniegelenk. Hefte Unfallheilkd 129:242–246

Glinz W (1979) Diagnostische Arthroskopie und arthroskopische Operationen am Kniegelenk. Huber, Bern Stuttgart Wien

Gschwend N (1976) Die Arthroskopie. Fortbildk Rheumatol 4:189–192

Hempfling H (1987) Die Endoskopie an großen Gelenken. Med Orthop Tech 107/2:73–78

Henche HR (1974) Indikation, Technik und Resultate der Arthroskopie nach Traumatisierung des Kniegelenks. Orthopäde 3:128–133

Henche HR (1976) Indikation und Technik der Arthroskopie des Kniegelenkes. Orthop Prax 2:165–167

Henche HR (1977) Die Arthroskopie des Kniegelenkes. Beitr Orthop Traumatol 24:217–220

Henche HR (1986) Von der diagnostischen zur operativen Arthroskopie des Kniegelenkes. Schweiz Rundschau Med 75/24:735

Henderson C et al (1982) Pneumoscrotum as a complication of arthroskopy. J Bone Joint Surg [Am] 64/8:1239

Henry A (1972) Arthroscopy in the management of internal derangements of the knee-joint. International Congress on the knee-joint, Rotterdam, pp 120–125

Hertel P, Schweiberer L (1980) Die Akutarthroskopie des Kniegelenkes als diagnostischer und therapeutischer Eingriff. Unfallheilkunde 83:233–240

Hertel P, Schweiberer L (1982) Die Arthroskopie des Kniegelenkes. Dtsch Ärztebl 79/19:29–38

Hey W, Henche HR (1984) Endoskopische Operationen am Kniegelenk. Chir Prax 33:491–496

Hofer H (1985) Fortschritte in der Arthroskopie. Enke, Stuttgart

Holder J (1982) Die arthroskopische Operation am Kniegelenk. Aktuel Traumatol 5:222–227

Holder J (1984) Arthroskopische Operationen am Kniegelenk. In: Buess G, Unz S, Pichlmaier H (Hrsg) Endoskopische Techniken. Deutscher Ärzte-Verlag, Köln, S 142–149

Holder J (1986) Technik und Ergebnisse der arthroskopischen Meniskotomie. Orthop Prax 22:115–122

Hurter E (1955) L'arthroscopie, nouvelle méthode d'exploration du genou. Rev Chir Orthop 41:763–766

Imbert R (1956) Arthroscopy of the knee; its technique. Marseille Chir 8:368

Imbert R (1957) Arthroscopy; significance of the method. Marseille Chir 9:676

Ino S (1939) Normal arthroscopic findings of the knee-joint in adults. J Jap Orthop Assoc 14:467

Jackson RW (1973) Arthroscopy of the knee. Curr Pract Orthop Surg 4:93–117

Jackson RW (1974) The role of arthroscopy in the management of the arthritic knee. Clin Orthop 101:28–35

Jackson RW (1975) Diagnostic uses of arthroscopy. Recent Adv Orthop 10:217–234

Jackson RW (1983) Arthroscopic surgery. J Bone Joint Surg [Am] 65:416–420

Jackson RW (1987) Memories of the early days of arthroscopy: 1965–1975, the formative years. J Arthrosk Rel Surg 3:1

Jackson RW, Abe J (1972) The role of arthroscopy in the management of disorders of the knee. J Bone Joint Surg [Br] 54:310–322

Jackson RW, Dandy DJ (1976) Arthroscopy of the knee. Grune & Stratton, New York

Jackson RW, De Haven KE (1975) Arthroscopy of the knee. Clin Orthop 107

Jackson RW, McCarthy DD (1971) Arthroscopy of the knee. University of Toronto Press, Toronto, pp 293–297

Jayson MI (1968) Arthroscopy; a new diagnostic method. Nurs Times 64:1002

Jayson MI, Dixon ASJ (1968) Arthroscopy of the knee in rheumatic diseases. Ann Rheum Dis 27:503–511

Johnson LL (1973) Diagnostic arthroscopy of the knee. International Congress on the knee-joint, Rotterdam, pp 131–139

Johnson LL (1981) Diagnostic and surgical arthroscopy. Mosby, St. Louis Toronto London

Johnson LL, Becker RL (1975) The role of the assistant in arthroscopy. 42nd Annual Meeting American Academy of Orthopedic Surgery, March 1975

Johnson LL, Becker RL (1976) Arthroscopy, technique and the role of the assistent. Orthop Rev 9:31–43

Johnson LL, Shneider DA, Becker RL (1976) Arthroscopy 76. 43rd Annual Meeting American Academy of Orthopedic Surgery, January–February 1976

Kawashima W (1943) Arthroscopy of the tuberculous knee in its early stage. J Jap Orthop Assoc 18:651

Kieser C, Rüttimann A (1976) Die Arthroskopie des Kniegelenkes. Schweiz Med Wochenschr 106:1631–1637

Klein W, Schulitz KP (1983) Arthroscopic Meniscotomy. Technique, problems, complications and follow up results. Arch Orthop Trauma Surg 101:231–237

Koike F (1943) Arthroscopic study of experimental suppurative arthritis. J Jap Orthop Assoc 18:656

Kreuscher P (1925) Semilunar cartilage disease, a plea for early recognition by means of the arthroscope and early treatment of this condition. IMJ 47:290–292

Lesky E (1966) Vom Lichtleiter zum Zystoskop. Med Monatsspiegel 4:76–80

Lipson RL, Clemmons JJ, Frymoyer JW (1967) Arthroscopy: Experience with percutaneous biopsy of intraarticular structures under direct vision. Arthritis Rheum 10:294

Löhnert J, Raunest J (1985) Arthroskopische Chirurgie des Kniegelenkes. Regensberg & Biermann, Münster

Marques J, Sanamaria A, Gomes, Martinez G (1971) Arthroscopy. Rev Esp Reum 14:47

Matsumo J (1959) Arthroscopic and histological studies of tuberculous and nonspecific chronic arthrides. J Jap Assoc Rheum 1:409

Mayer L, Burman MS (1939) Arthroscopy in the diagnosis of meniscal lesions of the knee-joint. Am J Surg 43:501

McGuire et al. (1986) Local anesthesia and arthroscopy surgery of the knee. Alaska Med 28/2:20

Mennet P (1971) Möglichkeiten und Grenzen der Kniearthroskopie. Schweiz Med Wochenschr 101:1591

Metcalf RW (1979a) Arthroscopic meniscectomy seminar, Salt Lake City, Utah, pp 21–22

Metcalf RW (1979b) Arthroscopic surgery technique: The bucket-handle meniscal tear. Am Acad Orthop Surg Proceedings

Metcalf RW (1984) Arthroscopic knee surgery. Adv Surg 17:197–240

Morscher E (1984) Erfindung und Entwicklung der Kniearthroskopie durch Eugen Bircher (1882–1984). Swiss Med 6:28

O'Connor RL (1973) The arthroscope in the management of crystal-induced synovitis of the knee. J Bone Joint Surg [Am] 55:1443

O'Connor RL (1974) Arthroscopy in the diagnosis and treatment of acute ligament injuries of the knee. J Bone Joint Surg [Am] 56/2:333–337

O'Connor RL (1977) Arthroscopy. Lippincott, Philadelphia Toronto

Ohnsorge J (1969a) Arthroskopie des Kniegelenkes mittels Glasfasern. Z Orthop 106:535–538

Ohnsorge J (1969b) Farbphotographie des Kniegelenkinnenraumes über ein neues Glasfiberendoskop. Langenbecks Arch Klin Chir 325:965–967

Ohnsorge J (1970) Die Arthroskopie des Kniegelenkes. Fortschr Endoskopie 2:29–34

Okamura T (1945) An arthroscopic study of the traumatic disorders of the knee-joint. J Jap Orthop Assoc 23:28

Robles Gil J, Katona G (1969) Arthroscopy as a means of diagnosis and research. Review of 80 arthroscopies. Proceedings of the 4th Panamerican Congress of Rheumatology. Excerpta Medica Amsterdam, p 209

Robles Gil J, Katona G (1971) Clinical and therapeutic usefulness of arthroscopy. Gazz Sanit 20:16

Robles Gil J, Katona G, Barroso MR (1968) Arthroscopy as an aid to diagnosis and investigation. Excerpta Medica International Congress Series 143

Sato K (1950) An arthroscopic study of knee-joint injury caused by dull force. J Jap Orthop Assoc 24:184

Sato K (1955) An arthroscopic study of knee-joint injury caused by dull force. J Jap Orthop Assoc 28:467

Shahriaree H (1984) O'Connor's Textbook of Arthroscopic Surgery. Lippincott, Philadelphia

Sommer R (1937) Die Endoskopie des Kniegelenkes. Zentralbl Chir 64:1692–1697

Sprague NF (1982) The bucket-handle meniscal tear: A technique using two incisions. Orthop Clin North Am 13:337–348

Suckert R (1960) Photoarthroskopie des Kniegelenkes. Z Unfallmed Berufskr 53:65–67

Takagi K (1933) Practical experience using Takagi's arthroscope. J Jap Orthop Assoc 8:132

Takagi K (1939) The arthroscope. J Jap Orthop Assoc 14:359–441

Tesson MC, Aignan M, Delbarre F (1970) Arthroscopy of the knee. Technique, indications, results. Presse Med 78:2467

Tiling T (1986) Arthroskopische Meniskuschirurgie. Enke, Stuttgart

Trickey, Hertel P (1986) Surgery and arthroscopy of the knee. Springer, Berlin Heidelberg New York Tokyo

Tsuyama N, Udagawa E (1966) Arthroscopy. Surg Ther (Osaka) 14:581

Vaubel E (1938a) Die Endoskopie des Kniegelenkes. Z Rheumaforsch 1:210–213

Vaubel E (1938b) Die Arthroskopie. Rheumatismus 9

Wagner H, Holder J (1982) Bericht über die 7. Murnauer Unfalltagung der Landesverbände der gewerblichen Berufsgenossenschaft am 15.5.1982

Watanabe M (1949) Arthroscopy of the ankle joint of the horse. J Jap Orthop Assoc 22:51

Watanabe M (1954) The development and present status of the arthroscope. J Jap Med Inst 25:11

Watanabe M (1974) Arthroscopy of the knee-joint. In: Helfet AJ (ed) Disorders of the knee. Lippincott, New York, pp 139–149

Watanabe M, Takeda S (1960) The number 21 arthroscope. J Jap Orthop Assoc 34:1041

Watanabe M, Takeda S, Ikeuchi H (1969) Atlas of arthroscopy, 2nd edn. Igaku Shoin, Tokio

Wilcke KH (1939) Endoskopie des Kniegelenkes an der Leiche. Bruns' Beitr Klin Chir 169:75–83

Wruhs O (1970) Die Arthroskopie und Endophotographie zur Diagnostik und Dokumentation von Kniegelenksverletzungen. Wien Med Wochenschr 8:126–133

Wruhs O (1972) Die Arthroskopie. Orthop Prax 9:75–78

Wruhs O (1973a) Die Endoskopie des Kniegelenkes zur Diagnostik und Dokumentation von Binnenschäden und Erkrankungen. Fortschr Endoskopie 4:225–226

Wruhs O (1973b) Endoskopisch faßbare Veränderungen des Femurpatellargelenkes. Z Orthop 111:525–526

Wruhs O (1973c) Die Arthroskopie des Kniegelenkes. Z Orthop 111:664–665

Wruhs O (1975a) Arthroskopische Befunde bei Vorverlagerung d. Tuberositas tibiae. Hefte Unfallheilkd 127:187–194

Wruhs O (1975b) Arthroskopie bei Schienbeinkopfbrüchen. Hefte Unfallheilkd 126:234–236

Zollinger H (1977) Indikation und Aussage der Gelenkendoskopie bei der Chondropathia patellae. Z Orthop 115:617

Subject Index

Page numbers in *italics* refer to passages of major importance

Acetylene 30
Aftertreatment 175ff.
Anatomy of the knee joint *43ff.*
Anesthesia *31ff.*, 94
Anterior horn flap 123ff.
Anterior horn resection, lateral 150ff.
Anterior horn section 111ff., 131, 144, 151, 155
Appointment 25
Appraisal 88f.
Approaches
– anterolateral 97
– anteromedial 97
– dorsolateral 37
– dorsomedial 37
– Gillquist's 36
– lateral 35
– medial 36
– Patel's 36
– posteromedial 97
– suprapatellar *36*
Aquarium effect *38f.*, 66, 179
Arthro-pneu 41
Arthroscope *6ff.*, 13
Arthroscopy, indication 24
–, operation 93ff.
Arthrotomy 93, 106,
Assessment 88f.

Bacterial filter 40
Basket forceps *99f.*, 109, 122
Bucket-handle tear *66f.*, 72, *108ff.*
– artificial 139
– displaced 108f.
– lateraler 141ff.
Bucket-handle tear medial
– repositioning 108f.
– resection 108f.

Carbon dioxide 40
Cartilage damage 39, 158
– arthroscopic treatment 158ff.

– degenerative 74f., 88
– traumatic 74f., 88
Cartilage fracture, classification 74, *76f.*
Cartilage shearing fractures 55
Charge-coupled camera 14ff.
Chondromalacia patellae *78f.*, 88, 158, 162
CLA model knee 18f.
Cold-light source 8f.
Collateral ligament, tibiae 97
Complications 178ff.
Condyle 43
– medial 48
Cruciate ligament
– anterior 35, 59, *81ff.*, 88
– posterior 35, 46, 59, *83ff.*,
– replacement 168
Cryotherapy 176
Cydex solution 30

Diathermy resection 10, 173f.
Discoid meniscus, lateral 71, *154ff.*
Dissecting scissors 99, 101, 111
Double Eyepiece Systems 12
Drainage cannula 98
Drape 28, *96*
Drawer sign, anterior 83

Effusion *47ff.*, 179
Empyema 178
Explanation 25ff.

Fat pad 33, 36, 43, 47f., 50, 53, 85, 166, 178
Femoral condyle
– lateral 35, 59, 62
– medial 35, 46, 50
Femorotibial joint 43
"figure 4" positioning 19, 35, 48, 62, 72
Flap tear 67f., *123ff.*
Fluid irrigation 96
Formalin vapor 30

Gas filling 96
Gas sterilization 30
General anesthesia *31*, 42, 81, 94
Glass fiber systems 6
Gouge 99, 101
Grasping forceps 99, 101, 102
Gripping forceps 99

Hooked scissors 101, 111
Horizontal tears 68
Hyperextension 94

Incision 35, *97*
Instability
– anteriomedial 51, 71
– anterior 82
Instruments breakage 178
Intercondylar fossa 95
Intercondylar region 35, *58f.*
Irrigation 48, 96, 175

Joint compartment
– lateral 95
– medial 95
Joint-filling
– fluid *38ff.*, 48, 96
– gas *40ff.*, 48, 96, 181
Joint irrigation 48f.

Lateral release 169
Leg holder 28
Leg support 94
Lens systems 6
Light sources 9
Linea terminalis 45
Local anesthesia *32,* 42, 81
Locking occurrs 37
Longitudinal tear *66ff.*, 72
Loose bodies 37, *102ff.*
Main tap 48, 49
Mattress sutures 169
Meniscal flaps 68
Meniscectomy
– partial 106
– subtotal 106, *139*

Meniscectomy
– total 106
Meniscus
– lateral 62, 71 ff.
– medial *51 ff.*, 61, 66 ff.
Meniscus fissures
– horizontal 134 ff.
– incomplete 134 ff.
– tangential 134 ff.
– transverse 129 ff.
Meniscus fraying 136 ff.
Meniscus lesions, degenerative 136 ff.
Meniscus operation
– lateral 141 ff.
– medial 108 ff.
Meniscus operations 106
Meniscus suture 168 f.
Meniscus tears, types of 67
Miniarthrotomy 182

Nitrous gas 40

Opening-up, medial 83
Operating arthroscope 13
Operation report 21
Operative equipment 99 f.
Optical system
– 30 ° *7*, 35 f.
– 70 ° *7*, 35 f., 84
– articulated 12
Osmium injection 66
Osteochondritis dissecans *80*, 88, 104, 162
– reattachment 80, 163
Outerbridge's ridge 55
Outer tube *8*, 46 ff., 50

Patella 53 ff.

– lateralization 169
Patella alta 88
Patellar abrasion 78 f.
Patellar facet 56, 169 ff.
Patellar ligament 97
Patella subluxation, habitual 172 f.
Pes anserinus 37
Photographic equipment 13 f.
Photographic documentation 13, 21
Plica
– alata *58*
– mediopatellaris 165 ff.
– synovialis 43, *58 f.*, *85*, 165 ff.
Plica syndrome 85
Polaroid camera 13
Popliteal hiatus 62
Popliteus tendon 62, 71
Positioning 28, 94
Posterior horn flap 123 ff.
Posterior horn lessions, longitudinal 116 ff.
Posterior horn resection, lateral 147 ff.

Rapid desinfection 30
Recessus
– dorsal 37, 48, 59, 83, 84
– lateral *62 f.*, 95
– medial 95, 111
– suprapatellar 35, 42, 43, 48, *58*, 95
Regional anesthesia 31 f.
Removal of metal 173
Ringer solution 38, 96, 175
Rod-lens systems 6, 13

Rotary instruments 9 f.
"rucked carpet" 53

Saline solution 38, 96, 175
Shaver systems 10 f.
Skin incision 35
Sterilization 30
Straight-line system 7
Stubs 115
Subcutaneous emphysema 40, 178
Synovectomy, arthroscopic 165
Synovial biopsy 165
Synovial fragments 38
Synovialis 35, 47, 51, *66*, 165
Synovial membrane 66, 165
Synovitis 38, 165
Synoviorthesis, chemical 66

Three-point technique 107
Tibial collateral ligament 81
Tourniquet 96
Transverse ligament 43, 51
Transverse tears 67, 71
Trocar *8*, 46
Trochlea *43*, 47
Tube cameras 14 ff.
Two-point technique 107

U-matic system 16, 17, 22

Valgus pressure 94
Varus pressure 94
Video recording 22
Video systems 14 ff.

Yttrium injection 66

Springer AV-Instruction Programme

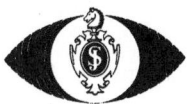

Slides

A. Gächter, F. Freuler

Arthroscopic Findings in the Knee Joint

260 slides (130 in color). Legends in English and German.
ISBN 3-540-92593-7

The usefulness of arthroscopic examination of the knee is not limited to revealing lesions of the meniscus: far more than this, the strength of the method, for a physician experienced in arthroscopy, lies in the possibilities it offers for identification of complex lesions as well. The combination of new traumatic damage with older, degenerative changes is a frequent finding. Ruptured ligaments also often occur in conjunction with other lesions; for instance, a rupture of the anterior cruciate ligament may be combined with damage to the cartilage of the medial condyle, avulsion of the posterior horn of the medial meniscus, or rupture of corner the semimembranous with concomitant dislocation of the patella. Arthroscopy also makes it possible simultaneously to carry out a test of function with the benefit of intraarticular vision; the implications of the injuries and the exact treatment procedure to be followed, operative or conservative, can thus be established.

For correct identification of injuries, clinical knowledge needs to be supplemented by familiarity with the visual findings. Recognition is dependent upon knowledge, and it is in order to deepen clinicians' knowledge of arthroscopy that this double series of slides has been created, in which *each* arthroscopic image is paired with an explanatory line drawing. Out of the 8000 arthroscopic examinations carried out at the University Orthopaedic Hospital in Basel, examples of important findings of types that are seen daily in arthroscopy were selected and photographed. The photographs are accompanied by a brief commentary linking the arthroscopic findings to clinical findings and differential diagnosis. The selection of clear and unambiguous images was a priority. All pictures were taken using the anterolateral approach and an optical angle of 30°. The use of carbon dioxide as a medium has made the pictures of the lesions very true to life, without synovial fluid obstructing the clear view. Where necessary, a series of photographs was taken of a single case in order to clarify the findings from different angles of vision.

Springer-Verlag
Berlin Heidelberg New York
London Paris Tokyo

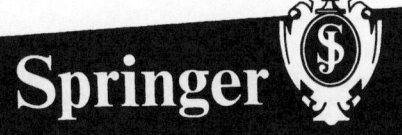

E. L. Trickey, P. Hertel (Eds.)

Surgery and Arthroscopy of the Knee

First European Congress of Knee Surgery and Arthroscopy, Berlin, 9.–14. 4. 1984

1986. 215 figures, 58 tables. XIX, 402 pages. ISBN 3-540-16274-7

This is an edited collection of papers presented at the First European Congress of Knee Surgery and Arthroscopy. Numerous experimental data, instrumental innovations, follow-up examinations, statistically assessed diagnostic and therapeutic measures, interpretations of pain problems, rare congenital phenomena, as well as questions of follow-up treatment are dealt with in depth, arranged according to lesions of ligaments, menisci, and cartilage. Another important chapter considers knee joint replacement. All topics bordering bone injuries of the knee joint are presented comprehensively.
Original contributions from numerous acknowledged and specially selected young research groups are published and underline the broad spectrum of ESKA's aims. The book is intended for specialists and physiotherapists involved in the theoretical experimental, or clinical problems of the knee joint who are looking for a current state of the art report.

W. Müller, W. Hackenbruch (Eds.)

Surgery and Arthroscopy of the Knee

Second Congress of the European Society of Knee Surgery and Arthroscopy
Basle, Switzerland, September 29–October 4, 1986

1988. Approx. 432 figures, 144 tables. Approx. 320 pages.
ISBN 3-540-17982-8
Distribution rights for Japan: Nankodo, Tokyo

This book contains the most important papers presented at the 1986 Congress of the European Society of Knee Surgery and Arthroscopy held in Basle, Switzerland.
In view of the international participation, the compilation offers an insight into the state-of-the-art of knee surgery both within and outside of Europe.
The emphasis in this volume is on the diagnostic and therapeutic issues in injuries to ligaments of the knee joint. Also covered are biomechanics, endoprosthetics, cartilage damage, and arthroscopy. The reports are based on developments that have taken place within the last 3 years.

Springer-Verlag
Berlin Heidelberg New York
London Paris Tokyo

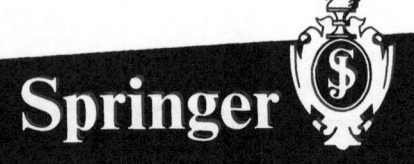